PSYCHIATRY AND THE CINEMA

PSYCHIATRY
AND THE CINEMA

Krin Gabbard and Glen O. Gabbard

THE UNIVERSITY OF CHICAGO PRESS   CHICAGO AND LONDON

The University of Chicago Press, Chicago 60637
The University of Chicago Press, Ltd., London
© 1987 by The University of Chicago
All rights reserved. Published 1987
Paperback edition 1989
Printed in the United States of America
96 95 94 93 92 91 90 89   5 4 3 2

Library of Congress Cataloging in Publication Data

Gabbard, Krin.
    Psychiatry and the cinema.

    Bibliography: p.
    Filmography: p.
    Includes index.
    1. Psychiatry in motion pictures.   2. Moving-pictures
—Psychological aspects.   I. Gabbard, Glen O.
II. Title.
PN1995.9.P78G3   1987   791.43'09'09353   86–25000
ISBN 0–226–27790–9 (cl.)
ISBN 0–226–27791–7 (pbk.)

TO OUR PARENTS

Contents

Illustrations   ix

Foreword   Irving Schneider, M.D.   xi

Preface   xiii

Introduction   xv

Part 1. The Psychiatrist in the Movies   1
     1. Typology, Mythology, Ideology   3
     2. The Alienist, the Quack, and the Oracle   44
     3. The Golden Age   84
     4. The Fall from Grace   115
     5. Countertransference in the Movies   145
     6. Clinical Implications   163

Part 2. The Psychiatrist at the Movies   175
     7. Methodology and Psychoanalytic Film Criticism   177
     8. Narcissism in the Cinema I:
        The Cinematic Autobiography   189
     9. Narcissism in the Cinema II: The Celebrity   204
     10. *Alien* and Melanie Klein's Night Music   226
     11. *3 Women:* Robert Altman's Dream World   240

Epilogue   252

Filmography   259

References   281

Index   289

Illustrations

1. Ginger Rogers with Barry Sullivan in *Lady in the Dark* (1944).
2. Timothy Hutton with Judd Hirsch in *Ordinary People* (1980).
3. Katharine Hepburn imprisoned by Freudian quack (Fritz Feld) in *Bringing up Baby* (1938).
4. Robert Cummings consults Hedy Lamarr in *Let's Live a Little* (1948).
5. Muckraking journalist Tony Curtis about to expose Natalie Wood, before falling in love with her, in *Sex and the Single Girl* (1964).
6. Mia Farrow as Dr. Eudora Fletcher, the savior and lover of Leonard Zelig in Woody Allen's *Zelig* (1983).
7. Hope Lange copes with Elvis Presley's transference in *Wild in the Country* (1961).
8. Herbert Grimwood attempts to drive Douglas Fairbanks to suicide in *When the Clouds Roll By* (1919).
9. Claudette Colbert and Theodore von Eltz minister to Nick Shaid in *Private Worlds* (1935).
10. Murderer (Chester Morris) arouses the curiosity and the sympathy but not the malice of oracular Ralph Bellamy in *Blind Alley* (1939).
11. Fred Astaire treats Ginger Rogers in *Carefree* (1938).
12. Claude Rains in *Now Voyager* (1942) joins Bette Davis for a hot dog.
13. Tyrone Power about to be outsmarted by Helen Walker in *Nightmare Alley* (1947).
14. Lew Ayres probes the mind of Olivia de Havilland and her "evil twin" in *The Dark Mirror* (1946).
15. Olivia de Havilland with caring, effective psychiatrist (Leo Genn) in *The Snake Pit* (1948).
16. Olivia de Havilland with incompetent quack (Howard Freeman) in *The Snake Pit* (1948).
17. Jimmy Piersall (Anthony Perkins) and his wife (Norma Moore) with faceless psychiatrist (Adam Williams) in *Fear Strikes Out* (1957).

18. Joanne Woodward as Eve Black, one of *The Three Faces of Eve* (1957), with Lee J. Cobb and Edwin Jerome.
19. Ginger Rogers with husband (Dan Dailey) and analyst (David Niven) in *Oh Men! Oh Women!* (1957).
20. Howard da Silva as Dr. Swinford in *David and Lisa* (1962).
21. Sidney Poitier, as the movies' first black psychiatrist, overcomes the racism of Bobby Darin in *Pressure Point* (1962).
22. Young Sigmund Freud (Montgomery Clift) with Cecily (Susannah York) in John Huston's *Freud* (1962).
23. Montgomery Clift's dream in *Freud* (1962).
24. Peter O'Toole details his sex life for Dr. Fritz Fassbender (Peter Sellers) in *What's New, Pussycat?* (1965).
25. McMurphy (Jack Nicholson) at odds with Nurse Ratched (Louise Fletcher) in *One Flew over the Cuckoo's Nest* (1975).
26. Bibi Andersson heals Kathleen Quinlan in *I Never Promised You a Rose Garden* (1977).
27. Ingrid Bergman nurtures Gregory Peck while her training analyst (Michael Chekhov) looks on: *Spellbound* (1945).
28. Saul Benjamin (Dudley Moore) succumbs to the transference wishes of his patient (Elizabeth McGovern) in *Lovesick* (1983).
29. Roy Scheider, Ben Vereen, Ann Reinking, and unidentified dancer in *All That Jazz* (1979).
30. Joe Gideon (Roy Scheider) choreographs his own death in Bob Fosse's *All That Jazz* (1979).
31. Woody Allen as Sandy Bates in *Stardust Memories* (1980).
32. Woody Allen with Anne de Salvo and Jaqui Safra in *Stardust Memories* (1980).
33. Robert De Niro in Martin Scorsese's *King of Comedy* (1983).
34. Zelig (Woody Allen) with Coolidge and Hoover in *Zelig* (1983).
35. Jeff Daniels and Danny Aiello in *The Purple Rose of Cairo* (1985).
36. Mia Farrow with Jeff Daniels in *The Purple Rose of Cairo* (1985).
37. The crew wakes up: Ridley Scott's *Alien* (1979).
38. Kane (John Hurt) explores the maternal body of a derelict ship in *Alien* (1979).
39. Sissy Spacek and Shelley Duvall in Robert Altman's *3 Women* (1977).
40. Edgar (Robert Fortier) and Pinky (Sissy Spacek) in *3 Women* (1977).

Foreword

If psychiatry had not existed, the movies would have had to invent it. And in a sense they did. *Psychiatry and the Cinema* tells the story of how the movie industry took the profession of psychiatry—its patients, theories, and explanations—and transformed it into a hybrid that joined the fantasies of the public with its own quest for profit in ways that were sometimes wondrous, but more often disappointing.

One could pair the history of the movies with the history of any profession, say an account of how the movies have depicted lawyers. Or a history of the cinema and dentistry could be traced from Gibson Gowland's painless dentist in Eric von Stroheim's *Greed* to Laurence Olivier's sadistic one in *Marathon Man,* with glances along the way at W. C. Fields, Bob Hope, and Alan Arkin, among many other screen practitioners. These histories would provide interesting and amusing insights into the vicissitudes of American film, the changes in the profession depicted, and the influence of popular culture on both.

But none would have the resonance and power of psychiatry and the movies, for to an uncommon extent the two have shared the same subject matter. Both have had as their prime focus human thought, emotions, behavior, and, above all, human motivation. In pursuit of their common subject, movies and psychiatry have frequently intersected. The two most explicit encounters are the subject of this book: psychiatrists have studied the movies, and the movies have depicted psychiatry.

The study of movies by psychiatrists has taken two major directions. Early in the history of the cinema, there was an attempt to understand the appeal and the power of the motion picture medium itself, apart from the specific content of any individual film. The outstanding example of this was Hugo Münsterberg's 1916 classic *The Film: A Psychological Study.* His central statement bears repeating: "The photoplay tells us the human story by overcoming the forms of the outer world, namely, space, time, and causality, and by adjusting the events to the forms of the inner world, namely, attention, memory, imagination, and emotion."

Ten years later, the eminent psychoanalyst Hans Sachs acted as consultant in Germany to the first movie on psychoanalysis, *Secrets of a Soul.* He went on to pursue his interest in movies in a series of articles in the English film journal *Closeup.* In a 1928 article he took Münsterberg one step further: "The film seems to be a new way of driving mankind to conscious recognition . . . by making the inexpressible expressible by means of displacements on to a small incidental action."

A number of interesting analyses have continued this approach, but the more popular direction in the psychiatrist's interest in movies has consisted of the uncovering of the covert message in individual movies or film genres. This has clearly arisen from the psychoanalytic approach to art and literature, much of it pioneered by Freud, himself not a movie fan but an avid interpreter of the arts. In recent years, the semiologists, with their merging of linguistic and psychoanalytic method, have come to occupy a central position in the effort to uncover the hidden messages in popular movies. The second part of *Psychiatry and the Cinema* presents illuminating examples of the interpretive methods psychoanalysts have brought to the study of the movies.

It is the movies' interest in psychiatry, however, that occupies the major part of this study, and it makes for a fascinating story. From the comic Dr. Dippy in the nickelodeons of 1906 to the heroic or evil psychiatrist in the movie currently playing in the nearest multiplex shopping mall theater, an interesting parade of mental health professionals has appeared on our screens. Their multiple personalities grace the pages of this volume. But above and beyond the depiction of psychiatrists themselves, one wonders what movie script writers would have done without dreams, amnesia, or homicidal maniacs, or where films, or psychiatrists for that matter, would have been without the ubiquitous traumatic event.

The French filmmaker Jean-Luc Godard once commented that "the cinema is neither art nor life, but something in between." Certainly very few psychiatric films have aspired to art, and even fewer have represented real life, but as Glen and Krin Gabbard so effectively demonstrate, that in-between area has yielded a series of films of great fascination, entertainment, dismay, and, one must even admit, educational value.

IRVING SCHNEIDER, M.D.

Preface

This book has been a cooperative project by writers from quite different intellectual backgrounds. The result has been a truly integrative effort to synthesize the relevant dimensions of film scholarship with those of psychiatry and psychoanalysis. Not only have we been able to avoid the all-too-obvious problems that might have confronted brothers engaged in a collaborative project of this kind, but we have also been able to reach a consensus on the many controversial issues raised by our study. Although both of us have contributed significantly to every chapter in this book, our own specialties have required each of us to contribute more to certain sections than to others. Most of chapters 1–4 were written by Krin Gabbard, while chapters 5, 6, 8, and 9 are primarily the work of Glen O. Gabbard. Chapters 7, 10, and 11 are true collaborative efforts to which both of us have contributed equally. If readers occasionally find differences of style or emphasis in the text, they may be sure these differences reflect no substantive disagreement between us.

The illustrations for this book also require a word of explanation. Many recent works about film have included frame enlargements from actual prints of movies. This convention puts on the page the exact image that audiences momentarily see during a screening of a film. We have chosen instead to rely upon the still photographs that studios have traditionally provided for promotional purposes. Although these stills seldom reproduce exact scenes from movies, they often reveal specific relationships among characters that the filmmakers—or, just as important, the studio executives—have tried to establish. In most cases we have chosen a still because it offers a striking example of how a film wishes to portray psychiatry even if the precise contents of the photograph never appear in the film.

Psychiatry and the Cinema could not have been written without the generous contributions of many friends and colleagues. We would especially like to thank Irving Schneider, Gerald Mast, Daniel M. Fox, Paul Fink, Robert Mugge,

Penelope Russianoff, Donald F. Muhich, Andrea Walsh, James Castrataro, Harriet Meier Castrataro, Jacob Lipkind, Louise Vasvari, and Carrol Lasker. We owe a special debt of gratitude to the staff of the University of Chicago Press. Like the authors of what must be 90 percent of the books about movies today, we received invaluable assistance from Charles Silver and Mary Corliss of the Museum of Modern Art. We also appreciate efforts on our behalf by the staff at the Library of Congress. Mrs. Faye Schoenfeld patiently typed numerous versions of the manuscript and was of invaluable assistance in organizing an enormous amount of correspondence. The State University of New York at Stony Brook and the Menninger Foundation provided both moral and financial support for portions of the project. Finally, we have been fortunate to receive exceptional tolerance and steadfast encouragement from two remarkable women, Paula Beversdorf Gabbard and Joyce Davidson Gabbard.

Shorter versions of chapter 5, "Countertransference in the Movies," and chapter 8, "Narcissism in the Cinema I: The Cinematic Autobiography," were published in *Psychoanalytic Review* 72 (Spring 1985): 171–84, and 71 (September 1984): 319–28. Chapter 10, "*Alien* and Melanie Klein's Night Music," appeared in *Psychoanalytic Approaches to Literature and Film,* ed. Maurice Charney and Joseph Reppen (Madison, N.J.: Fairleigh Dickinson University Press, 1987). An earlier version of chapter 11, "*3 Women*: Robert Altman's Dream World," was published in *Literature/Film Quarterly* 8 (1980): 258–64.

Introduction

They grew up together. Cinematic art and modern psychodynamic psychiatry, both still in their infancy, were brought to America from Europe at the turn of the century and were firmly established within a few decades. The relationship has been complementary and also hostile. As cooperative endeavors, both psychiatry and the cinema strive to cut through the seemingly random content of everyday life and reveal the secrets of the human character, and since curing and entertaining are often related in our culture, movies as well as psychiatry have been regarded as therapeutic. Psychiatry has provided filmmakers with abundant material, even if we consider only the psychoanalytically derived "motivations" that have driven actors in every genre of film, from musicals to westerns (Holland 1959). Movies have become the great storehouse for the images that populate the unconscious, the chosen territory of psychoanalytic psychiatry. Irving Schneider (1985) has pointed out that as early as 1900 a writer would describe his psychotic episode in terms of the "magic lantern" effects of the first nickelodeons. Early surrealist filmmakers even saw the production of dream images in the human unconscious as fundamentally analogous to the "cutting" process by which movies are made (Williams 1981), and the American film industry was being called a *Traumfabrik,* or "dream factory," as early as 1931 (Ehrenburg). More recently, psychoanalytically inclined students of film have made persuasive connections between the language of the cinema and Freud's account of the dream-work (Metz 1982).

Because of the special opportunities they have provided for filmmakers, psychiatrists and psychiatry have played roles in almost every type of film, including silent farces like *Plastered in Paris* (1928), early gangster films like *Blind Alley* (1939), classic tearjerkers like *Now Voyager* (1942), teen exploitation horror flicks like *I Was a Teenage Werewolf* (1957), Doris Day sex farces like *Lover Come Back* (1961), low-budget art films like *David and Lisa* (1962), and contemporary Hollywood "bio-pics" like *Frances* (1982). In fact, there are well over two hundred films across the spectrum of Hollywood genres that make some use of psychiatry. This figure does not include numerous English and other foreign films in American circulation dealing with the subject, nor does it include innumerable "B" movies—forgotten quickies from the 1940s, nudies from the 1960s, and adult films from the 1970s and 1980s—many of which have found a place for psychiatrists in their mise-en-scènes. Nevertheless, whether movies are A, B, or triple-X, they present few psychiatrists who do not belong to a fairly limited range of stereotypes. In addition, there are only a few basic conventions that characterize how American films have dealt with psychiatry and its practitioners. Schneider (1985), for example, has divided all movie psychiatrists into three categories: Dr. Dippy (after a film we will discuss in chapter 2), Dr. Evil, and Dr. Wonderful.

Even though these stereotypes and conventions offer filmmakers the opportunity to produce fantastic dream sequences or logical explanations for the otherwise inexplicable behavior of their characters, practitioners of psychiatry have seldom found reason to applaud the images of themselves appearing on the screen. For reasons that are not difficult to understand, the motion picture industry has shown only a passing interest in the more complex aspects of psychiatric treatment. The one hundred minutes of the average American film have only rarely provided an insider's view of World War II, space exploration, or even baseball. We can scarcely expect the medium to provide balanced insights into the multifaceted, constantly evolving questions of psychotherapy: any serious attempt at such an undertaking would probably bore audiences silly. Filmmakers and their audiences are, of course, much more interested in the compelling, arousing, and/or consoling entertainment that is usually characterized, perhaps unfairly, as "escapist." For a variety of reasons, which we will address in this work, psychiatry has regularly been exploited for purposes quite inconsistent with the loftier goals of the profession.

In our attempts to sort out the various relationships between movies and psychiatry, we will often be concerned with the stereotypical characters and conventions dominating the presentation of movie psychiatrists. We have found that the predominance of certain stereotypes over others changes, often dramatically, from one historical moment to the next and that the portrayal of psychiatrists is best understood in terms of the largely mechanical needs of the films in which they appear, particularly the conventions of genre. Also, we are often able to identify a relationship between historical changes in the mental health profession and its image on the screen: some of the more negative portrayals can be blamed on psychiatrists themselves, and some cannot. Chapter 1 is an overview of the most common stereotypes and of the film genres in which these stereotypical characters and plots are ensconced. Because we are primarily concerned with cultural/historical patterns in the American view of psychiatry in the movies, we have confined ourselves to theatrically released American-made films. In spite of their immense appeal and importance, we will not engage in extended analyses of Robert Wiene's *The Cabinet of Dr. Caligari*, G. W. Pabst's *Secrets of a Soul*, Fritz Lang's *The Testament of Dr. Mabuse*, Liliana Cavani's *The Night Porter*, or Ingmar Bergman's *Face to Face*. The discussion of psychiatrists in foreign films, as well as in American television programs, would require more elaborate methodologies and would expand our subject beyond manageable proportions. We will make reference to these only when our inquiry into the American cinema demands it. After we have established the familiar stereotypes and genres and the problems of their interpretation, we will devote three chapters to what appears to be a historical pattern in the evolution of cinematic depictions of psychiatry.

The term *psychiatrist* is used generically in this study to represent all mental health professionals, particularly psychotherapists. To attempt further distinction among the various mental health disciplines would be to go far beyond the efforts of filmmakers themselves. Significantly, American films have never completely succeeded in distinguishing psychiatrists from psychoanalysts, psychologists, social workers, and other therapists. In *The Dark Mirror* (1946), for example, the door to Lew Ayres's office bears the inscription, "Dr. Scott Elliott, M.D., Ph.D., M.S., Psychologist." This confusion may also represent a more deeply rooted perception, one which effectively segregates movie psychiatrists from other medical doctors such as surgeons or pediatricians. Throughout our research for this study, we have found that the work of psychiatrists in the cinema is frequently indistinguishable from that of clergymen, caseworkers, school guidance counselors, or even newspaper advice columnists. At least since the 1930s, the American cinema has focused so heavily on simplified versions of the psychiatric "talking cure" that the profession has in effect become demedicalized in the movies.

In our survey of how movies have portrayed psychiatrists (chapters 2–4), we have attempted to tie these changing images to American cultural history. While it is true that the Hollywood cinema "reflects" American attitudes, it is also true that it reflects them selectively. We will attempt to identify both the popular notions that become manifest in films as well as those which appeared either belatedly or not at all. After we have completed this historical survey, we will devote a chapter to the phenomenon of countertransference, one of the most exploited and misunderstood aspects of psychiatry that has regularly appeared in American films, especially in the last few years. We will also devote a chapter to the clinical implications of our study, particularly the impact that the cinematic mythology of psychiatry has had and can have on the relationship between patient and therapist.

Part 1 of this study addresses how movies have looked at psychiatrists. We occasionally make use of the insights of Freud and his followers to account for these cinematic images, but our principal subject in part 1 is the changing image of the psychotherapist in American movies, an image which may or may not accurately reflect American attitudes. In part 2 we adopt the reverse perspective and look at movies with psychiatrically informed eyes, thus completing our study of the complementary relationship between psychiatry and the movies. One reason for the ubiquity of psychiatrists in the American cinema may be their profession's relevance—in the imaginations of both moviemakers and movie consumers—to how film affects the mind. Even the most naive statements about movies "warping" the minds of young people acknowledge the profound and mysterious impression that the cinema has on its viewers. We feel that an inquiry into images of psychiatry in films ought also to examine the relationship of movies to the workings of the unconscious. Further, we believe that psychoanalytically informed criticism can be an extremely important aid to understanding the special hold that the movies have on audiences.

Applying psychology to the movies is by now a familiar pursuit, one that goes back at least to 1916 when Harvard psychologist Hugo Münsterberg (1970) published his thoughts on how "the photoplay" can replicate the actual workings of the mind more successfully than conventional narrative forms. Modern psychoanalytic film criticism probably began in 1950 when Martha Wolfenstein and Nathan Leites (1970) realized that films repay psychological scrutiny just as richly as the plays of Sophocles, Shakespeare, and Ibsen, to which Freud had once applied his substantial skills as a literary critic. Since the appearance of Wolfenstein and Leites's work, mental health professionals have frequently written about movies, and the bibliography of psychoanalytic film criticism is now much too expansive to summarize here. We mention only Dr. Harvey R. Greenberg's *The Movies on Your Mind* (1975) as an excellent and readable example of the psychiatrist at the cinema. In colleges and universities, psychoanalytic criticism, or something very much like it, is as familiar to students of film as the Odessa Steps or Rosebud.

In the first chapter of part 2 we will attempt a brief survey of the important developments in psychoanalytic film criticism that have taken place since the 1970s. The remarkable ascendancy of Jacques Lacan as a key figure in film theory has brought together a substantial community of scholars who draw upon linguistics, feminism, Marxism, and semiotics as well as psychoanalysis.

Although we owe a debt to these writers, we have relied more upon the literature of clinical psychoanalysis and less upon semiotic theory for our analyses of the films addressed in part 2. In particular, we have chosen to illustrate a number of methodologies based on different theoretical frameworks that we find particularly suited to several interesting films. All of the movies in part 2 repay psychoanalytic scrutiny although most have yet to be systematically illuminated in terms of this tradition.

Few of the movies we discuss in *Psychiatry and the Cinema,* especially in part 1, are masterpieces of the art. With the prominent exceptions of Alfred Hitchcock and Woody Allen, few of the American "pantheon" directors are well represented in our filmography: Orson Welles, Fritz Lang, John Ford, and Josef von Sternberg never made American films that deal directly with psychiatry even though their mastery of character and mise-en-scène places them among the most psychologically sophisticated directors. In the chapters that follow, we are much more likely to encounter the films of Anatole Litvak, Mark Robson, Curtis Bernhardt, or Edward Dmytryk, directors whose works were long ago confined to the oblivion of occasional broadcasts on late-night television. Perhaps the mere presence of a psychiatrist in an American film signals that it contains a thematic shortcut, that the filmmaker has severed some Gordian knot by inserting the brief but authoritative pronouncements of a psychiatrist. The French critic Marc Vernet has made a somewhat different observation: "The great contribution of psychoanalysis has been to provide a new alibi for the structure of the American narrative film" (1975, 233). Even Hitchcock—some would say *especially* Hitchcock—has made awkward use of psychoanalytically engineered plot mechanics, for example, in *Marnie* (1964), a film that does not even include a psychiatrist in its cast of characters. We will have a good deal more to say about Hitchcock, whose use of psychiatry requires special attention to the complex means by which his films are "enunciated." But most of the films we address in part 1 are less challenging, inviting cultural/sociological treatment more often than close reading. By the same token, most of these films are relatively unsophisticated from a cinematographic point of view—inevitably employing the "invisible style" of classical Hollywood (Bordwell, Staiger, and Thompson 1985)—and do not demand the kind of shot-by-shot analysis that can illuminate more complex films.

The mediocrity or obscurity of most of the films we discuss in this book should in no way undermine the validity of our argument. If the questions of genre, historicity, and interpretation that we raise in chapters 1–4 are valid, we should be able to apply them to the whole range of American films, not just to those that have been canonized by box-office receipts or critical acclaim.

Our principal interest in these movies is not, after all, whether they are aesthetically or commercially successful. All were created with the intention of returning at least some money to the studio, and all were tailored to closely studied populations of ticket-buyers. With few exceptions, the films were made according to well-established formulas that only a handful of filmmakers were willing to modify to any substantial degree. Consequently, our interest is most aroused when the portrayal of psychiatrists changes dramatically over a short period of time or when a certain character type suddenly begins to appear more frequently. Our goal is first to identify these changes in the movies and second to offer some means of accounting for them. In doing so, we may mention the most cynical exploitation films in the same sentence with an Academy Award winner (assuming for the moment that the latter type of film is qualitatively different from the former). But by concentrating almost entirely on a film's relationship to psychiatry, we may also develop new criteria for thinking about these films. Even when a film touches only briefly on psychiatry, its treatment of the subject can tell us a great deal about the film's attitudes and intentions, including those that the film's makers may not have articulated elsewhere.

PART · ONE
The Psychiatrist in the Movies

Typology, Mythology, Ideology   1

■ The changing images of psychiatry during eighty years of American cinema
offer a unique opportunity to assess the complex interactions between different currents in twentieth-century American culture. Part 1 of this book addresses the strange relationship between movie "mythology" and the history of psychiatry in America. In chapters 2, 3, and 4 we will consider the history of cinematic representations of the psychiatrist in terms of three periods: one before, one after, and one during a Golden Age in the late 1950s and early 1960s when psychiatrists were almost consistently idealized. Negative stereotypes predominate during the periods before and after this Golden Age, though for quite different reasons. To understand these historical changes, we must first consider the kinds of movies that have established themselves in our culture and the special needs that psychiatrists answered in these films. We will see that the myths embedded in American movies offered only a few highly conventionalized niches for doctors of the mind. We will devote special sections to the narrowly circumscribed role of the female psychiatrist in the movies as well as to the handful of generic therapies available to the movie psychiatrist. In this present chapter we are concerned with *continuity* in images of psychiatry over time: our thesis here is that a film's handling of psychiatry presents an especially useful stance for "decoding" that film, even when a psychiatrist appears to be a strictly marginal character.

In his consideration of movie mythology, Michael Wood (1975) has observed that American films, especially those made prior to the 1960s, involve frequently contradictory assumptions about our most important worries. He suggests that entertainment does not so much present an escape from problems as it does a "rearrangement of our problems into shapes which tame them, which disperse them to the margins of our attention" (p. 18). Problems in movies, whether world wars or juvenile delinquency, can appear quite real at some times, though ultimately they are revealed to have little importance. Wood continues: "The mythological function of the movies is to examine these problems without seeming to look at them at all. Movies assuage the discomforts of blurred minds; but they also maintain the blur" (p. 21). One of the major blurs that Wood finds in the American spirit as reflected in movies is the indiscriminate equation of "assertions of the self" with issues of the greatest national or international importance. At the beginning of *Casablanca,* for example, Rick (Humphrey Bogart) is basically an American isolationist, unwilling to become involved in world politics. When he finally does take action and shoots Strasser (Conrad Veidt), he is still acting from personal feelings for Ilsa (Ingrid Bergman) and Victor Laszlo (Paul Henreid) rather than from any patriotic motives. And yet the film is clearly intended as an endorsement of the American policy that brought us into World War II.

Robert B. Ray (1985) has expanded this interpretation of *Casablanca,* applying to the film a methodology that has greatly influenced our argument in this book. Ray argues that *Casablanca* successfully transforms world conflict into the conventional problems of melodrama because it appropriates the traditional story of "the outlaw hero versus the official hero" that Americans knew well from years of being exposed to movies about the Old West. The character of Rick (Bogart) looks back to a tradition of uniquely American heroes (including, for example, Huck Finn) and ahead to the Shane of Alan Ladd and director George Stevens. All are reluctant heroes who exist on the fringes of society and the law, struggling with conflicts which approximate but eventually replace the larger political questions. Ultimately, "the self-determining, morally detached outlaw hero came to represent America itself" (Ray 1985, 91). The outlaw hero is usually at odds with an official hero, who represents a parallel tradition in American mythology with roots in parental figures such as George Washington and Abe Lincoln. Ray even points out the striking resemblance that Victor Laszlo (Paul Henreid), the "official hero" of *Casablanca,* bears to George Washington (1985, 98). Although our sympathies are with the outlaw hero, American movies of the "classic" period usually find ways of sparing the audience the psychological agony of choosing him over the official hero. At the climax of *Casablanca,* Rick and Laszlo find themselves working toward the same goal much in the same way that Shane avoids conflict with that film's official hero (Van Heflin) by joining him in the fight against the bad guys.

We have simplified Wood's and Ray's readings of *Casablanca,* but their thesis should be clear: America's most popular films frequently avoid answering the most troubling questions by displacing them into melodrama, where solutions are found more easily. Drawing upon the work of Charles Eckert (1974), who has compared this displacement to Freud's account of displacement in the dream work, Ray finds *reconciliation* to be the most important psychological element in classical Hollywood's "thematic paradigm." Because melodrama throws a film's center of gravity onto the decisions of a single individual, American movies reinforce the often paradoxical belief that the answer—and, ultimately, the solution—to just about anything lies within ourselves. Wood (1975) cites the end of *The Best Years of Our Lives* (1946), in which Dana Andrews only has to pull himself together in order to get a job, even though the film grimly argues that there are no jobs for him in the difficult years after World War II. Wood mentions psychoanalysis, "which is easily cast as a doctrine of self-help," as a means for preparing the self for the inevitable victory over what lies outside (1975, 38). But Wood does not mention how psychoanalysis, which also says that deep-seated problems have been with us since childhood and may even be intractable, becomes an easy target for films that deny the realities behind our worries. The long-standing ambivalence toward psychiatry in American movies grows naturally out of an optimistic mythology that uses psychiatrists in two quite dissimilar ways.

Throughout this study, we will use the term *ideology* in much the same sense as does Louis Althusser (1977), who defines it as "a system . . . of representations (images, myths, ideas, or concepts, depending on the case)" (p. 231). As many film critics have discovered, this definition is ideally suited to the study of movies. Although he is reluctant to use the term as prominently as other critics, Robert Sklar (1975) has convincingly traced the dominant ideology implicit in American films. Sklar observes that for all its affronts to traditional values, Hollywood's major contribution was essentially the affirmation of familiar American beliefs about, for example, "the virtues of deferred gratification and the assurance that hard work and perseverance would bring success" (p. 196). He shares Wood's thesis that American films made prior to the 1960s seldom venture outside received cultural myths. However, Sklar is more interested in how these myths are related to economics and power than to the half-conscious workings of "blurred minds" that Wood addresses. Like Ray, Sklar quotes Roland Barthes, whose book *Mythologies* describes "collective representations" such as movie myths, and he joins Barthes in the call to "go further than the pious show of unmasking them and account *in detail* for the mystification which transforms petit-bourgeois culture into a universal nature" (p. 197). Sklar attempts such an accounting with the great master of these mystifications and transformations, Frank Capra. Following Sklar, we will show in the next chapter how in *Mr. Deeds Goes to Town* (1936) Capra used an absurd psychiatrist from Vienna as a foil for that most natural of men, Gary Cooper, who in this film carries a name that suggests his uniquely American talents and desires, Longfellow Deeds.

Another way of thinking about psychiatrists in American movies suggests something other than the ideologically charged transformations of which Barthes speaks in the passage cited by Sklar. Quite apart from what would seem to be an ideological function in the movies, psychiatrists have often provided a convenient means for effecting the mechanics of plot, regardless of what that plot may be. In one sense, the people who have written stories for fiction, drama, television, or movies have found the psychiatrist to be as important an invention as the telephone. Before the telephone, dramatists had to establish background information by arranging characters and settings in awkward patterns. In act 1 of Ibsen's otherwise gracefully crafted masterpiece of 1884, *The Wild Duck,* one by one each of the major characters crosses the stage as he is identified in the conversation of two servants. After Alexander Graham Bell had made his contribution to civilization, a playwright could accomplish just as much with a phone call in the first scene. An actor could then stand alone on stage and quickly supply crucial information while talking to an imaginary character on the other end of the line. Amanda Wingfield's telephone conversations in Tennessee Williams's *The Glass Menagerie* present a good example of this technique: her unsuccessful attempts to sell magazine subscriptions are a poignant character revelation.

Like telephone conversations, psychiatric consultations have offered filmmakers the perfect device for unearthing dark secrets and simplifying exposition. As early as 1922 an individual resembling a psychiatrist sets up key scenes in *The Man Who Saw Tomorrow,* a silent film in which the hero goes to a psychologist/mesmerist to find out which of two women he should marry. Once the man is hypnotized, the film cuts to a pair of dream sequences foretelling events in the hero's life with each of the two women. Of course psychiatrists are on hand for flashbacks much more frequently than flashforwards, as for example in Curtis Bernhardt's *Possessed* (1947). The film begins with an incoherent and delirious Joan Crawford wandering alone through city streets. Placed under the care of psychiatrists, who are initially incapable of learning her identity, she soon reveals the information they (and the audience) require when she is injected with a truth drug, part of a process called "narcosynthesis," a favored technique in the films of the late 1940s. Although the psychiatrists make elevated pronouncements about what they learn of her story (and although their patriarchal account of the heroine's condition has a definite ideological component), their major function in the film is to provide a bridge into flashbacks containing the Crawford character's life story.

More recently, psychiatrists as movie characters have become subtler, though no less conventionalized, vehicles for exposition and character development.

Playing the expensive call girl Bree Daniels in Alan Pakula's *Klute* (1971), Jane Fonda engaged in two quite different styles of acting. As the plot of the film takes her through scenes of romance and suspense, she is confident and smooth. But in scenes with her female psychiatrist (Vivian Nathan), Fonda uses the improvisational techniques of "method acting" to express the inner thoughts of her character, and she becomes hesitant and uncertain. Psychotherapy offered Pakula the opportunity to reveal vulnerability and complexity in the self-confident Bree Daniels that might otherwise have been lost to the melodramatic demands of the scenario. In the same year as *Klute,* a psychiatrist performed a quite similar function while listening to the confessions of George C. Scott in the first moments of Arthur Hiller's *The Hospital* (1971). The psychiatrist (David Hooks) appears only in this introductory scene so that the audience can establish early on that Scott's character is depressed and contemplating suicide.

A formalist critic might say that a psychiatrist used in this fashion functions principally as what Henry James (1934) has called a *ficelle*. Literally the strings with which a puppeteer controls his puppets, a *ficelle* has the same role as the colorless confidants and confidantes to which several centuries of stage heroes and heroines have explained their thoughts for the benefit of the audience. For James, a *ficelle* is of special importance in fiction when the author chooses to write in a self-effacing voice or to emphasize the complexity of the central characters by juxtaposing them with minor, one-dimensional characters. The invention of psychotherapy has presented filmmakers with the ideal *ficelle,* one that need not even speak, yet whose presence allows a character to engage in intense self-scrutiny before the cameras.

So far we have touched upon the ideological and "mythological" forces that shape the role of the cinematic psychiatrist and upon the less ideologically charged formal necessities they are often called upon to effect. We now offer a reading of a film that provides a good example of these and other forces in action as well as a model for interpreting them. Falling midway through the eighty years of psychiatry in American movies, Mitchell Leisen's *Lady in the Dark* (1944) unassumingly introduces conventions we will encounter repeatedly throughout this study: the "faceless" psychiatrist, the psychiatrist as plot ex-pediter, the psychiatrist as spokesman for the dominant ideology, as well as the psychiatrist with the ability to effect a dramatic cure after the resurrection of a repressed trauma from childhood. *Lady in the Dark* was based on a 1941 Broadway musical hit (467 New York performances) written and directed by Moss Hart with music by Kurt Weill and lyrics by Ira Gershwin. The film version was also a box office success even though it omits many of the Weill/Gershwin songs including the haunting "My Ship," which is only hummed a few times by the eponymous lady played by Ginger Rogers. The film, however, does not lack production numbers, almost all of which originate in Ginger Rogers's analytic sessions much in the same way that the narcosynthesis sessions in *Possessed* provide the frame for flashbacks.

Lady in the Dark begins with Liza Elliot (Ginger Rogers) suffering a malaise for which her doctor can find no medical explanation. When he suggests that she see a "psychoanalyst," she interjects, "You're not serious. You don't really believe in that?" Liza is the editor of *Allure*, a popular fashion magazine, and although Ginger Rogers is made up to be an attractive woman, her character dresses in rather severe business attire. Charlie Johnson (Ray Milland), an employee at the magazine who makes her the butt of his frequently cruel jokes, has suggested that holding down a man's job has made Liza too masculine and that he would like to have her position at the magazine. Two other men in Liza's life are Kendall Nesbitt (Warner Baxter), a wealthy older man who has given Liza her editor's job and who would marry her if his wife would give him a divorce, and Randy Curtis (Jon Hall), a popular young movie idol who much prefers Liza to the mobs of squealing women who crowd around him when he arrives for a photo session at Liza's office. She seems unwilling to accept his dinner invitation, however, and cannot even recall that they had met on a previous occasion.

When Liza reluctantly arrives at the office of psychoanalyst Alexander Brooks (Barry Sullivan), her first session soon gives way to a balletic dream sequence working several characters from her life into a highly stylized setting. In a second session, after Nesbitt has told Liza that his wife will divorce him and that they can marry, Liza dreams up a wedding that is an elaborately costumed medieval pageant. After a long dance number featuring Munchkin-like figures, the royally clad Liza and Nesbitt approach the altar, but before the dream is over she has embraced not Nesbitt but Randy the movie star.

The analyst's interpretation of Liza's dream ignores the Munchkins and goes right to the resemblance between Nesbitt and Liza's father. In a surprisingly frank exposition of psychoanalytic theory (and one that suggests Freud's 1916 reading of Ibsen's *Rosmersholm*), the psychoanalyst tells Liza that she is reluctant to marry Nesbitt because she fears violating the oedipal taboo. Liza bristles at the suggestion, but Dr. Brooks authoritatively says,

> If it's not true, then why do you reject Randy Curtis? . . . Most women would be very interested in Randy Curtis.
> LIZA: I am not most women. . . . I can think of nothing I'd hate more than a lot of men chasing after me making love to me.

BROOKS: Aren't you rejecting his invitation because you're afraid of competing with other women?

We soon learn that Liza's beautiful but aloof mother had made Liza feel like an ugly duckling. Once when Liza tried to perform a song ("My Ship") that she had carefully prepared with her father, the mother ignored the child while flirting with one of her admirers. The mother died while Liza was still in her childhood, and one day the little girl put on a blue dress that was a favorite of her father whenever her mother wore it. Still grieving over his beautiful wife's death, the father flew into a rage when he saw his daughter in the dress, an incident which Liza had repressed but which ultimately caused her to suffer anxiety and depression. After learning all this, the psychoanalyst lectures Liza on her flight from femininity, finally concluding that she needs "some man to dominate" her.

Smiling, Liza walks out into the sun a changed woman. Almost immediately she encounters Randy (Jon Hall), the boyishly handsome movie star who has already expressed more than a passing interest in her. Liza seems to enjoy his attentions as well, especially now that she can hold her own with a man whom many other women find attractive but who is not a surrogate father. Randy soon asks her to marry him, but only after he has unsettled her a little by telling her how much he needs her to run the new movie production unit he is planning. He concludes his marriage proposal with the words: "Don't worry. You're still going to be the boss." Liza is agonizing over a marriage proposal for the second time in a few days when Charlie (Ray Milland) enters her office to apologize for the numerous times he has insulted and ridiculed her. He explains that he behaved badly because he wanted power. Liza then realizes that Randy is much too submissive for her and that she has found the necessary dominant male in Charlie. The film ends as they embrace.

Lady in the Dark is most memorable for its production numbers, despite its introduction of psychoanalytic dream interpretation into the unlikely genre of musical comedy. Perhaps as a result, the analyst who serves primarily as the triggering device for these set pieces is something of a cipher, quite detached from any other character, including the heroine (plate 1). However, the detachment of Dr. Brooks (Barry Sullivan) need not characterize a film of this type. Compare, for example, Sullivan's character in *Lady in the Dark* with the psychiatrist played by Yves Montand in Vincente Minnelli's *On a Clear Day You Can See Forever* (1970). The Montand character performs the same function of listening to the heroine, in this case Barbra Streisand, so that the film can cut to flashy production numbers, which in this film illustrate the reincarnated

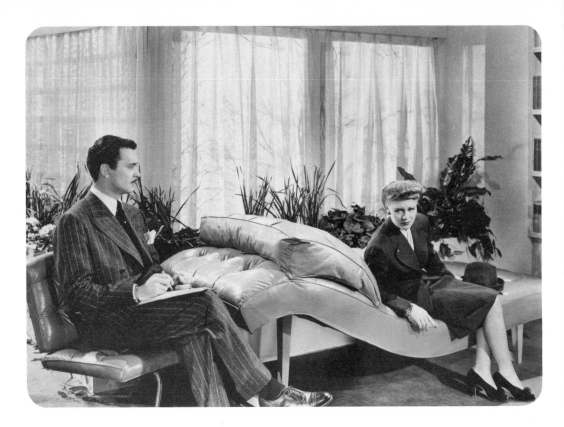

PLATE 1. Ginger Rogers with Barry Sullivan in *Lady in the Dark* (1944). Paramount Pictures. The Museum of Modern Art/Film Stills Archive.

heroine's past lives. But although Montand is frequently pushed into the penumbra by the formidable Streisand, his suave, Continental character is much more substantial than Sullivan's. Montand even becomes a principal player in the reconstruction of Streisand's previous lives. The neutral attitude affected by Sullivan in *Lady in the Dark* is of course quite consistent with the professional conduct expected of "real life" psychiatrists. In the movies, however, his colorlessness is unusual.

In one sense, Dr. Brooks in *Lady in the Dark* can be understood as a special kind of *ficelle*—the analyst-as-plot-mechanism—a recurrent phenomenon in American films before and after this one. His flat character would seem to result logically from his perfunctory presence as a device for facilitating plot and exposition. We call this character type *the faceless psychiatrist* after his peculiar lack of identifying traits. Even facelessness, however, can be understood in terms of the historical interactions between movies and psychiatry. In earlier films such as *The Front Page* (1931) the problem of how to present an interesting psychiatrist in a bit part was solved (as it had been in the stage play of 1928) by introducing the stereotypical Viennese with tails, pince-nez, and a vaudeville version of a *Mittel Europa* accent. Although this figure has persisted to the present, Americanized psychiatrists first began to appear in the mid-1930s, especially when the presentation was intended to be positive. Hollywood was acknowledging that psychoanalytic psychiatry was no longer the exclusive province of European immigrants.

Schneider (1977) has reported that Moss Hart wrote *Lady in the Dark* as a tribute to his own analyst, and perhaps for this reason the handsome and poised Barry Sullivan was given the part of Dr. Brooks in the film. The work of a sympathetic psychiatrist, however, is somewhat more obscure than that of a Viennese quack, and many people, then and now, believe that therapists deliberately wear expressionless masks for their patients. Consequently, Dr. Brooks has few of the distinguishing qualities that characterize bit players such as the wisecracking cab drivers, the diplomatic policemen, or the effeminate sales clerks who regularly populated films of this period. Barry Sullivan, a relatively unknown actor working in films for only the second time in *Lady in the Dark,* is almost a stand-in for the *idea* of a psychiatrist. He has moments of compassion as well as authority, but unlike almost every other character in the film, he has few, if any, human qualities. We have no idea what kind of husband or father he is, or even if he *is* a husband or father. Nor do we have any idea what personal feelings he may hold for his patient.

Facelessness has continued to be part of the typology of the movie psychiatrist even though the significance of this kind of character seems to have changed. In more contemporary films the facelessness of psychiatrists is often a function of their ineffectiveness: if they had more character, they might be able to help people. In Michael Pressman's *Some Kind of Hero* (1982), Richard Pryor plays a returning Prisoner of War whose best friend was killed in Vietnam, whose wife has just left him, and who laughs hollowly when a faceless shrink lamely asks him if he has "any problems." An almost identical scene occurs in a more serious film, Michael Cimino's *The Deer Hunter* (1978), when an Army psychiatrist mechanically asks dehumanizing questions of Christopher Walken, who responds with grim humor. This myth of the ineffectual or out-of-touch psychiatrist has been especially well represented in movies during the last twenty years: in a subsequent chapter we will discuss the various ideologies that emerged from the 1960s along with this character type.

The psychiatrist in *Lady in the Dark,* however, is characteristic of the quite different movie myths of the 1940s. We have already quoted Michael Wood on the consoling function of classic American movies, which acknowledge our deepest anxieties while at the same time making them seem marginal. Liza Elliot's depression is rooted in painful childhood memories, but most of her therapy is dramatized as charming musical pageantry. Even the Munchkins in one of her dreams provide a consoling counterpoint, evoking the child's fantasy of *The Wizard of Oz,* a film released just five years before *Lady in the Dark.* The earlier film was about an orphan who, as Harvey Greenberg (1975) has persuasively argued, heroically overcomes her adolescent anxieties. The rejection that Liza Elliot suffered at the hands of both her mother and her father is not only softened by this reference to *The Wizard of Oz* and the possibilities of transcending orphanhood, but the effects of this rejection are soon dispelled entirely by her psychoanalyst.

The myth of psychiatry expressed in *Lady in the Dark,* as well as in other films from the early forties such as *Now Voyager, Spellbound,* and *Since You Went Away,* is rooted in a cinematic romance with psychoanalysis that looked forward to what we have called the Golden Age of psychiatry in the movies (1957–63). During World War II, the wondrously soothing message that personal problems are easily solved was well received, and all four of these films were box office winners. Psychiatry offered the perfect means for disposing of a problem by wrapping it in mystifying, pseudoscientific trappings and then sending it away cheerfully. The facelessness of Dr. Brooks in *Lady in the Dark,* as well as his function as a kind of elaborate song cue, reflects the film's preference for denying the pain of childhood rejection over a more unsettling inquiry into how a patient comes to terms with the family romance.

Feminist analysis has concentrated on another side of Dr. Brooks's function in *Lady in the Dark.* Even women who have embraced few of the goals of the women's movement might today object to the "you need a man to dominate you" message that *Lady in the Dark* offers them. Molly Haskell (1974) has found the film to be a good example of the limited and limiting roles that women are asked to fill, even in what have been called "women's films." The message of many Hollywood films from the thirties through the fifties is that women cannot and should not have it all. According to Haskell, in the "sacrifice" category of women's film, a woman must give up "(1) herself for her children—e.g., *Madame X, The Sin of Madelon Claudet;* (2) her children for their own welfare—e.g., *The Old Maid, Stella Dallas, To Each His Own;* (3) marriage for her lover—e.g., *Back Street;* (4) her lover for marriage or for his own welfare—e.g., *Kitty Foyle* and *Intermezzo,* respectively; (5) her career for love—e.g., *Lady in the Dark, Together Again;* or (6) love for her career—e.g., *The Royal Family of Broadway, Morning Glory"* (1974, 163). As Haskell points out, the theme of these films is that women are only "complete" when they surrender to the roles that conventional middle-class ideology assigns to them. When a sophisticated Manhattan psychoanalyst verifies these attributes in *Lady in the Dark,* we have an excellent example of what Barthes means when he suggests that institutions such as movies can transform "petit bourgeois" homilies into "nature."

Andrea Walsh (1984), who characterizes *Lady in the Dark* as "rabidly" antifeminist, observes that the film was made in a decade that began and ended with the equally popular films *His Girl Friday* (1940) and *Adam's Rib* (1949), both of which suggested that achievement and femininity can be compatible. *Lady in the Dark,* presenting the opposite view, can nevertheless coexist with these films because all three compellingly address the same problems of social roles confronting women in the 1940s. Walsh has also brought the history of American psychoanalysis into a discussion of *Lady in the Dark,* specifically the "biologically determinist Freudianism à la Helene Deutsch and the notorious Lundberg and Farnham" (1984, 161). These last two authors used a popularized version of Freud's writings to discourage women from remaining in the workplace. She argues that in spite of the new independence that women began to experience as they entered the work force during World War II, the dominant ideology of America in the 1940s drifted toward a "feminine mystique" that was instrumental in justifying the massive demobilization of women after the war. This ideology, supported by American government and industry, found its intellectual validation in books such as Lundberg and Farnham's *Modern Woman: The Lost Sex* (1947). Walsh does not point out the extent to which the fear of a potentially explosive army of jobless male veterans lay behind the postwar demobilization of women. She is right, however, in refusing to characterize Freud's work as antifeminist even though popularized Freudianism easily lends itself to the perpetuation of traditional female stereotypes. *Lady in the Dark* is an excellent case in point.

What then do we make of Dr. Brooks in this film? The film presents him much as Schneider (1985) has described him: "a compassionate, intelligent, sophisticated man." Through his efforts, we are told, the Ginger Rogers character overcomes her depression and lives happily ever after in a necessary surrender to domesticity. With a few changes, however, this same scenario can turn sinister, as in fact it does in a 1970 film, *Diary of a Mad Housewife,* the story of a frustrated woman (Carrie Snodgress) whose psychiatrist urges her to find fulfillment as a wife and mother even though the film portrays his suggestions as grotesquely inappropriate to her actual situation.

Unlike the psychiatrist in *Diary of a Mad Housewife,* Dr. Brooks in *Lady in the Dark* invites quite different interpretations. The question of his "meaning" becomes especially problematic when we are concerned with the ideologically explosive issue of the role of women but also when the subject is embedded in a film such as *Lady in the Dark* that does not fit neatly into a single category. Both Haskell and Walsh have called it a "women's film" even though it may be the only musical that they include in this category. Musicals make different demands on their audiences than women's films, and any interpretation of *Lady in the Dark* ought to address the genre to which it belongs. Although Ginger Rogers had recently won an Academy Award for her performance in an *echt* women's film, *Kitty Foyle* (1940), she had also danced her way through no less than ten musicals with Fred Astaire—not to mention several other musicals including two choreographed by Busby Berkeley—and she surely carried this association for audiences in *Lady in the Dark.* Following a pattern that Mulvey (Mast and Cohen 1985, 803–16) has identified in musicals, *Lady in the Dark* often stops its "diegetic," or conventional, narrative flow for production numbers in which the audience is invited to examine Rogers's body. In women's films, stars such as Colbert, Crawford, Hepburn, and Fontaine usually carry less of the theatricalized glamor that Ginger Rogers possesses, and their bodies are seldom presented for the audience's visual pleasure outside a strictly narrative context. If *Lady in the Dark* exists primarily for its music and spectacle, we are even more inclined to see the psychiatrist simply as a *ficelle* and a means for introducing production numbers. If we focus more on the dilemma facing Ginger Rogers as the heroine of a women's film, his function is more important, and he becomes her liberator or her enslaver, depending upon what a critic such as Stanley Fish (1976) would call "the interpretive community" to which the viewer belongs.

We have begun this chapter with a discussion of *Lady in the Dark* because it easily invites several modes of analysis. An attempt to account for the psychoanalyst in *Lady in the Dark* raises historical questions not only about psychoanalysis itself but also about American movies, about American culture in general, and about American myths that underlie them all. Coexisting with these historical questions, and to a certain extent overlapping with them as well, are problems of film genres, styles, and stereotypes. *Lady in the Dark* is not a very good film (Walsh is probably correct in calling it "an aesthetic disaster") but it does introduce important conventions such as the faceless *ficelle,* the psychiatric agent for society, and the simple cure based on the recall of childhood memories. The rest of this chapter will be devoted to a survey of the character traits assigned to psychiatrists in American films and of the film genres which give life to these stereotypes. A special section will be devoted to the even more rigidly defined conventions that films impose when women play psychiatrists, and another section will explore "the cathartic cure," which quite a few characters besides Liza Elliot have undergone when psychiatrists are nearby.

DOUBLE-EDGED STEREOTYPES

Movie myths from America have much in common with myths from worlds even more exotic than Hollywood. Film scholars interested in myth have appropriated some of the same methodologies used by classicists and anthropologists. Wood (1975) cites the work of G. S. Kirk (1970), a classicist who has studied myth in a variety of cultures. Drawing upon the binary analytic method of Claude Lévi-Strauss, Kirk sees myth as a mediation between opposites that allows for the coexistence of seemingly incompatible truths. For example, from the eighth through the fourth century B.C., the Greeks possessed two completely different myths about the centaurs, beasts half man and half horse that lived outside society in purely natural surroundings. One group of centaurs were savages who routinely attempted to rape human women and battle their protectors. Another type, including Chiron, the tutor of heroes such as Achilles and Jason, was wiser and gentler than most mortals. Kirk suggests that the Greeks reconciled themselves to the paradox of a natural world that could be both fierce and gentle by creating two corresponding models of man quite literally *in nature,* that is, attached to an animal. Horses, after all, can be fierce in action but gentle in repose.

Kirk's structuralist model of mythmaking is quite compatible with the apparently paradoxical way in which movie myths treat our problems: "Myth offers an apparent way out of the problem, either by simply obfuscating it, or making it appear abstract and unreal" (1970, 21). The myths in American movies serve the ancient function of allowing us to live with the contradictory, to keep our illusions at the same time that we acknowledge our limitations. Or as Ray has observed, "The great Hollywood czars became naive, prodigious anthropologists" (1985, 13).

Movie psychiatrists may offer the film student a privileged view of cinematic mythmaking in action. Each of their attributes can be divided into good and bad halves, producing complementary pairs of "good" and "bad" psychiatrists. Like the two classes of centaurs through four centuries of Greek civilization, paired stereotypes of psychotherapists have coexisted comfortably throughout the history of American cinema. We offer table 1 as a basic guide to movie

TABLE 1 Cinematic Stereotypes of the Psychiatrist

Attribute	Good Psychiatrist	Bad Psychiatrist
Faceless	Cures by presence	Ineffectual
Active	Effective and caring	Manipulative, criminal, or vindictive
Oracular	Omniscient; good detective	Arrogant but misguided
Social agent	Reconciling	Repressive and malevolent
Eccentric	Human and fallible	Neurotic and ridiculous
Emotional	Compassionate	Psychotic
Sexual	Healing lover	Exploitative lecher or libidinous clown

stereotypes of psychiatrists, reserving for later a discussion of the more complex cases. Each of the attributes to the left is a constant that movies present differently in good and bad psychiatrists.

We have already suggested that the idea of the "faceless" psychiatrist in more recent American films reflects his ineffectuality or helplessness before insuperable problems such as those experienced by the victims of America's adventure in Vietnam. On the other hand, the ideology of Robert Mulligan's *Fear Strikes Out,* the 1957 film about baseball player Jimmy Piersall, clearly allows for the success of psychiatry, and the faceless doctor in that film (Adam Williams) seems to work his cure simply by being near. When a film is sympathetic to psychiatry, the faceless psychiatrist usually accomplishes his work quickly, as if the filmmakers were anxious to get on with the business of the plot. This seems to be the case both in a comedy like Norman Jewison's *The Thrill of It All* (1963) as well as in a more earnest film such as Elia Kazan's *Splendor in the Grass* (1961): in both these films from the Golden Age, protagonists conquer their problems after less than two or three minutes of screen-time with their psychiatrists. The logical extension of the faceless psychiatrist is, of course, the invisible psychiatrist: *Diary of a Mad Housewife* ends with a tight close-up of the heroine as she listens quietly to a chorus of self-involved characters at what is apparently a group therapy session presided over by a therapist who is neither seen nor heard. The same practice of holding the camera on an actor's face while he or she talks to an invisible psychiatrist has been used by Woody Allen in *Interiors* (1978) and by Ken Russell in *Crimes of Passion* (1984). In Arthur Hiller's *The Lonely Guy* (1984), Steve Martin speaks to his analyst exclusively through an intercom.

When "good" psychiatrists play more important roles, and the audience has the opportunity to see them working actively, they are deeply involved with their patients, and their cures usually work even if the psychotherapists function as little more than advice-dispensing guidance counselors. Consider as examples the following films spanning four decades: classic forties films such as *Now Voyager* and *Lady in the Dark;* Golden Age films such as *The Three Faces of Eve* (1957) and *David and Lisa* (1962); and more recent films such as *I Never Promised You a Rose Garden* (1977) and *Ordinary People* (1980). When we see "bad" psychiatrists actively pursuing their work, they can be manipulative like James Earl Jones in Aram Avakian's *End of the Road* (1970), vindictive like Lane Smith, the pencil-sharpening quack in Graeme Clifford's *Frances* (1982), or avariciously crooked like Helen Walker in Edmund Goulding's *Nightmare Alley* (1947).

One of the most common charges made against psychiatrists is that they pretend to knowledge they do not have (Freedman and Gordon 1973). Accordingly, the movies have given us a great variety of oracular psychiatrists, although they too exist as mythological pairs. When a psychiatrist's oracularity is regarded as a positive trait, the psychiatrist will appear to know everything about a case in a dazzling display of brilliance. When asked to make discoveries outside the confined world of doctor and patient, psychiatrists can be intrepid detectives like Ralph Bellamy in Charles Vidor's *Blind Alley* (1939) and Simon Oakland in Alfred Hitchcock's *Psycho* (1960), who leave behind few mysteries for the police to solve. A negative psychiatrist with oracular pretensions is likely to be a pompous know-it-all who is in fact misinformed or misguided.

The convention of the psychiatrist as society's agent deserves a more detailed discussion, especially when the films portray society negatively. In films such as *Lady in the Dark,* in which we are asked to accept the dominant ideology, psychiatry helps confused individuals to live more happily in a benevolent society. Much the same can be said of the supremely compassionate psychoanalyst bearing the formidable name Sigmund Gottlieb Golden in John Cromwell's *Since You Went Away* (1944), who heals the spirits of wounded veterans and helps Jennifer Jones find sense in her life after the death of her fiancé. The other side of this myth presents psychiatrists as coconspirators and willing accomplices in crimes against sensitive and vital individuals. Milos Forman's Academy Award–winning *One Flew over the Cuckoo's Nest* (1975) has become the most prominent among numerous films that portray psychiatry as a weapon in the substantial arsenal that society uses against its nonconforming members. The protagonist of *Cuckoo's Nest*, Randall McMurphy (Jack Nicholson), becomes a Christ figure for whom shock therapy is the crown of thorns and lobotomy the cross.

American movies frequently portray psychiatrists as eccentric or weird on the assumption that one must be a bit crazy oneself to become a psychiatrist. Many real-life psychiatrists have grown accustomed to hearing the double-edged compliment, "You don't act like a psychiatrist." Hence, the popular stereotype of the eccentric psychiatrist is well represented in the movies. If the psychiatrist is portrayed in a positive light, his tendency to be different becomes refreshing and human, as with Dr. Berger (Judd Hirsch) in Robert Redford's *Ordinary People* (1980). His messy office (plate 2), disheveled manner of dress, and informal, if not brusque, style of speaking make him a pleasant contrast to the orderly but sterile environment presided over by his patient's mother (Mary Tyler Moore). Dr. Berger is weird and "psychiatrist-like," but also human and fallible.

When eccentric psychiatrists are seen in a more negative light, they are portrayed as more neurotic than their patients and in need of treatment themselves. Ridiculous psychiatrists can be traced back at least to 1938, when Fritz Feld added a nervous tic to the Viennese stereotype in Howard Hawks's *Bringing*

PLATE 2. The disorder of this man's office reflects his ability to help his patients: Judd Hirsch with Timothy Hutton in *Ordinary People* (1980). Paramount Pictures. The Museum of Modern Art/Film Stills Archive.

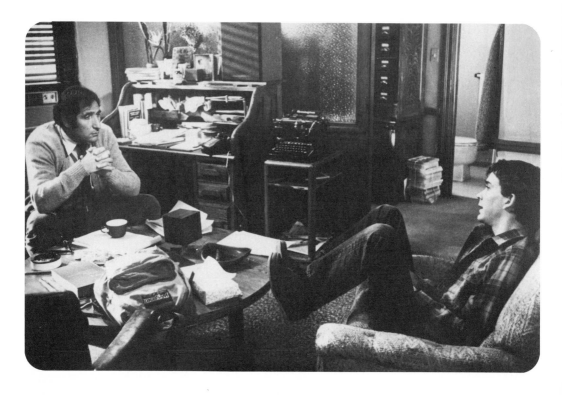

up Baby (plate 3). The sanitarium doctor who menacingly wags his finger in the face of Olivia de Havilland (plate 16) in Anatole Litvak's *Snake Pit* (1948) fits into the same category, as does the misguided doctor in Gilbert Cates's *Oh God! Book II* (1980), who looks at his diplomas on the wall to shore up his fragile self-esteem. Later on, *Oh God! Book II* features an entire room full of self-inflated, humorless psychiatrists, at least one of whom has a pronounced tic, recalling Fritz Feld's from forty years earlier.

If the movie psychiatrist departs from emotional neutrality, our scheme becomes a little more complex. In *Agnes of God* (1985), Jane Fonda throws herself into her work, risking her professional and personal security for the sake of a naive young nun (Meg Tilly) who believes that she was impregnated by an angel. Outside the office, a psychiatrist can get falling-down drunk, as does Gregory Peck in *Captain Newman, M.D.* (1963), and still be as charming as Peck's leading lady (Angie Dickinson) seems to find him as she lovingly sees him safely home. In *Starting Over* (1979), Charles Durning goes to great lengths to help his brother (Burt Reynolds) overcome a serious case of premarital anxiety. Just as often, however, the movies present negative images in which the emotional psychiatrist is substantially more disturbed than his patients or simply psychotic. In addition to psychiatrists who actually murder their patients— Peggie Castle in *I, the Jury* (1953), Maximillian Schell in *St. Ives* (1975), and Michael Caine in *Dressed to Kill* (1980)—we might also mention Rip Torn, who films his own breakdown in *Coming Apart* (1969). In one of the first cinematic depictions of psychiatrists, the mind doctor (Herbert Grimwood) in Victor Fleming's *When the Clouds Roll By* (1919) turns out to be an escaped lunatic (plate 8).

A psychiatrist's emotional life is judged less clearly in the movies when he or she falls in love with a patient. It is much more difficult here to separate the "good" psychiatrists from the "bad" ones because audiences are seldom asked to find fault with therapists who help their patients by giving them love. As anyone familiar with psychiatric ethics knows, however, acting on countertransference sexual wishes is strictly forbidden. The prohibition is spelled out quite clearly to Ingrid Bergman in Alfred Hitchcock's *Spellbound* (1945), to Jason Robards, Jr., in Henry King's *Tender Is the Night* (1962), and to Dudley Moore in Marshall Brickman's *Lovesick* (1983), films that span a period of forty years. In each case a former mentor warns the romantically inclined psychiatrist about the dangers of falling in love with a patient. Yet in each film the audience is invited to sympathize with the lovers and to applaud the actions of the emotionally involved psychiatrist. These and other films contribute to the demedicalization of psychiatry, suggesting that disturbed people only need love

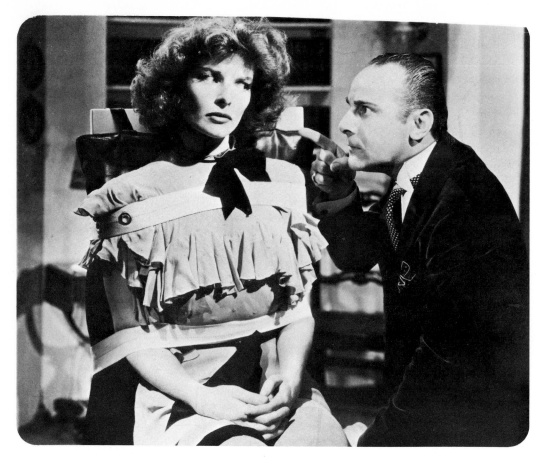

PLATE 3. Even a quack like Fritz Feld in *Bringing up Baby* (1938) can tell that Katharine Hepburn has been behaving strangely. RKO. The Museum of Modern Art/Film Stills Archive.

and that, if psychiatrists really care, they can save their patients by supplying that love, even if they must also give up their profession and the possibility of healing anyone else. In chapter 5 we will discuss in more detail the issue of countertransference in the movies.

When films portray psychiatry more negatively, the romantically inclined psychiatrist is often held up to ridicule: for example, the sexually jealous Richard Benjamin in Stan Dragoti's *Love at First Bite* (1979) and the lecherous Peter Sellers in Clive Donner's *What's New, Pussycat?* (1965) (plate 24). Even in a film such as Philip Dunne's *Blindfold* (1966), a tongue-in-cheek spy mystery about a psychiatrist (Rock Hudson) who uses psychiatric as well as detective skills to outsmart a group of enemy agents, Hudson is nevertheless shown to have been through a long list of failed relationships with women: as each engagement is announced in newspaper social columns and then called off, reporters begin referring to him as "Dr. Bluebeard." In a less comic setting, Tom Conway in *The Cat People* (1942) attempts to seduce Simone Simon even though her husband (Kent Smith) is his friend. The reverse situation is represented in Otto Preminger's *Whirlpool* (1950): although the psychoanalyst played by Richard Conte is idealized in every other way, he cannot devote enough attention to his troubled wife (Gene Tierney), who wanders into the clutches of a murderous hypnotist/astrologer (Jose Ferrer). But when it comes to a psychiatrist's romantic inadequacy, the sex of the psychiatrist is usually female.

THE FRAGILE CAREERS OF FEMALE PSYCHIATRISTS IN THE MOVIES

When women are cast as psychiatrists, they are almost always portrayed as effective professionals whose "inadequacy as women" emerges as a central theme in the film. One of many female psychiatrists in love is played by the Swedish actress Mai Zetterling in Norman Panama and Melvin Frank's *Knock on Wood* (1954). In this combination of spy melodrama, musical comedy, and Freudian romance Danny Kaye plays Jerry, a ventriloquist whose suppressed thoughts are spoken by his dummy and who consequently has trouble staying engaged to women, who take issue with his dummy's statements. Eventually his case is turned over to the beautiful, European-accented psychiatrist Ilse Nordstrom (Mai Zetterling), who quickly determines through hypnosis that Jerry associates marriage with the constant fighting he witnessed between his parents. The session is barely over before the ventriloquist has learned, through Dr. Nordstrom's didactic, guidance counselor presentation, that all marriages need not involve the same kind of strife that his parents endured. Jerry (Kaye) has already told his doctor that he finds her attractive, and in a second session, Dr. Nordstrom acts out a scene that occurs repeatedly in movies whenever beautiful psychiatrists treat leading men: she explains to him about transference. Jerry, however, has found in her office a picture of a man in uniform whom he soon discovers to be the doctor's fiancé, killed in the war while she was a nurse. The film has nothing else to say about Ilse's progress from nurse to psychiatrist, another good example of how movies make little distinction between psychiatry and less technical helping professions. Jerry immediately jumps to the conclusion that she has responded to her fiancé's death by withdrawing from life and becoming a psychiatrist. The ventriloquist then makes advances, telling her

that there is more wrong with her than with him. The doctor loses her professional composure and desperately suggests that Jerry see another psychiatrist.
That night, Jerry sits up reading Freud (the camera reveals that he has acquired
a volume of *A General Introduction to Psychoanalysis*), and the next morning he
assaults Dr. Nordstrom with a jargon-laden speech, insisting that she has a
"guilt complex" because her man died and not her. She has denied herself
fulfillment as a woman by becoming a psychiatrist.

KAYE: It's like punishing yourself because you didn't die too. Don't you
      see that? It's true, isn't it?
ZETTERLING: (looking down pensively and nodding as music swells): I
      just didn't think it showed.
KAYE: Maybe you'll feel better if you talk about it.

Knock on Wood shows Hollywood mythmaking in action. On the one hand,
we have the conventional solution to psychological problems, which demands
only a little magic—in this case hypnosis—and a short conversation. Psychiatry
works, or at least a cinematic brand of psychiatry that is almost entirely divorced
from medicine. On the other hand, audiences need not take the profession's
more problematic aspects seriously, since its practitioners are the ones who
actually need help, and a quick reading of Freud is all the hero needs to cure
his therapist. More specifically, the audience is freed of the even more troubling
ramifications of a *female* psychiatrist. Barbara Melosh (1983) has tied fictional
portraits of aggressive nurses, specifically "Hot Lips" Hoolihan in *M*A*S*H*
and "Big Nurse" Ratched in *One Flew over the Cuckoo's Nest,* to the greater
visibility of professional nurses in hospitals during the postwar years. Middle-
class patients, once treated almost exclusively by male doctors and student
nurses, were unsettled when more authoritative female nurses began regularly
to appear at their bedsides. After World War II, fictional stereotypes of docile
and devoted nurses began to give way to the officious, threatening images
represented by Hot Lips and Nurse Ratched. Although the movies have seldom
dealt with female medical doctors, films like *Knock on Wood* could acknowledge
the significant number of women who had for a long time practiced psychiatric
specialties largely because psychiatry was not perceived as medicine. The film,
however, also obscures the implicit threat of female professionalism by exposing
it as a neurotic denial of feminine domesticity.

Portraits of female psychiatrists in love were largely unchanged from the
forties through the sixties: almost all of the actresses even had foreign accents.
Like Ingrid Bergman in *Spellbound* (1945) (whose case we will discuss in the
next chapter), Hedy Lamarr in *Let's Live a Little* (1948) (plate 4), and Mai
Zetterling in *Knock on Wood,* the beautiful psychiatrist in Michael Gordon's *A*

Very Special Favor (1965) is also played by a European woman, in this case the French actress Leslie Caron. In this film, Lauren (Caron) is at first engaged to her hairdresser, played with exaggerated effeminacy by Dick Shawn. When Lauren's disapproving father, a traditional Old World male played by Charles Boyer, enlists Paul (Rock Hudson) to make his daughter a "real woman," Hudson first appears in her office with a story about how he has been unable to resist the constant attentions of women ever since an affair ended tragically. He then takes her out to dinner, where he discovers that he can easily manipulate her by appealing to her vanity and jealousy and also that she cannot hold her liquor. Paul takes Lauren home to his apartment after she has become intoxicated at the restaurant, and the next morning he attempts to convince her that she had made advances to him the previous evening. When his initial plans for seducing Lauren fail, Paul eventually succeeds by pretending to have homosexual tendencies. He even goes so far as to arrange a meeting with a young man (actually his female secretary in drag), a meeting which Lauren breaks up by rushing in and eventually collapsing in Paul's arms. This shot dissolves into the final scene, showing the former psychiatrist in a maternity ward holding a baby. The camera then pulls back to reveal Paul and, apparently, five more of their children

PLATE 4. Robert Cummings consults Hedy Lamarr in *Let's Live a Little* (1948). Eagle-Lion Productions. The Museum of Modern Art/Film Stills Archive.

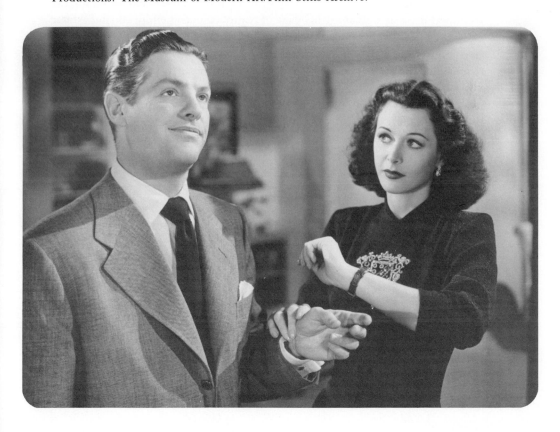

looking in from the other side of the glass. Caron's face suggests that the psychiatrist has given up psychiatry for the more fulfilling occupation of motherhood. Once she meets the right man, the formerly repressed therapist becomes not just feminine but ultrafeminine.

This idea that a male patient can cure a female psychiatrist occurs frequently in films of the forties and fifties, but it also shows up as recently as 1971 in Anthony Harvey's *They Might Be Giants.* Joanne Woodward plays a psychiatrist who is called in to examine a wealthy man named Justin (George C. Scott), a respected judge who suffered a breakdown after the death of his wife and became convinced that he was Sherlock Holmes. At an early stage in the psychiatrist's relationship with this "classic paranoid," Justin uses his Holmesian powers of deduction to describe her: "You tint your hair and have a vitamin deficiency. You were a tomboy and an only child. Your adolescence was a nightmare, and you didn't lose your acne until your middle twenties. You can neither cook nor sew, and your apartment needs a thorough cleaning. You suffer from insomnia and sometimes drink yourself to sleep. You think you're homely, and you're glad you're growing old. You bite your nails; you're frightened that you're a failure; but you're lost without your work. . . . You've never been engaged. No one you've loved has ever loved you back." As if this were not sufficient, Woodward vividly confirms his assertions, at least about her inability to cook, by making a botch of a meal after she has invited Justin to her apartment for dinner. By the end of the film she has put on a prom dress and fallen for the pseudo-Holmes as well as for his view of reality, and as the film concludes, the two face the imagined appearance of Holmes's archnemesis Moriarity with equal conviction. The Woodward character, by the way, is named Dr. Watson, fated by name to be Holmes's intellectually inferior companion.

These films suggest a pattern of growing resistance to the notion that women can or should help male patients. Although in 1971 *They Might Be Giants* at last acknowledges that an *American* woman (Joanne Woodward) can practice psychiatry in the United States, each film imposes progressively greater humiliations upon the female psychiatrist as the price of her desire to practice her craft. Like other heroines of the 1940s, such as Katharine Hepburn and Rosalind Russell, Ingrid Bergman in *Spellbound* (1945) retains both her dignity and her femininity before and during her love affair with Gregory Peck. Mai Zetterling in the fifties film *Knock on Wood* is much more the cool Swede than Bergman but also more the passive object of her lover's attentions. Janet Leigh, portraying an Army psychologist romanced by Tony Curtis in *The Perfect Furlough* (1958), keeps her cool except when she is dumped gracelessly into a vat of wine. By the sixties, Caron in *A Very Special Favor* is subjected to outright ridicule, as is Natalie Wood, who, as Helen Gurley Brown in *Sex and the Single Girl* (1964), attempts to practice psychotherapy on Tony Curtis (plate 5). Neither Wood nor Caron, however, endures anything like the constant humiliations suffered by Woodward in *They Might Be Giants*. Although the women in all these films are returned to the submissive roles demanded by the dominant ideology, the movies become more aggressive in the methods they use to effect this return.

Laurel Samuels (1985) has compiled a long list of films and novels in which women portray psychiatrists. Almost without exception the women are either corrupt—as in *Nightmare Alley* (1947), *Shock Treatment* (1964), and the two versions of *I, the Jury* (1953 and 1982)—or inadequate as women—as in *A Very Special Favor* and *They Might Be Giants*. Occasionally, they are simply faceless, like Annie Hall's analyst, who appears on a split screen with the equally ineffectual male analyst treating the Woody Allen character in this 1977 film. It is true that in Jack Hofsiss's *I'm Dancing as Fast as I Can* (1982), a competent therapist (Dianne Wiest) definitely helps Jill Clayburgh's character, and that Kathleen Quinlan is clearly saved by the analyst (Bibi Andersson) based on Frieda Fromm-Reichman in Anthony Page's *I Never Promised You a Rose Garden* (even though the film cannot resist pointing out that the analyst is childless). But, according to our research, in only two American films does a woman successfully treat a man without succumbing to his sexual appeal: In Gregory La Cava's *Private Worlds* (1935), the male patient appears only briefly, while in the other, Jonathan Demme's *The Last Embrace* (1979), the female therapist is a minor character. When a beautiful psychiatrist and her male patient are central, however, the prognosis is more dubious. In Jack Gold's *The Medusa Touch* (1978), Lee Remick is sought out by Richard Burton, the unwilling possessor of telekinetic powers that can be used only for destructive purposes. When she realizes that psychiatry cannot change him, the female psychiatrist attempts to kill the Burton character, and when that fails, she takes her own life. In Roger Christian's *The Sender* (1982), Kathryn Harrold is another beauty who finds herself in a position much like Remick's when she is unable to stop her male patient (Zeljko Ivanek) from sending his nightmares into the minds of other people, usually with disastrous results. The psychiatric arts practiced by the women in these two films are no match for the extraordinary powers of the male characters.

A quantitative analysis helps to put the matter of women psychiatrists in the movies into perspective. First, we can identify only eight American films in which male psychiatrists fall in love with their female patients: *Carefree* (1938), *Condemned Women* (1938), *The Dark Mirror* (1946), *Tender Is the Night*

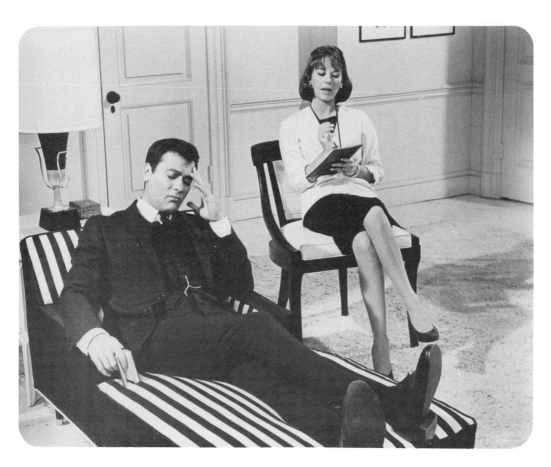

PLATE 5. Muckraking journalist Tony Curtis is about to expose Helen Gurley Brown (Natalie Wood), before falling in love with her, in *Sex and the Single Girl* (1964). Warner Brothers. The Museum of Modern Art/Film Stills Archive.

(1962), *Lilith* (1964), *What's New, Pussycat?* (1965), *Love at First Bite* (1979), and *Lovesick* (1983). There are at least a dozen films in which the wives of male psychiatrists are introduced, and at least twelve more in which unmarried male psychiatrists carry on romantic relationships with women other than their patients. However, we cannot identify *any* American films in which a female therapist's husband or male lover appears (unless he is a former patient), but in at least seventeen American films women psychiatrists fall for male patients or men for whom they play some kind of therapeutic role: *The Flame Within* (1935), *Spellbound* (1945), *She Wouldn't Say Yes* (1946), *High Wall* (1947), *Let's*

Live a Little (1948), *Shadow on the Wall* (1950), *Knock on Wood* (1954), *The Perfect Furlough* (1958), *Wild in the Country* (1961), *Sex and the Single Girl* (1964), *A Very Special Favor* (1965), *Dead Heat on a Merry-Go-Round* (1966), *A Fine Madness* (1966), *They Might Be Giants* (1971), *Zelig* (1983), and *The Man Who Loved Women* (1983). Jerry Lewis's *Three on a Couch* (1966) is a feminist's nightmare, but it does allow the heroine (Janet Leigh) to go on practicing psychiatry after her marriage. In this film, Leigh has married the hero (Lewis) after he had quit a high-pressure job and, with her encouragement, had become a successful painter. When Lewis wins the opportunity to study in Paris, Leigh says she cannot go with him, because her three patients need her. The purpose of their therapies is unclear, however, since the film reveals all three to be beautiful young women whose troubles are due entirely to their inability to find the right men (once again, the psychiatrist as guidance counselor). In an effort to remove the obstacle preventing his wife from accompanying him to Paris, Lewis implements the scheme of posing as an appropriate Mr. Right for each of the women. *Three on a Couch* is slightly more sophisticated than most of Jerry Lewis's films, but it is nevertheless a Jerry Lewis film: in spite of the questionable charms of each of the grotesque characters Lewis plays, all three girls decide that they no longer need therapy once they meet the appropriate incarnation of his character. Ideologically, the film has neutralized the unsettling idea of a female psychiatrist by transforming her into a mother surrogate for three lovesick daughters, just as it has relegated psychotherapy to the level of a dating service.

Female therapists have fallen for male patients in every decade since the advent of talking pictures, and the convention is still alive today: two such pictures were released in 1983 alone. In Blake Edwards's *The Man Who Loved Women* Julie Andrews falls in love with Burt Reynolds even though as an analyst she should have had no difficulty seeing him as a rather pathetic womanizer. Edwards's film is a remake of a French film directed in 1977 by François Truffaut, which succeeds much better in finessing the problem of making the hero's insatiable desire for women seem understandable and sympathetic. Significantly, the psychiatrist played by Julie Andrews in the remake corresponds in the original to a female editor who reads the male protagonist's life story, often setting up flashbacks. To a large extent, Andrews functions in the role of analyst-as-plot-device. The second film is Woody Allen's *Zelig* (plate 6), in which Mia Farrow's performance is a deadpan parody of the female psychiatrist who succumbs to the transference wishes of her patient, in this case the Chameleon Man, Zelig (Allen). The growing acceptance of less limiting roles for women has clearly had some effect on these more recent films: Allen's treatment of the subject seems primarily ironic, and in both films the male protagonists experience substantially more humiliation than their more dignified therapists.

In the list of films featuring female psychiatrists, there is an intriguing gap between the years 1958 and 1964, the Golden Age of psychiatry in the movies. Even during this period, when psychiatrists were regularly canonized as pipe-smoking saints, we can locate only one sympathetic female psychiatrist, surprisingly in a film made for the specialized audience of Elvis Presley fans. In Philip Dunne's *Wild in the Country* (1961), Hope Lange plays another de-medicalized psychiatrist—she works for the parole board—who is assigned to the case of a sensitive but rebellious young man played by Presley. Dr. Irene Sperry (Lange) deals effectively with his hostility and later encourages his talent for writing fiction before she becomes emotionally involved with him. The psychiatrist is a widow who has been dating at least one other man (John Ireland) since her husband's death, and the film never suggests that she is sexually inadequate, even if it observes the entrenched tradition of depicting female therapists exclusively as spinsters or widows. Perhaps because the script for *Wild in the Country* is by no less a talent than Clifford Odets, the film lacks

PLATE 6. Mia Farrow as Dr. Eudora Fletcher, the savior and lover of Leonard Zelig in Woody Allen's *Zelig* (1983). Orion Pictures Company/Warner Brothers. The Museum of Modern Art/Film Stills Archive.

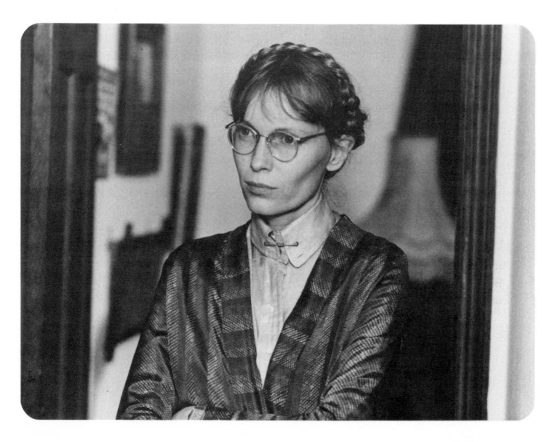

much of the anti-intellectualism and good old boy mystique that characterize Presley's films, especially the later ones. There is even a likeable English professor (Alan Napier), who invites Presley to come study with him at the state university. Consistent with other films of the period, Lange's character is meant to be as sympathetic as possible, and she is almost entirely professional as she attempts to deflect Presley's first expressions of love with the inevitable mention of "transference." Presley, however, dismisses her statements as "book talk" and proceeds to romance her (plate 7). Before the film is over she has saved his life by attempting suicide, thus setting off a chain of events that results in manslaughter charges against him being dropped. At the end of the film, she puts Presley on a train and sends him off to college. She will presumably go back to a satisfying career as something akin to a caseworker, helping more young men like Presley even if she has to take the kind of risks that she barely survived with him.

The sexual contact between female psychiatrist and male patient in *Wild in the Country* consists of a few chaste kisses, but it is clear that both characters must exercise considerable restraint to prevent their strong feelings for each other from extending the sexual component of their relationship. The Production Code was, after all, still in effect. In addition, the film dwells on the intense feelings that Presley felt for his mother before her death. In the film, the woman psychiatrist, who is supposed to be about ten years older than the Presley character, performs a maternal, nurturing role. Lest by some fluke there are psychologically sophisticated individuals in Presley's audience, the film allays any suspicions about his sexuality by offering both Millie Perkins and Tuesday Weld for more traditional love interest. *Wild in the Country* is remarkable, however, for avoiding the more familiar stereotype of the unfulfilled woman who renounces her career when the right man comes along. Nevertheless, the positive effects that Lange has on Presley are not really the result of professional efforts but largely the issue of a loving, potentially sexual relationship. Furthermore, like the other female psychiatrists in films from the fifties, sixties, and seventies that we have discussed, Lange is regularly subjected to public scorn and humiliation, although she bears it with the kind of grace we associate with an earlier breed of therapeutic heroine such as Ingrid Bergman.

PSYCHIATRY AND FILM GENRES

If the comparison between Hope Lange in *Wild in the Country* and Ingrid Bergman in *Spellbound* is valid, the reason probably lies in the shared concerns of the two films: the participation of women in the psychiatric profession,

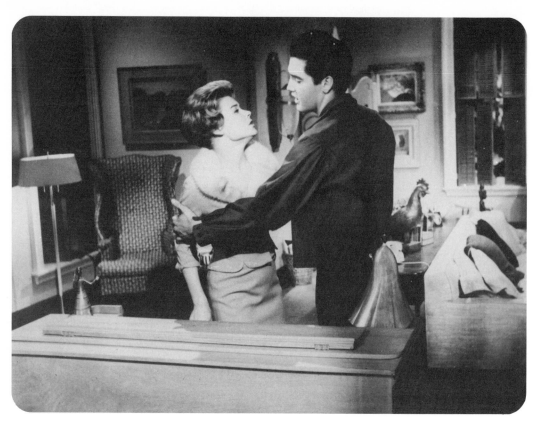

PLATE 7. Hope Lange copes with Elvis Presley's transference in *Wild in the Country* (1961). Twentieth Century–Fox. The Museum of Modern Art/Film Stills Archive.

especially when movies divorce psychiatry from scientific medicine and its technical trappings, can be an extension of women's nurturing instincts rather than an unseemly encroachment into a male profession. This view of psychiatry is rooted more in the special conventions of the two films than in their historical contexts. Films such as *Knock on Wood, Sex and the Single Girl,* and *A Very Special Favor,* in which the heroines lose a good deal of the dignity they possessed initially, belong to a quite different genre: farce/comedy can afford to be less veiled in its antagonism to female achievement. Or as Freud has written, we are often most serious when we are joking. We have already suggested that the interpretation of a film such as *Lady in the Dark* can be strongly influenced by a priori assumptions about the genre to which it belongs. We will now attempt to catalog the various genres in which movie psychiatrists are likely to appear and to assess the effect that the concerns of these genres can have on the portrayal of mental health professionals.

Although movies of more recent vintage are sometimes more difficult to classify as "'melodrama," "romantic comedy," "psychological thriller," or even "western" than are earlier films, the most financially successful movies still seem to lend themselves to one-sentence descriptions. Audiences would rather know that they are about to sit through a "scary movie about a man-eating shark" or a "funny/inspirational film about a cute creature from outer space" than pay money for an experience they cannot quite label. Consequently, Hollywood films have almost always fallen into easily identifiable categories, many of which were already available in dime-store novels, newspapers, and the theater when the first filmmakers began looking around for plots. This is not to suggest, however, that film genres are monolithic and unchanging. On the contrary, film genres have always responded to social change as well as to audience expectations, with firmly entrenched genres rising and falling in popularity and subgenres arising out of larger traditions (Braudy 1977). Moreover, in the last twenty years, some kinds of films have moved from large screen to small screen, adapting themselves along the way to the demands of serial drama, commercial interruptions, smaller budgets, and varying production techniques. One example is the "mother film," a type of movie that makes heroic figures out of women who make sacrifices for their children and that has evolved from the likes of *Stella Dallas* (1937) to the numerous melodramas now seen almost exclusively on television. Of course, even attempts by filmmakers such as Robert Altman to undermine genres merely serve in the end to broaden and perpetuate those very traditions (Self 1984); and though these genres may continue to evolve, certain characters within them must continue to play stereotypical roles or else the pieces of a genre film, almost by definition, will not fit together.

Musicals and romantic comedies may seem not to take issues very seriously, but as we have seen when women therapists appear in these films, ideology can often operate most directly when it is softened by the film's lighter tone. As Braudy (1977) points out, a major goal of musicals and comedies is to "puncture pretension," exactly what they do in films from *The Front Page* (1931) to *The Gay Intruders* (1948) to *Lover Come Back* (1961) to *High Anxiety* (1977). All of these films take comic advantage of the distinguished air that psychiatrists affect or that society has bestowed upon them. But when psychiatrists are central in comedies and musicals, they are usually united with a lover by the end, countertransference notwithstanding. The singing, tap-dancing psychiatrist played by Fred Astaire in Mark Sandrich's *Carefree* (1938) wins Ginger Rogers; the handsome psychiatrist played by Charles Drake is united with his nurse (Peggy

Dow) in the conclusion to Henry Koster's *Harvey* (1950); and Dudley Moore gives up everything for Elizabeth McGovern at the end of *Lovesick* (1983).

In crime-and-detective movies, psychiatrists divide along the same lines we identified for films emphasizing their oracular abilities. In films such as *Blind Alley* (1939), *The Dark Mirror* (1946), *High Wall* (1947), *Blindfold* (1966), and *Still of the Night* (1982) psychiatrists are as successful at their own profession as they are in detective work. In almost all of these films, the brave and ingenious hero also wins a lover at the end, just as we might expect from stories about all but the most hard-boiled private detectives. When psychiatrists are bad or misguided, they stand in the way of the detective work practiced by the heroes in films such as *I, the Jury* (1953 and 1982), *Mirage* (1965), *The Detective* (1968), and *The Boston Strangler* (1968). Needless to say, there is no romantic reward for the psychiatrists in these films.

We have already mentioned films of the science fiction, horror, and fantasy traditions such as *The Medusa Touch* and *The Sender* that put psychiatrists— often very sympathetic ones—up against supernatural obstacles. In Sidney J. Furie's *The Entity* (1983), Ron Silver plays one of several dedicated psychiatrists trying to help Barbara Hershey. If the film did not argue that the heroine actually is the victim of an invisible demon rapist, the efforts of the psychiatrists would seem perfectly valid if not heroic. Here, as in many films of this type, the scrupulously rational and earthbound work of psychiatrists makes them the perfect foil for the generic conceit of the unknown, the unseen and, the unimagined. This tradition may have begun with Jacques Tourneur's *The Cat People* (1942), in which the suave English psychiatrist played by Tom Conway refuses to believe that Simone Simon can actually turn into a panther. However, we might want to go back even further to the naive sanitarium doctor (Herbert Bunston) in Tod Browning's *Dracula* (1931), who, unlike the otherworldly-wise Professor Van Helsing (Edward Van Sloan), finds the vampire count to be a charming if eccentric aristocrat. Later on, the rational psychiatrist rendered impotent by the supernatural becomes a crucial ingredient in *Miracle on 34th Street* (1947), *Zotz!* (1962), *Oh God! Book II* (1980), and *The Terminator* (1984).

In Don Siegel's original 1956 version as well as in Philip Kaufman's 1978 remake of *Invasion of the Body Snatchers,* a psychiatrist becomes one of the "pod people." We are never sure at what point the transformation takes place, but the well-established theme of the psychiatrist's inadequacy in the face of supernatural phenomena is enhanced by the suggestion that his familiar statements— the mind has the power to create illusions, etc.—originate not from professional conviction but actually from a conspiracy to conceal the horrible truth of an alien invasion. The psychiatrist played by Patrick Macnee in *The Howling* (1981) serves the identical function by first explaining the werewolf phenomenon in rationalist terms and then revealing himself to be one. John Boorman's *Exorcist II: The Heretic* (1977) is rather incoherent on most levels, but it is quite clear in juxtaposing the impotent gestures of a psychiatrist (Louise Fletcher) against the heroic posturings of the priest played by Richard Burton. The priest frequently responds to Fletcher's liberal humanist account of the world with Manichaean lectures about "Evil," the existence of which the film goes to some lengths to verify.

John Carpenter's *Halloween* (1978) may be unique in giving speeches about Evil to the psychiatrist played by Donald Pleasence. He alone has looked deeply into the eyes of the killer and seen the Devil, or, in the words of a terrified child, "the Bogeyman." The police and the psychiatrist's nurse see the killer as just another crazy, but Pleasence's convictions are verified when the villain's corpse disappears after stopping five bullets from the psychiatrist's revolver. *Halloween* is a rare example of a horror/science fiction film in which a psychiatrist is not the last to recognize the existence of unnatural forces. This apparent anomaly has been explained by Robin Wood, who calls Pleasence's statements "surely the most extreme instance of Hollywood's perversion of psychoanalysis into an instrument of repression" (1986, 194). Wood's critique of *Halloween* involves the film's unwillingness to come to terms with the sexual and social themes that it engages. The opening shots of the film, in which a confused six-year-old boy is revealed to be the killer of his sexually active older sister, contain the seeds for "the definitive family horror film": "the child-monster, product of the nuclear family and the small-town environment; the incest taboo that denies sexual feeling precisely where the proximities of family life most encourage it. Not only are those implications not realized in the succeeding film, their trace is obscured and all but obliterated" (Wood 1986, 194). When Pleasence identifies the killer as the Devil, an unchanging source of evil, *Halloween* has compromised the one figure who should be able to understand the forces of repression that drove a child to murder his sister. As the film stands now, there is little to separate it from the mass of mad-slasher films (all of them in fact inspired by the box-office success of *Halloween*), which seem to argue that sex among teenagers ought to result in death. Although the plot suggests that the psychiatrist is uniquely aware of the nature of evil, *Halloween*'s subtext reveals that the psychiatrist is just as out of touch with the important issues as were his cinematic predecessors who denied the existence of vampires, invisible demons, and invading armies from outer space. Horror and science fiction films invariably suggest, in one way or another, that psychiatry cannot penetrate beyond the superficial.

Beginning with the first loosenings of the Production Code in the 1950s, the film industry found that psychiatrists could legitimize sexuality in films. Before the new ratings system opened the floodgates of sexuality in 1968, a number of films appeared with titles like *Three Nuts in Search of a Bolt, Suburbia Confidential, The Twisted Sex, Ragina's Secrets,* and even *Loves of a Psychiatrist.* These films were part of a rash of "nudies" that used psychiatry largely to set up sex scenes but also to give the film some semblance of "redeeming social value." In at least one film, the off-screen words of a psychiatrist provided an easily ignored jargonistic sound track to go with the moans and cries of the actors. Not surprisingly, psychiatry became much less important to the adult film industry when the Supreme Court removed social redemption from its test for pornography.

Psychiatrists performed the same basic function on an only slightly more sophisticated level in the more socially acceptable "sex comedies" of the late fifties and early sixties. The profession gave a veneer of legitimacy to sexual leering in films such as *The Perfect Furlough* (1958), *Who's Been Sleeping in My Bed?* (1963), *Sex and the Single Girl* (1964), and *A Very Special Favor* (1965). However, Hollywood also created a genre of more serious "sex" films—more commonly referred to as melodramas—in which psychiatrists played a role. In *Splendor in the Grass* (1961), the audience knows that Deanie (Natalie Wood) is having a breakdown when she jumps out of a bathtub and exposes a good deal of her naked back. Presumably the scene was a legitimate portrayal of mental illness, soon to be cured, and not subject to the same strictures as less ambitious subjects. George Cukor's *The Chapman Report* (1962), based on Irving Wallace's novel about Alfred Kinsey's research, cast Andrew Duggan as a faceless researcher doing psychoanalytically informed work in a community where the women (Jane Fonda, Claire Bloom, Glynis Johns, and Shelley Winters) engage in sexual activities not often suggested (and not actually seen even today) in family films. Duggan interviews the women from behind a room divider, thus exploiting the same voyeuristic fantasies that scenes in confessional booths had previously supplied to audiences. *The Chapman Report* provided titillation but all in the inquiring spirit of social science. In case the psychiatric sanction was not sufficient, the film ended on the reassuring note that these women were not typical and that almost every other wife in the community was actually quite normal. A psychiatrist was also on hand to put the confessions of a prostitute into a more acceptable context in *Girl of the Night* (1960). Although it hardly fits into the genre of "sex film," John Huston's *Freud* (1962) was, after all, rereleased with the subtitle, *The Secret Passion,* and Susannah York expresses more sexual energy in this film than was ordinarily permitted in the early 1960s.

Especially during the 1940s and 1950s, Hollywood turned its attention to the "social problem" film. Along with issues such as alcoholism, racism, and homosexuality, mental illness was explored and often exploited in this film genre even though the subject was usually treated with deadpan earnestness. Consistent with the patterns of Hollywood mythmaking, films of this type often ended on an optimistic note so that audiences could leave the theater reassured, their anxieties eased out to the margins. But as Ray (1985) has written, many of these films were less convincing than their prewar counterparts, largely because Hollywood's thematic paradigm had lost much of its ability to obscure effectively the difficult questions that Americans confronted after World War II. Although social problem films about mental illness desperately needed psychiatric cures, and although mental health professionals became the most active element in society's solution to its problems, the endings of these films were seldom satisfying. Faceless healers became a staple of the American cinema, beginning with Dr. Kik (Leo Genn) in *The Snake Pit* (1948) (plate 15). Within a few years, audiences could witness the achievements of psychiatry in *The Three Faces of Eve* (1957), *Fear Strikes Out* (1957), *The Mark* (1961), and *David and Lisa* (1962). Sometimes more than one social problem was addressed in the same film: for example, *Home of the Brave* (1949) and *Pressure Point* (1962), both produced by Stanley Kramer, explored mental illness and racism simultaneously, although, as we shall see later, with varying degrees of equivocation.

Another genre seldom acknowledged but ideally suited to our study is the mental institution film, a subgenre of the prison movie. This genre has little in common with general hospital films, such as *Men in White* (1934) and *The Interns* (1962), which, with a few rare exceptions like *The Hospital* (1971), consistently idealize the healing powers of an institution's staff. The most famous example of the mental institution film is *One Flew over the Cuckoo's Nest* (1975), in which an institution is explicitly portrayed as worse than a prison. In fact, almost all of the films in this genre suggest that institutions are the last place we should go if we wish to be "cured" of our emotional problems. Often the most sensational elements of psychiatric treatment are central in these films: *Shock Corridor* (1963), *Shock Treatment* (1964), *The Fifth Floor* (1980), and *Frances* (1982) as well as *Cuckoo's Nest* all make the most of electroconvulsive therapy and insulin injection. *Snake Pit* can fit into this category as well as the social problem genre, although it is one of the few mental institution films in which a patient actually recovers. Even when patients are not shocked or lobotomized in these films, they are not likely to benefit from their confinement. Like prison movies, institution films engage American myths of freedom, easily lending themselves to plots in which innocent people must face drastic curtailment of their liberties. This is certainly the case with the Jose Ferrer character in *The Shrike* (1955), who, according to the film, never should have been committed in the first place. The year 1967 saw the release of two completely different films that nevertheless belong to the institution film genre: in both the documentary *Titicut Follies* and the "theater of cruelty" *Marat/Sade* there is little suggestion that the inmates of the asylums will benefit from their institutionalization.

THE CATHARTIC CURE

Stereotyped portrayals of psychiatrists lead to stereotyped portrayals of psychiatric treatment. Consistent with their tendency to demedicalize psychiatry, movies have almost always presented a striking overrepresentation of "the talking cure" and an equally striking underrepresentation of treatments such as electroconvulsive therapy (ECT) and pharmacotherapy. Even though the introduction of effective medications has revolutionized American psychiatry, movie psychiatrists seldom prescribe medication. In fact, American psychiatry during the last two decades has been characterized by a strong movement toward "remedicalization." Interest in psychoanalytic psychiatry has declined while psychopharmacology, brain chemistry, and neurosciences have received more attention. We can speculate that this trend is related to the consistently negative portrayal of verbal therapies in films of the sixties and seventies, but there is no question that psychotherapy is still portrayed as the predominant or exclusive therapeutic practice of the vast majority of movie psychiatrists. ECT has been depicted somewhat more often in movies, usually as punishment. In institution films such as *One Flew over the Cuckoo's Nest* and *Frances* ECT is used malevolently to produce socially appropriate behavior, lobotomy standing in reserve as the final solution to the nonconformist problem. In *The Snake Pit* (1948), ECT is made to appear grotesque by means of camera angles and orchestral crescendos on the sound track. To emphasize the excruciating pain of the process, the film focuses on the contraption forced into the mouth of the victimized patient (Olivia de Havilland) as if it were a bullet that cowboys bite during an operation on the prairie with only a slug of whiskey for an anesthetic. However, after exploiting the melodramatic aspects of electroshock, *Snake Pit* goes on to endorse its positive effects: after a few sessions, the patient's condition begins to improve, and soon she is able to reap the benefits of psychotherapeutic interventions. As we approach the Golden Age, and ECT is portrayed as effective, it usually occurs off-camera, as in *Fear Strikes Out* (1957), where we see the treatment room only from the outside.

The talking cure of psychotherapy and psychoanalysis seems more favored by moviemakers even though it holds much less dramatic power than ECT. Consequently, filmmakers have developed a convention that cuts across all periods of psychiatric films: the *cathartic cure,* the sudden and dramatic recovery from mental illness. This convention has also been noted by Vernet (1975) and Eber and O'Brien (1982), who emphasize that the formula lends itself well to the building of dramatic tension and its climactic release. There is no corresponding method by which a medical, rather than a mental, patient can dramatically recover from, say, an infectious disease unless the film appropriates more fantasy-oriented types of movie magic. Often a simple montage sequence can make a long period of recovery take up very little screen time, but this convention cannot compete with the drama of the cathartic cure. As is the case with other conventions, the psychiatrist is not really essential for these cathartic cures, variations of which appear frequently in films even when some kind of therapist is completely absent. Consider the sudden recovery of Dorothy McGuire in *The Spiral Staircase* (1946), of Jane Wyman in *Johnny Belinda* (1948), or of Heather Sears in *The Story of Esther Costello* (1957). But when the recovering patient is not deaf, dumb, or blind, psychiatrists are frequently nearby.

Few practicing therapists report moments of catharsis such as those depicted in films. More importantly, instances in which the sudden recovery of repressed memories is *curative* are even rarer. Many American films conventionally reflect one historical moment in the development of psychoanalysis, when Freud himself was attempting to cure his hysterical patients with this method. In his seminal 1895 work, *Studies on Hysteria,* Freud hypothesized that the conversion symptoms of hysterics were caused by repressed traumatic memories. The cure, in his view, was to derepress these memories. Hypnosis and suggestion were both means of removing the repression barrier and allowing these memories to surface. Freud soon learned, however, that the mere recovery of these memories was not in fact curative. He went on to develop the much more sophisticated and complex technique of analyzing resistances and transference as they developed in the analytic situation.

If filmmakers have studied the history of the psychoanalytic movement, it would seem that they stopped reading Freud's works at this particular historical point. Most of the positive portrayals of psychotherapy or psychoanalysis revolve around the derepression of a traumatic memory. The classic example is Nunnally Johnson's 1957 film *The Three Faces of Eve.* In this supposedly true story of a woman suffering from multiple personality, Joanne Woodward is cured by a caring and effective psychiatrist, Dr. Luther, played by Lee J. Cobb. As Dr. Luther becomes aware that he is dealing with a rare multiple personality syndrome, he searches the patient's past for an explanation of the illness. He apparently regards the cure and the discovery of the etiology of the illness as virtually synonymous. Dr. Luther laments how normal her childhood was and expresses a wish that he could find some shocking traumatic episode in her past, implying that such a trauma would be the key to unlock the mystery of both the etiology and the means of cure.

To assist the search, Dr. Luther employs hypnosis, another technique that is greatly overrepresented in the movies in proportion to its actual use by therapists and psychoanalysts. Prior to his use of hypnotic methods, Joanne Woodward displays two personalities, Eve White, a depressed, withdrawn housewife, and Eve Black, a seductive, histrionic floozy (plate 18), whose emergence is usually accompanied by a jazzy clarinet on the sound track. When the psychiatrist begins to use hypnosis, Jane, a third personality, emerges as the integration of the two selves represented by Eve White and Eve Black. Woodward plays Jane by adopting better posture and, consistent with Hollywood's regional stereotyping, by dropping her Southern accent. Through further hypnosis Jane is able to recover a repressed traumatic memory of an episode in her childhood when her parents forced her to kiss her dead grandmother prior to her burial. After this memory is derepressed, Eve White and Eve Black are absorbed by the healthy and well-integrated personality of Jane, who discovers that she now has complete memory of her past. Jane quickly reconstitutes after the emotional catharsis associated with recovering the memory and happily drives off with her new husband and daughter as the film ends. How the childhood trauma has caused the problem of multiple personality remains a mystery, as does the relationship between remembering the incident and curing the illness.

Although *The Three Faces of Eve* is based on a true account, it fits much more neatly into the mythological functions of psychiatry. Most psychiatrists never see anything approaching a cure as dramatic as this one, let alone a multiple personality. In fact, when the real-life "Eve," Chris Costner Sizemore, published her autobiography (1977), she revealed that the cathartic recovery of the repressed traumatic memory did not lead to a lasting resolution of her multiple personality syndrome. Following the treatment depicted in the film, more personalities appeared—a total of twenty-two in all—over the ensuing years. Sizemore finally achieved what she perceived to be a lasting recovery in 1974 following a suicide attempt and intensive therapy. Moreover, she reveals that there were other significant traumatic incidents in her childhood besides the one depicted in the movie. This revelation is much more in keeping with our current understanding of multiple personality, that it is a pattern of repetitive incidents, rather than a single traumatic incident, that produces the syndrome.

Whether or not the depiction of the psychotherapeutic cure in *The Three Faces of Eve* is historically accurate, the point to emphasize here is that such a cure is the preferred account of the mechanism of psychotherapy in the movies. Sometimes cathartic cures do not even involve the derepression of a traumatic childhood memory. In the first scenes of Mark Robson's *Home of the Brave* (1949), a black serviceman named Moss (James Edwards) returns from a World War II battle and says that he cannot walk even though doctors can find no physical disabilities. An Army psychiatrist (Jeff Corey) is first introduced for the familiar purpose of plot mechanics ("What happened on that mission?"), but he soon discovers the source of Moss's problem. In a series of flashbacks we learn that Moss was close friends with a white soldier, Finch (Lloyd Bridges), who eventually died on the mission. Just before he was shot, however, Finch called Moss "a dirty, yellow-bellied nig—" and then corrected himself by saying "nitwit." Moss becomes afflicted with hysterical paralysis because he cannot cope with the realization that he *wanted* Finch to die. Once all this is explained to him, Moss says that he understands, but he still cannot walk. Finally, the psychiatrist begins taunting him, even calling him a "dirty nigger." This does the trick, and Moss rises to attack the psychiatrist only to realize that he has been cured. *Home of the Brave* was produced by Stanley Kramer, one of Hollywood's most outspoken liberals, and Carl Foreman's script was daring in its overt treatment of racism, especially for 1949. The cathartic cure is central to the film, and not just because it provides a dramatic climax. The way in which the cure is administered asks the audience to confront the harsh effects of racial prejudice upon black people while at the same time supporting the politically complementary idea that something can be done to heal the wounds inflicted by racial hatred. Nora Sayre (1982), however, is correct when she argues that the film badly confuses Moss's sensitivity to racism with racism itself and that by basing much of Moss's cure on the realization that he is "just like everybody else," the film denies the real problems of American racism, much as it submits psychiatry to the familiar optimistic conventions of movie myths. Consistent with the Hollywood paradigm of reconciliation, the cathartic cure in *Home of the Brave* provides an effective cinematic means for displacing the overwhelming problems of racism with an uplifting story of one soldier's dramatic recovery from paralysis.

Instant cures also appear in Charles Vidor's gangster film *Blind Alley* (1939), as well as in its remake, Rudolph Mate's *The Dark Past* (1948). A good deal of primitive psychoanalytic theory is bandied about in the story of a gangster (Chester Morris in *Blind Alley,* William Holden in *Dark Past*) who killed because of a desire to destroy his father. By coincidence he finds himself in the house of a psychiatrist (Ralph Bellamy in the original, Lee J. Cobb in the remake) after escaping from jail. Holding the household hostage while waiting for members of his gang to arrive, the gangster is interrogated by the psychiatrist, whose interest in his captor seems purely scientific (plate 10). At first the gangster dismisses the doctor's questions with comments such as "Ah, you're a screwball," but he soon begins recounting a nightmare that has been keeping him awake for years. Using Freudian dream analysis, the psychiatrist identifies various displacements in the criminal's dream, finally explaining his antisocial behavior as a continuing desire to destroy his father. When he is finished, the doctor assures the gangster that he will no longer be able to kill, now that he understands his darker impulses. Like many other oracular psychiatrists in the movies, the doctor has done his job so well that when the police arrive, they easily shoot down the killer, who cannot bring himself to return their fire.

It is tempting to dismiss the preeminence of the cathartic cure as simply emblematic of a particular historical period in the cinematic treatment of psychiatry, but a quick look at a recent Academy Award–winning movie reveals that this is not the case. The sudden recovery of Conrad Jarrett (Timothy Hutton) in *Ordinary People* (1980) is closely related to a moment of catharsis. Released from an institution after a suicide attempt, Conrad is brought closer to health by the parallel efforts of Dr. Berger (Judd Hirsch) and his girlfriend (Elizabeth McGovern). He cannot, however, quite overcome the hostility of his mother (Mary Tyler Moore), and when he learns that a girl he knew in the institution (Dinah Manoff) has killed herself, he slips back into suicidal depression. In desperation he calls Dr. Berger in the middle of the night and arranges to meet him at the psychiatrist's office. In a few minutes, Berger has fixed on the guilt that afflicts Conrad over the death of his brother—also his mother's favorite child—when both boys were involved in a boating accident. Conrad is out of control in Berger's office, screaming and crying as he thrashes about the room. Raising his own voice to get Conrad's attention, Dr. Berger forces him to confront the memory of the boating accident. He asks Conrad what he did wrong, and after resisting the question, Conrad shouts at him, "I hung on!" With this catharsis Conrad's survivor guilt is relieved, but he tells Berger that being alive does not feel good. The intense but unsentimental monotone delivery of Judd Hirsch makes the following exchange particularly effective:

BERGER: It is good, believe me.

CONRAD: How do you know?

BERGER: Because I'm your friend.

CONRAD: I don't know what I would have done if you hadn't been here. Are you really my friend?

BERGER: I am. Count on it. (Hutton reaches out and they embrace.)

Free of his depression, Conrad arrives at the house of his girlfriend with every indication that he is prepared to start life anew. After this scene, the film need only dispose of its villain, Conrad's mother (Mary Tyler Moore), who soon drives away and leaves her son with his father—a postfeminist revision of the *Stella Dallas* cliché of the mother who sacrifices all to save her child.

The unlikely cathartic cure in *Ordinary People* did not prevent the film from receiving an Oscar for best picture. In fact, the film's popularity was probably due in large part to the positive feelings audiences experienced after witnessing the swift and total exorcism of the film's two major demons—Conrad's depression and Mary Tyler Moore. No one can discount the fact that Judd Hirsch was portrayed as a caring and effective psychiatrist. Nor can one dismiss the curative power of a genuine relationship between therapist and patient where the patient feels he is valued. The more interesting dynamics of Conrad's depression, however, such as the obvious sibling rivalry and his consequent but unconscious death wish toward his brother, are left largely unexplored in therapy. Similarly, as Robin Wood has observed, there is no examination of the overtly oedipal process that replaces the mother with a more compliant female (Elizabeth McGovern) in order to facilitate the patriarchal reconciliation of father and son—a process in which, at least on the subtextual level, the psychiatrist is complicit (Wood 1986, 263). The cathartic cure in *Ordinary People* may not have alienated filmgoers, but it did inspire a parody in Jerry Lewis's *Cracking Up* (1983). When the comic protagonist (Lewis) and his analyst (Herb Edelman) finally solve the patient's problems, analyst and patient bound across the office into each other's arms in slow motion à la *Elvira Madigan*.

Electroconvulsive therapy and the cathartic cure are not the only treatments that have become conventionalized in American movies. Simple, commonsense advice is also frequently depicted as essential to psychotherapeutic technique. In the popular film *Now Voyager* (1942), Dr. Jaquith (Claude Rains) is never actually seen in the act of psychotherapy although, as in plate 12, he occasionally mixes with his patients on an elemental level. Basically, he conceptualizes the problem of Charlotte Vale (Bette Davis) as overexposure to an unsympathetic parent, and the therapy he recommends is a South American cruise. This kind of guidance counseling may take the form of telling a woman that she needs a man to dominate her, as in *Lady in the Dark,* or it may be somewhat more sophisticated, as in *Fear Strikes Out* (1957). Like *Three Faces of Eve* this film was based on a true story, the psychiatric struggles of baseball player Jim Piersall, played by Anthony Perkins. The film, however, portrays the recovery of Piersall solely in terms of reconciliation with the male parent. The film argues that Piersall's domineering father (Karl Malden) caused his son's eventual breakdown by withholding love from the boy in order to drive him to higher levels of athletic achievement. After his psychotic depression is relieved through ECT, we see a number of sessions between a faceless psychiatrist played by Adam Williams (an extremely active but virtually anonymous actor) and Piersall (plate 17). The cure is a three-part process in which the psychiatrist first demonstrates that Piersall's father has pushed him into unhappiness and mental illness, then helps the patient to understand that he must keep his father out of his life until the treatment is over, and finally leads Piersall to forgive his father and to leave the institution in a spirit of reconciliation.

This treatment, which results in patients blaming and then forgiving their parents, is an almost generic cure that movie psychiatrists dispense like aspirin. It is consistent with movie myths of self-help, but more specifically with the notion that patients have no responsibility for their illness. Psychiatric disorders are caused by bad parents, and cure is effected by convincing the blameless offspring that he must forgive his parents. While variants of this view of psychiatric illness persist in psychiatry today—for example, Kohut's (1971) view that empathic failures of the mother result in narcissistic disorders in the child—etiological theories have for the most part abandoned the formula of the schizophrenogenic mother and the victimized child. Modern psychiatry is much more likely to view most mental illnesses in terms of a complex interplay among biological, intrapsychic, and environmental factors, with a particular emphasis on the adequacy of the "fit" between child and mother (Thomas and Chess 1984).

In this chapter we identified typological and generic patterns in the portrayal of psychiatry in the movies. Sometimes these patterns result from the simple solutions they offer filmmakers who wish to cut from the present to the past. At other times they are tied in with rigidly prescribed conventions of specific genres that audiences are content to encounter again and again throughout their lives as moviegoers. These patterns are also strongly related to cultural myths, many of which perform the seemingly contradictory functions of acknowledging our problems while simultaneously denying their importance. The mysterious curative powers of psychiatrists can help facilitate this kind of paradoxical mythmaking, but they can also become myths themselves. The ability of cultural myths to tolerate diametrically opposed images accounts for parallel traditions of good and bad psychiatrists.

On the other hand, conventions of plot and character are not always evenly distributed throughout cinematic history. And as we have seen with *Lady in the Dark,* questions of interpretation depend on the historical context of the film. We have been able to link some of the conventions of psychiatry in the movies to specific historical eras, dividing psychiatric films into three historical periods. The first stretches from the earliest turn-of-the-century caricatures in crude one-reelers about escaped lunatics to about 1957. The second and shortest period, from 1957 through 1963, is the Golden Age of psychiatry in the cinema, in which the effectiveness and benevolence of psychiatry fully realized its mythic potential. Third is the period of almost consistently negative depictions beginning almost immediately after the Golden Age ended. Although it may be too soon to tell, a fourth period may have begun in 1980 with the nearly simultaneous appearance of the homicidal transvestite psychiatrist in Brian De Palma's *Dressed to Kill* and the heroically compassionate therapist Dr. Berger in *Ordinary People.* In the three chapters that follow we will chart the changes in the image of the movie psychiatrist and attempt to account for these historical patterns.

The Alienist, the Quack, and the Oracle

2

So far as we can tell, a psychiatrist first appeared in an American film in 1906. *Dr. Dippy's Sanitarium*, the prototype for the genre of mental institution films, evoked vaudeville stereotypes of madness and portrayed a sanitarium as a bedlam subject to sudden takeovers by inmates. When Dr. Dippy's patients overwhelm a newly hired attendant in this twenty-minute feature, they gleefully torment him by rolling him down a hill in a barrel and then by hurling knives at him in the style of the familiar knife-throwers in the circus. The inmates are easily brought under control, however, when Dr. Dippy arrives with a picnic lunch of pie, and as the film ends they all turn their undivided attention to the lusty enjoyment of their meal.

This crude entertainment was probably not created in the interest of dramatizing the work of a psychiatrist. More likely the intention was to capitalize on the great success of a 1904 one-reeler, *The Escaped Lunatic*. A publicity bulletin for the film describes it as "the escapades of an insane man who imagines himself to be Napoleon I. He escapes from the asylum by a miraculous jump from a third story window, and is pursued across the country by the keepers through a series of ludicrous adventures, until finally disgusted at the chase, he jumps back into the window of the asylum, and is very comfortably reading a newspaper when the tired and mud-spattered keepers enter." (Niver 1971, 130). Schneider (1985) has identified several other films that attempted to duplicate the success of this film, but *Dr. Dippy's Sanitarium* is the only one in which a mental health professional, other than a "keeper," actually appears. Dr. Dippy's role in this particular version of a lunatic's antics seems to have been an afterthought, and it may partially explain why we have been unable to locate another film with a psychiatrist until thirteen years later in *When the Clouds Roll By* (1919).

Some American physicians had specialized in the treatment of mental disorders since the 1830s, and idealized portraits of fictional psychiatrists appeared at least as early as 1861 in the novels of Oliver Wendell Holmes, Sr. (Guthmann 1969). If nothing else, the first identifiable psychiatrist in American movies

44

reveals the vastly different audiences to which novels and early films appealed. *Dr. Dippy's Sanitarium* also serves as the earliest example of an ambivalence toward psychiatry that runs through the entire history of the American cinema: primitive as it is, the film establishes some basic patterns that recur regularly. Dr. Dippy's institution is clearly not designed for the cure of its patients, but the director does not abuse his patients and in fact treats them with a certain amount of respect when he politely introduces them one by one to the new attendant. He is also able to bring his charges under control with dispatch and effectiveness even if his pie treatment is rather unorthodox. The doctor is "dippy" apparently because he lives and works around crazy people whose childish and erratic behavior he cannot always control.

Dr. Dippy's Sanitarium also relies heavily on the received stereotypes of the day: like the protagonist in *The Escaped Lunatic*, one inmate dresses as Napoleon while another, a sleepwalker out of Gothic romance, is clad in a flowing white nightgown, a candle and its holder in her extended arm. Dr. Dippy himself is the embodiment of a nineteenth-century medical stereotype: he has a beard, a pince-nez, tails, and a portly bearing. Although this image could fit many middle-class American doctors at the turn of the century, it was soon to be associated almost entirely with psychiatrists, particularly those with foreign accents. The stereotype is still present, by the way, in a film as recent as Billy Wilder's 1974 remake of *The Front Page*.

With easily recognizable characters and with a plot designed for action, the film need not concern itself with the nature of psychiatry and the character of psychiatrists. In fact, even with the limited number of genres available to American filmmakers in the first decade of this century, a similar film could have been made about unruly children in a reform school—or about cannibals in the jungle—or about Indians in the Old West. The real importance of the institution is that it provides a recognizable background for slapstick comedy. As critics since Aristotle have observed, ridiculous characters are suitable subjects for comedy even when real danger and violence are possible, and the 1906 audience laughed at *Dr. Dippy's Sanitarium* knowing that nothing bad was going to happen to anybody they really cared about. Crazy people were fair game as comic subjects and so were their keepers. Insane asylums and their occupants easily met the demands of one of the earliest types of film comedy.

EXPLORATION, EXPLANATION, AND EXPLOITATION

For all its shortcomings, *Dr. Dippy's Sanitarium* was at least able to associate a certain kind of doctor with mentally disturbed patients in an institution. During

the early days of the American cinema, however, the proper domain of psychiatrists was regularly confused with that of hypnotists, clairvoyants, and other
assorted specialists with obscurely defined credentials, setting a pattern for the
demedicalization of psychiatry in hundreds of films yet to be made. In 1919,
the same year as the revolutionary *Cabinet of Dr. Caligari* appeared in Germany,
Douglas Fairbanks starred in *When the Clouds Roll By*, a film that is memorable
if only as the first directorial effort of Victor Fleming, who would later receive
credit for directing both *The Wizard of Oz* and *Gone with the Wind*. *When the
Clouds Roll By* is tailored primarily to the jumping-jack exuberance of Fairbanks,
but its plot also involves a mysterious "doctor of the mind" who seeks to drive
the hero to suicide as part of a scientific experiment. Dr. Ulrich Metz, played
by Herbert Grimwood with what appears to be a large false nose (plate 8), is
first introduced lecturing to an audience of his colleagues. A title card reads,
"Here he confirms the popular prejudice of the time against the mushroom
growth of dubious psychologists." In one of the most interesting scenes in the
film, Fairbanks is given a meal specially prepared by Dr. Metz and his valet to
produce nightmares. The resulting dream sequence, probably inspired by Edwin
S. Porter's *Dream of a Rarebit Fiend* (1906), represents one of the first instances

PLATE 8. Herbert Grimwood is attempting to drive Douglas Fairbanks to suicide in *When the
Clouds Roll By* (1919). The Museum of Modern Art/Film Stills Archives.

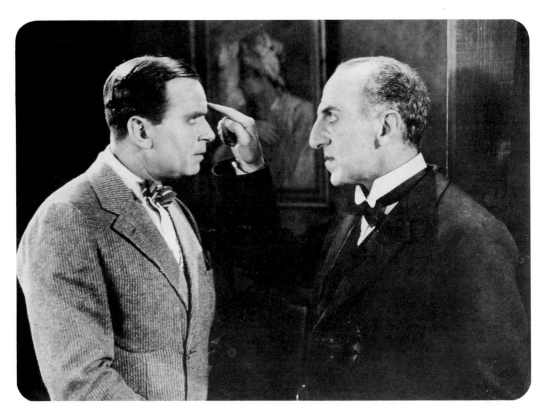

in American film of the creative use of special effects to replicate the dream world. The film concludes as Fairbanks triumphs over several villains, including the mind doctor, who is discovered to be an escapee from an insane asylum.

Only a handful of films appeared in the 1920s with characters resembling psychiatrists. *The Case of Becky* (1921) involves a "nerve specialist" who saves his daughter from an evil hypnotist so that she can marry a nice young man. In *The Man Who Saw Tomorrow* (1922) a psychologist uses hypnosis to enable his clients to see into the future. Also in 1922, Will Rogers played a mild-mannered psychology professor in a film called *One Glorious Day*. He tells the spiritualist society that he chairs that he is about to leave his body and reappear as a spirit. Instead, an aggressive entity takes over his body and does basically what the hero would have done were he not too meek. In *Boomerang* (1925) a doctor in need of patients sets himself up as the director of a mental institution, where he is joined by a female clairvoyant who signs on as his nurse. Surprisingly, the institution is a success, and the two get married. In the 1928 silent film *Plastered in Paris*, a "specialist" fails to cure a World War I veteran's kleptomania, an affliction which the film attributes to a war wound.

The scarcity of psychiatrists in films of the silent era does not, however, reflect their lack of importance in American culture. John Gach has chronicled the early history of psychiatry in America and concluded that "by 1920 the Freudian revolution had succeeded. Psychoanalysis . . . by then assured of its cultural niche . . . verged on orthodoxy" (1980, 155). Burnham (1979) has even unearthed a popular song of 1925 with the prolix title "Don't Tell Me What You Dreamed Last Night, for I've Been Reading Freud." Movies did not fully exploit the abundant cinematic possibilities offered by psychiatry, perhaps because of their conservative nature: in spite of the success of a film like *When the Clouds Roll By*, the movie industry could flourish by continuing to rely on the conventions of vaudeville, the dime novel, and the stage melodrama, forms that had developed in the nineteenth century and that seldom needed psychiatry. Furthermore, the most ambitious producers, such as Cecil B. DeMille, found that the most lucrative formulas lay in biblical epics and spectacles rather than in genres like the social problem film, which might at this time have provided a niche for a psychiatrist. Even when psychiatrists began appearing more regularly in the talking films of the 1930s and 1940s, they were almost always embedded in scripts adapted from plays and novels. This may reflect the slow westward move of psychoanalysis: an accredited psychoanalytic institute was not established in the Los Angeles area until 1946. The playwrights and novelists in the Northeast may have been well acquainted with the profession of psychoanalysis, but the creative members of the movie industry were probably unfamiliar with the new breed of talking doctor because the film industry had been firmly based in the vicinity of Los Angeles since 1915.

However, even sophisticated playwrights like Ben Hecht and Charles MacArthur were willing to use psychiatry mostly for laughs even though Hecht, who would later contribute to Hitchcock's *Spellbound,* was clearly fascinated by the institution. Hecht and MacArthur's 1928 work *The Front Page* featured the appearance of an "alienist," as did the two film versions of the play, which mark both the beginning and the end of the 1930s. During the nineteenth century, "alienist" was one of several names variously assigned to doctors in mental institutions, including those accepted by courts to testify on the mental competence of defendants and witnesses. By the 1920s psychiatrists had for some time been established as replacements for such experts. The Hecht and MacArthur stage play provided the basis for Lewis Milestone's 1931 film of the same title as well as for Howard Hawks's *His Girl Friday* (1940). In *The Front Page* of 1931 a motley collection of cynical reporters awaits the execution of Earl Williams (George E. Stone), the convicted, but unlikely, killer of a policeman in Chicago. One of the reporters (Edward Everett Horton) calls his editor to announce that an alienist named Max J. Egelhofer of Vienna has been called in to examine the convicted man. When the effeminate Horton character adds that Egelhofer has written a book called *The Personality Gland*, one of his colleagues adds, "And where to put it." The film also offers this exchange on the subject:

REPORTER 1: That doctor's the fourteenth pair of whiskers they've sent in on this case.

REPORTER 2: Say, those alienists make me sick. All they do is goose you and then send you a bill for five hundred bucks.

When we meet Egelhofer, he is directing a large dentist's light at the befuddled killer. His pince-nez is on a chain attached to his vest, and a medal hangs on a ribbon around his neck. The alienist also has a stylized beard and an accent that suggests Bela Lugosi more than a denizen of Vienna. When he interviews Earl Williams, he asks that he reenact his crime, even insisting that the sheriff hand the convict a gun for a more precise re-creation. When Williams reaches the crucial moment in his reenactment, Egelhofer asks, "And then what did you do?" Obligingly, the prisoner shoots him in the leg. As the alienist falls to the floor, he exclaims triumphantly, "Dementia praecox!" The movies had at last found a use for psychiatry.

Nine years later, in *His Girl Friday*, little has changed except that the alienist has become a beardless American. Still named Egelhofer, he is portly, wears a pince-nez, and the sheriff calls him both "Professor" and "Doctor" even though the filmmakers have also retained the obsolete title "alienist." For some reason the number of alienists in *His Girl Friday* who have been called to examine Earl Williams has been reduced by four. The relevant exchange between reporters is more typical of 1940, but the spirit is roughly the same as in *The Front Page*:

REPORTER 1: Must be about the tenth alienist they've put on Williams. If he wasn't crazy before, he would be by the time ten of those babies got through psychoanalyzing him.

REPORTER 2: Is this guy Egelhofer any good?

REPORTER 3: Figure it out for yourself. He's the guy they sent to Washington to interview the brain trust. He said *they* were sane.

The 1940 version of Egelhofer also asks Earl Williams to reenact the shooting, but the audience does not actually see Williams shoot the alienist. However, we are told by the heroine (Rosalind Russell) that Egelhofer has been taken "to the County Hospital, where they're awfully afraid he'll recover."

The 1931 and 1940 versions of *The Front Page* make a fascinating comparison with chronologically parallel versions of Clemence Dane's play *A Bill of Divorcement*, George Cukor's original film adaptation dating to 1932, and John Farrow's faithful remake to 1940. Although this family melodrama raises biological questions about mental illness as well as moral questions about granting a divorce on the grounds of insanity, the only doctor in both films is a family physician. While the alienists in *The Front Page* and *His Girl Friday* are comic figures treating a completely sane individual, the crisis of mental illness in historically parallel versions of *A Bill of Divorcement* is presided over by a physician in general practice.

In spite of the ridicule and neglect suffered by the profession during this time, the 1930s also saw the first attempts to deal seriously with psychiatry in American film, *Reunion in Vienna* (1933) and *Private Worlds* (1935). These two films provide excellent examples of what Robert Sklar has called the two "golden ages" of the American cinema, one of "turbulence" and one of "order" (Sklar 1975, 175). Inspired by the new possibilities of sound and determined to engage audiences with controversy, filmmakers spent the years 1930–34 producing a body of work that succeeded so well in titillating and provoking Americans that it caused the creation of the Breen Office. Founded in 1934, the Breen (or Hays) Office strictly administered the movie industry's system of self-censorship, a Production Code that remained strong until the late 1950s. In his psychoanalytically astute study of the American cinema, Robin Wood has suggested that the code represented the purest example of how the forces of sexual repression operated on the powerful "drives" of the American cinema to produce a body of work consistent with dominant ideology (Wood 1986, 48). But although the code proscribed the sex and violence that had outraged religious groups since the earliest nickelodeon peep shows, it was also designed to bring back a lost audience of moviegoers who had been alienated by the film industry's fascination with social complexities during the early years of the depression. Almost immediately, vigilant enforcement of the Production Code worked alongside the New Deal administration to "boost the morale of a confused and anxious people by fostering a spirit of patriotism, unity and commitment to national values" (Sklar 1975, 175).

The social criticism and sexual license of Sidney Franklin's *Reunion in Vienna* (1933) is typical of what Sklar has called "the first golden age" (not to be confused with what we have called the Golden Age of psychiatry in the movies that began twenty-five years later). Based on Robert E. Sherwood's stage play, *Reunion in Vienna* centers around the dilemma of Elena (Diana Wynyard), once the favorite mistress of Archduke Rudolf Maximillian von Habsburg (John Barrymore) but now the wife of eminent Viennese psychiatrist Anton Krug (Frank Morgan). The action begins in 1929, ten years after the Habsburgs were expelled from Vienna. Elena first appears in the Schonbrunn palace, taking the official tour of rooms where she once carried on her affair with the charming but wildly irresponsible Habsburg aristocrat (Barrymore). When she returns home to her psychiatrist husband, we learn that she misses the romance which the practical and often didactic Dr. Krug openly preaches against. The thera-peutic romance of Freud's Vienna cannot compare to the Old World romance of Habsburg Vienna.

The psychiatrist, however, is surprisingly tolerant when Rudolf flaunts Aus-trian law by returning from exile to resume his love affair with Elena. Krug clearly articulates the theme of the film, that the Habsburgs represent an obsolete order—a romantic dream—which has been replaced by rational values embodied most perfectly by psychoanalysis. When Rudolf arrives at Dr. Krug's door and offers to fight him for the favors of Elena, the psychiatrist's first impulse is to remove his glasses and fight the archduke with his fists. But the psychiatrist quickly comes to his senses and realizes that Rudolf has succeeded in making him appear a fool in the eyes of his wife. At this moment, Elena rises, apparently to choose between her two suitors. Before she can announce her choice, however, word arrives that the police are waiting outside to arrest Rudolf. Krug is unwilling to turn his rival over to the authorities and even departs to entreat the prefect of police to allow Rudolf to leave the country gracefully. In doing so, Krug intentionally leaves his wife alone with the archduke for the duration of the night, urging her to see him for what he is, a dream of her past.

Reunion in Vienna even suggests that Krug is willing to offer his wife a final sexual encounter with Rudolf—an opportunity that she does in fact appear to seize—so that she can more easily bring to a close an old chapter in her life. The film ends the next morning with Rudolf gallantly taking his leave and Elena happily accepting her husband as the man most deserving of her love. The reunion of husband and wife becomes an allegory for the inevitable rise of reason, science, education, and psychoanalysis after the eclipse of Old World decadence. On the other hand, the film's rhetoric contradicts its own message, making Rudolf an infinitely more interesting figure than Krug. Similarly, the screenplay cannot resist applying religious, rather than rationalist, metaphors to psychiatry, even allowing Krug to refer to himself unashamedly as a "messiah." Yet *Reunion in Vienna* is primarily a lighthearted costume drama, which does not always spare psychiatry from the same satiric eye it directs toward the Habsburgs and their world. Krug's practice appears to be limited entirely to women who, as Krug's father (Henry Travers) explains, "tell him their dreams, and he tells them what to do about them."

A quite different brand of psychiatry is practiced in a more earnest film, *Private Worlds* (1935), directed by Gregory La Cava and produced by Walter Wanger. The seriousness of this film has much more to do with the Breen Office than it does with a dramatic change in American attitudes toward the profession. As Sklar has written (1975, 175), 1934 marked the beginning of "the second golden age of the American cinema." Turning away from satire and the sexual themes of early talking films such as *Reunion in Vienna*, Hollywood created a glamorous, consoling (and profitable) world of upbeat values, but it also attempted to shake off its somewhat disreputable image by connecting its product with highly respected and/or popular novels. This was the period of *The Barretts of Wimpole Street* (1934), *Les Miserables* (1935), and *A Tale of Two Cities* (1935).

It was also the period of *Private Worlds*, based on a novel by Phyllis Bottome, who later became Alfred Adler's biographer. In keeping with the new seriousness, the film was made with a Dr. Samuel Marcus acting as "technical adviser." Set in "Brentwood Hospital," *Private Worlds* involves the interactions of the staff with each other more than with their patients. The plot involves the love affair between the new director of the institution, Charles Monet (Charles Boyer), and the protagonist, a soon-to-be-familiar female psychiatrist who is out of touch with her emotions, played here by Claudette Colbert. Dr. Monet (Boyer) arrives at the sanitarium to tell Dr. Jane Everest (Colbert) that he strongly disapproves of women in the profession, thus arousing the anger of Jane's steadfast colleague Alex MacGregor (Joel McCrea), who also dislikes the new director because he wanted the job for himself. MacGregor seeks revenge on Monet by carrying on an affair with Monet's sister (Helen Vinson), eventually causing his own wife Sally (Joan Bennett) to attempt suicide. The main plot, however, focuses on the relationship between Colbert and Boyer, who proclaim their love for one another only after she has stepped down from her position at the hospital. Nevertheless, the film does not adhere completely to the antifeminist values we identified in chapter 1 as central to the ideology of the vast majority of American films with female psychiatrists. The McCrea character is capable of maintaining a professional and mutually respecting relationship with Jane Everest (Colbert) throughout the film, and in one early scene, the female doctor even bids farewell to a male patient who heartily thanks her for curing him and then disappears for the duration of the film. Furthermore, Dr. Everest is not required to give up her profession for marriage: at the film's conclusion, the formerly misogynist Dr. Monet (Boyer) asks her to stay on at the institution after she has resigned. Perhaps Colbert's character was given greater latitude as a professional in 1935 because the American public and the film industry were not yet as concerned about the "proper" role of women as when female workers began leaving the home in great numbers in 1942.

Nevertheless, *Private Worlds* is primarily an awkward ninety minutes of melodrama, exploiting adultery as much as insanity but always staying within the limits of the Production Code. The film even looks back to old silent films about escaped lunatics in several scenes with a violent patient whose outbursts can only be controlled by the soothing words of Dr. Everest. The film also offers an early example of the American cinema's difficulty in conceptualizing psychiatrists as medical doctors (plate 9). Both Colbert and McCrea wear white coats throughout most of the film and carry on a long-term, though obscure, experiment involving microscopes, mathematical equations, and conversations about "neurons." They are scientific doctors in the same tradition as the medical paragons in *Magnificent Obsession, The Story of Louis Pasteur*, and *Disputed Passage*, but when the psychiatrists actually treat patients, they are little more than "keepers," restraining the violent ones and consoling the depressed ones. McCrea even has a scene in which he successfully brings a smile to the face of a suicidal young woman by telling her that "life's a lot of fun when you find the joy of living." It did not take the movies long to learn that simplified talking psychiatry offers more drama and consolation than the scientifically technical aspects of the profession.

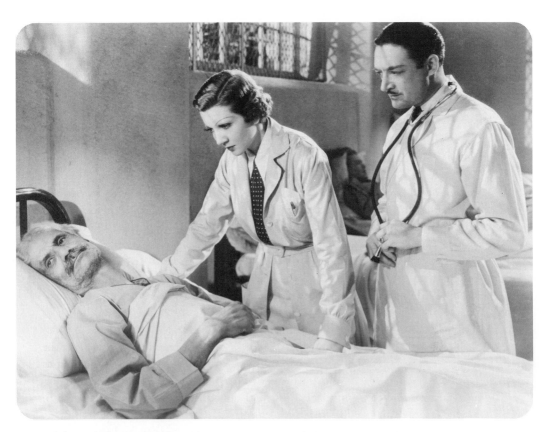

PLATE 9. Two of the first—and last—medicalized psychiatrists in American movies: Claudette Colbert and Theodore von Eltz with Nick Shaid in *Private Worlds* (1935). Warner Brothers. The Museum of Modern Art/Film Stills Archive.

By 1939 the image of the oracular, demedicalized, and godlike psychiatrist had fully emerged in *Blind Alley* with Ralph Bellamy's portrayal of Dr. Shelby. Based on a play by James Warwick, the film begins as "Far above Cayuga's Waters" plays on the sound track behind an establishing shot of a college campus. As the camera enters Dr. Shelby's classroom, he is lecturing authoritatively on the thin dividing line between madness and sanity. He even offers a kind of cultural relativism in his discussion of insanity by asking what Norwegians would think of "jitterbug jive" and what the Chinese might make of women's hats. He then turns Platonic and suggests that even love is a kind of madness. Returning home from the classroom that evening, his foreign-accented wife greets the doctor in their comfortable lakeside house. ("Cayuga's

Waters" and the lake suggest Cornell although its medical school is 350 miles away. Once again, the absence of medical imagery in a psychiatric film is striking.) The picture that emerges in the first minutes of this film suggests that Dr. Shelby combines two quite different roles that, according to Burnham (1979), psychiatrists often filled in the 1930s. According to Burnham, the earliest American psychoanalysts saw themselves as "avant-gardists," disseminating Freud's revolutionary ideas, while later practitioners assumed a less controversial role as advocates for traditional Western values. The character that Ralph Bellamy plays in *Blind Alley* is both a professor and a psychiatrist; he upsets the parochial preconceptions of his students but argues for tolerance and pluralism; and he leads a traditional family life though his wife is European. To use Burnham's terms, he is both a member of the social and intellectual avant-garde and a spokesman for "the rational and the humane," the latter role having been "superimposed" on the former during the 1930s. Bellamy's Dr. Shelby represents a synthesis of the avant-garde psychiatrist (represented negatively in *The Front Page*) with images of psychiatry based on enlightened rationalism (as in *Reunion in Vienna* and *Private Worlds*).

Nevertheless, the doctor in *Blind Alley* is not out of place in the genre of gangster movies, maintaining his intellectual composure even when his house is invaded by an escaped killer (Chester Morris). Although the villain actually shoots down one of his students, fear and doubt never enter the mind of Dr. Shelby (plate 10). The cure that he administers, and that is responsible for the death of the gangster, seems to emerge from Shelby's scientific and professional mission rather than from any stratagems to eliminate his unwanted houseguest. Smoking the inevitable pipe, Bellamy lectures Morris on dream interpretation and unconscious motivation in the same spirit that he instructs his students. He even tells the killer, "You interest me."

The overall image of psychiatry which emerges in the movies of the 1930s is even more diffuse than *Reunion in Vienna, Private Worlds,* and *Blind Alley* might suggest. In fact, a comprehensive cinematic "myth" of psychiatry, built on a tension between diametrically opposed images, was already established by this time. For example, the idealization in *Private Worlds* and *Blind Alley* must be understood alongside the negative portrayals of psychiatrists in *The Front Page* and in a film like Hobart Henley's *Free Love* (1930). Based on a play by Sidney Howard, the latter film introduces us to another avant-garde quack who is more out of touch with reality than his patients could possibly be. The constant bickering between Stephen and Hope Ferrier (Conrad Nagel and Genevieve Tobin) finally drives Hope to a psychiatrist. For a fee of $800 she learns that she is an "intuitive introvert" and that Stephen is an "infantile extrovert."

This diagnosis is all Hope needs to collect her belongings and her children and leave her husband. She even goes to Atlantic City with her husband's best friend, thus inspiring Stephen to punch the man in the jaw. Stephen fails to bring his wife home until he recalls the advice of a casual acquaintance, a drunk he met in a speakeasy. "You should not have punched your best friend," the barroom philosopher tells him, "you should have punched your wife." When Stephen finally does exactly that, his wife recovers her senses and, without recriminations, falls into his arms as a repentant and faithful wife. Unlike *Lady in the Dark, Free Love* casts a psychiatrist as a force opposed to the received notions of femininity upheld by the film.

A blow to the jaw also plays a prominent role in one of Ginger Rogers's last films with Fred Astaire. As the dancing psychiatrist in *Carefree* (1938), Astaire is little more than a glorified hypnotist, but he is also one of the first stereotypical shrinks to save a patient by falling in love. Astaire even does a dance with Rogers in which he performs the conventional coaxing, arm-waving gestures of the show business hypnotist. Ralph Bellamy is also in *Carefree* but this time as Rogers's befuddled fiancé, who takes her to his friend the psychiatrist because

PLATE 10. Murderer Chester Morris arouses the curiosity and the sympathy but not the malice of oracular Ralph Bellamy (with Rose Stradner) in *Blind Alley* (1939). Columbia Pictures. The Museum of Modern Art/Film Stills Archive.

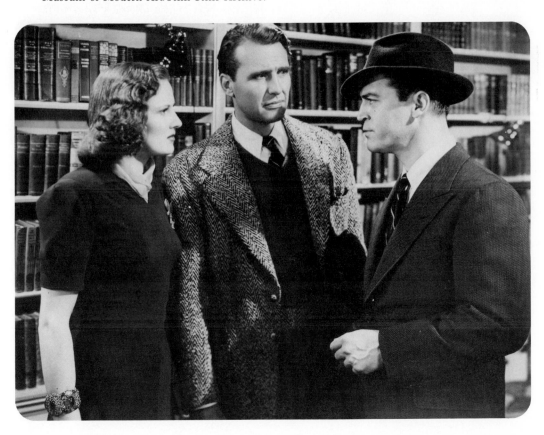

she keeps breaking off their engagement. In accord with the Astaire/Rogers formula, she falls in love with the psychiatrist instead of with Bellamy although Astaire has yet to succumb to her allure. Quickly circumventing the problems raised by Rogers's passion for him, Astaire hypnotizes her and plants the conviction in her mind that she loves Bellamy. To make certain that she abandons her feeling for him, the psychiatrist even tells her that men like himself should be shot down like animals. Before Astaire can bring her out of the trance, however, she wanders out of his office, acquires a gun from her skeet-shooting fiancé, and does in fact attempt to shoot Astaire. By the time Astaire realizes that he is in love with Rogers, he is incapable of getting close enough to hypnotize and reprogram her. Finally, he crashes the ceremony just prior to Rogers and Bellamy's wedding, and after a blow to the jaw, Rogers returns to her trance. Astaire then quickly transforms her back into the woman who loves him. Clearly, there was no psychiatric adviser on the set of *Carefree*.

The pairing of Astaire and Rogers in *Carefree* must not, however, be dismissed so lightly. On the one hand, Ginger Rogers presents a curious case in the history of psychiatry in the movies, having played more analysands than probably any other actress: after *Carefree* (plate 11), she appeared in *Lady in the Dark* (plate 1) and, in 1957, *Oh Men! Oh Women!* (plate 19). And yet there is practically nothing in Rogers's screen persona that suggests anything but wholesome American normality. In *Carefree*, as in *Free Love* and *Reunion in Vienna*, psychotherapy is primarily a pastime for members of the idle rich who are a little short on common sense. Rogers ends up in Astaire's office because she only partially understands the not-so-awful truth that audiences at Leo McCarey's *The Awful Truth* (as well as Howard Hawks's *His Girl Friday*) would soon learn: marriage to Ralph Bellamy may offer security but certainly not excitement (Cavell 1981b). On the other hand, the casting of Astaire as a psychiatrist suggests something a little different. While it is true that the great leading men of Hollywood—from John Wayne and Henry Fonda to Dustin Hoffman and Robert De Niro—have never played psychiatrists, it is also true that Astaire is, in the words of Michael Wood, "our enduring dream of the effortless conquest of recalcitrant circumstance" (1975, 150). When Astaire lends his aura to psychiatry, the profession becomes more than a little magical. Although *Carefree* was intended as just another container for the Astaire/Rogers formula, the tension between the perfectly healthy analysand and the perfectly graceful psychiatrist was an appropriate complement for the more fundamental tension in their relationship: "while the aristocratic, urbane Astaire was frequently called on to play musical versions of the outlaw hero . . . the saucy, down-to-earth Rogers appeared in parts that called for her to assume

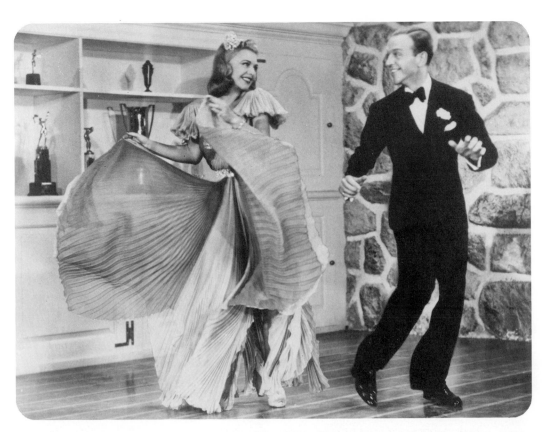

PLATE 11. Therapy in the thirties: Fred Astaire treats Ginger Rogers in *Carefree* (1938). RKO. The Museum of Modern Art/Film Stills Archive.

airs. . . . The plots that kept them apart, therefore, nearly always turned on mistaken identities, and it gradually became clear that the two were perfectly compatible" (Ray 1985, 166). On its subtextual level, *Carefree* also presents a perfect compatibility between Rogers's message that psychiatry is unnecessary and Astaire's that it is as graceful and effortless as his dancing. No better pair could have exemplified the split mythology of psychiatry that Hollywood had absorbed in the 1930s: the studios may not have understood the strange profession, but they knew exactly what to do with it.

Nevertheless, Astaire is regularly referred to as a "quack" in *Carefree*, even by some ducks he encounters in a bicycle tour of Central Park. More familiar stereotypes of the middle European quack in the 1930s are present in W. S. Van Dyke's *After the Thin Man* (1936), Ernst Lubitsch's *Bluebeard's Eighth Wife* (1938), Anatole Litvak's *The Amazing Dr. Clitterhouse* (1938), and Howard

Hawks's *Bringing up Baby* (1938). In the second of the *Thin Man* features, George Zucco plays "a crackpot psychologist" with thick glasses who at one point accuses a seemingly pleasant young man (James Stewart) of being crazy. When Nick Charles (William Powell) reveals that the Stewart character is a murderer, Stewart bursts into a wild confession of his hatred for various characters, deceased and otherwise, revealing himself to be quite mad. In one of the final shots in the film, the camera closes on Zucco, who exclaims, "Good heavens, I was right. The man is crazy." In *Bluebeard's Eighth Wife*, Lawrence Grant plays Professor Urganzeff, another bespectacled, goateed middle European eccentric, who runs a sanitarium to which Gary Cooper is briefly committed. When one of the doctor's patients is released, presumably after being cured of the conviction that he is a chicken, the patient takes one look at the stock market quotations in the newspaper and exclaims, "Cock-a-doodle-doo." Even more ridiculous is the psychiatrist in *The Amazing Dr. Clitterhouse* (1938), who appears briefly in a courtroom scene and succeeds in confusing everyone, including himself. In chapter 1 we discussed the comic figure played by Fritz Feld in *Bringing up Baby* (1938): although the psychiatrist does offer the heroine (Katharine Hepburn) and the audience a crucial bit of psychological information ("The love impulse in men very frequently reveals itself in terms of conflict"), he is eventually shown to be as easily deluded as the bumbling sheriff he assists. In all three of these 1938 films, as in many to come, the audience can sustain ambivalent attitudes toward psychiatry by watching exotic psychiatrists demonstrate competence and then suffer devaluation.

This kind of mythmaking is used to greatest effect in Frank Capra's *Mr. Deeds Goes to Town* (1936), written by Capra's regular collaborator Robert Riskin from a short story by Clarence Budington Kelland. Gary Cooper plays the "Capracorn" hero from a small town who embodies the American values that Sklar (1975) has called "Jeffersonian agrarian." When Deeds decides to distribute his multimillion dollar inheritance among the depression army of common men like himself, the New York bankers and lawyers protect their investments by enlisting the services of Emile von Haller (Wyrley Birch), "the most eminent psychiatrist in the world." Complete with pince-nez and thick accent, von Haller testifies in court that Deeds is insane and therefore not fit to spend his own money. Even though von Haller has never examined Deeds, he demonstrates the hero's "manic-depressive" qualities with a chart showing that Deeds vacillates in and out of a "sane and normal" range into "abnormal" and "subnormal" extremes.

Mr. Deeds's enemies in the film argue that his hobby of playing the tuba proves that he is insane. When the hero rises to defend himself, he argues that tuba-playing helps him to relax and concentrate in much the same way that other people are served by their nervous habits. Von Haller, as Deeds points out, is a doodler. When the court confiscates the psychiatrist's notepad, the camera reveals that von Haller has doodled a childish rendering of a grotesque face. In spite of his august stature, the doctor's more revealing practices show that he is quite different from what he pretends to be. His credibility destroyed, the doctor throws down his pencil petulantly.

The Viennese fraud in *Mr. Deeds Goes to Town* is the perfect foil for the virtues that Capra endorses in this film. Sklar describes the director's vision: "Capra's social myth, it's true, required turning back the clock to an imagined past social stability founded upon an image of the American small town, with comfortable homes, close-knit families, friendly neighbors—a modest but prosperous community with bountiful farms and a benign wilderness nearby" (1975, 210). Capra knew that audiences could accept this myth when presented with a world in which the only dissenting voices are easily discredited. At one point during his testimony, Dr. von Haller turns to one of the other court psychiatrists and asks if he recalls "the case of the young nobleman." How can we believe a man who comes from a world so distant and socially askew that it can include "a young nobleman"? As the psychiatrist continues to spout jargon and mystification, Capra's camera shows a courtroom gallery full of humbly dressed but respectfully silent spectators, one of whom scratches his head in confusion. As the film's audience regards itself in this mirror, it can believe that mental illness and the doctors who treat it are entirely out of place in America. In fact, the craziest people in the film are the charming and harmless Faulkner sisters from Deeds's home town, who are convinced that everyone except themselves is "pixilated."

The 1930s end with a curious example of psychiatry in the cinema, *Children of Loneliness*. Filmed in 1939 but denied a license for exhibition until the 1950s because of its attention to forbidden subjects, *Children of Loneliness* uses a psychiatrist to link two vignettes about homosexuality. A psychiatrist who "aids the police in cases of abnormal sexuality" narrates the film and appears in both episodes when characters concerned about their sexuality visit him. In the first episode, the doctor tells a young woman not to submit to the sexual advances of her girlfriend, and in the second he counsels a male painter who fears that the "femininity" of his work reveals sexual abnormality. This plot summary, however, does not capture the tone of the film, which is closer to *Reefer Madness* than to *Making Love* and was clearly intended to exploit the issue of homosexuality rather than to educate the public. Nevertheless, the film is one of the first to present a psychiatrist entirely without avant-garde or exotic associations and in the new role as a spokesman for "normality." *Children of Loneliness* was eventually resurrected and released in the same year as *Glen or Glenda?* (1953) to capitalize on the enormous publicity surrounding the sex change operation of Christine Jorgensen in 1952 (Russo 1981).

THE FORTIES: DR. JAQUITH, DR. KIK, AND THE SINISTER DR. RITTER

One of the most influential cinematic psychiatrists from the 1940s was Dr. Jaquith (Claude Rains) in *Now Voyager* (1942). The character looks back to the pipe-smoking oracle played by Ralph Bellamy in *Blind Alley*, but like many of the idealized psychiatrists of the early 1940s, he is entirely rooted in a straightforward rationalism with none of the avant-garde trappings of the psychiatrist in *Blind Alley*. Dr. Jaquith runs a clinic called Cascade, which resembles a country manor much more than an asylum and where he is right at home with his air of easy grace and authority (plate 12). He also exudes an ethereal kind of sexuality even though the film does not allow him to focus his sexual emanations on any one character. Bette Davis (Stine 1974) has said that she believes a continuation of the incidents in *Now Voyager* would have shown her married to Jaquith and helping him at Cascade after she realizes that she cannot marry Jerry (Paul Henreid). It would be difficult, however, to imagine Dr. Jaquith coming down to earth long enough to become romantically involved with a woman. Furthermore, when Charlotte Vale (Davis) takes over the treatment of the daughter of her married lover (Henreid), Jaquith accepts it with good humor even though the film suggests that the girl needs mothering more than the conventional, perhaps cold treatment that Jaquith administers.

The exact nature of Dr. Jaquith's treatment is uncertain since we never really see him working with a patient. Unlike *Blind Alley* with its crude Freudianisms, *Now Voyager* contains nothing reminiscent of psychoanalytic theory or technique. Instead, Dr. Jaquith dispenses homilies such as "independence is reliance upon one's will and judgment." He tells Charlotte that people come to him when they are "tired" or "confused," and when he first encounters Charlotte in her domineering mother's house, he tells Charlotte, "You don't need my help," and he scolds her mother. *Now Voyager* did a great deal to domesticate and demystify the image of the psychiatrist in America, but it did so by shying away from any real confrontation with the technical aspects of psychiatry, even avoiding the expressionistic dream sequences of *Blind Alley*, which were rapidly becoming conventionalized in films of the 1940s. Here as in several films we discussed in the portion of chapter 1 devoted to the "cathartic cure," mental illness is presented as overexposure to an unsympathetic parent, and the cure is a cruise on a luxury liner and a new boyfriend. Later on, when Charlotte blames herself for her mother's death and returns to Jaquith's sanitarium, the main reason is the plot necessity of bringing her together with Jerry again. Other than that, she commits herself because she is a little sad.

Now Voyager is one of several "women's films" that comfortably provide a niche for psychiatrists, involved as these films are with the problem of identity that women faced during the upheavals of the 1940s (Walsh 1984). We have already discussed *Lady in the Dark* (1944) in this context; we should also mention *Since You Went Away* (1944), *Possessed* (1947), and the English *Seventh Veil* (1945) as films that also appropriate psychiatry as an important element in women's search for identity. Alfred Hitchcock's *Spellbound* (1945) fits into this category as well despite the picture's more ambitious scope and the casting of a woman as a psychiatrist. Like *Now Voyager* and *Since You Went Away*, *Spellbound* was based on a novel, still the major source for movie plots with psychiatrists in the 1940s.

At one point in *Spellbound*, Dr. Bruloff (Michael Chekhov), the crusty old analyst who trained Constance Peterson (Ingrid Bergman), says, "Women make the best psychoanalysts until they fall in love. Then they make the best patients."

PLATE 12. Claude Rains in *Now Voyager* (1942) is almost godlike, but he is not above joining Bette Davis for a hot dog. Warner Brothers. The Museum of Modern Art/Film Stills Archive.

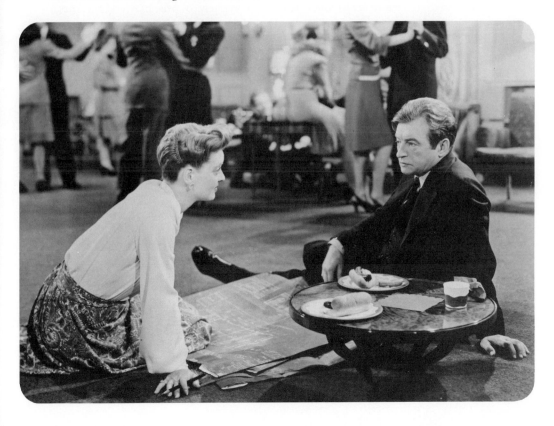

Actually, at least in *Spellbound*, he is wrong. Women make mediocre analysts *until* they fall in love. Then they become superb analysts, detectives, and, of course, helpmates. Dr. Peterson (Bergman), a psychoanalyst on the staff of a clinic called Green Manors, first appears as a somewhat mousey woman, hiding her beauty behind a long white coat, a cigarette holder, glasses, and an un-flattering coiffure. As if to emphasize her lack of femininity, her first patient is a flamboyantly beautiful woman (Rhonda Fleming) who plays out her sexual passions by first enticing and then physically attacking the male members of the clinic's staff. Bergman accomplishes virtually nothing with the Fleming character, and their brief session together ends with the patient throwing a book at the psychoanalyst before being taken away by an orderly. A male psychiatrist on the staff of Green Manors then lectures Dr. Peterson on her icy conduct as both an analyst and a woman. He is clearly interested in forming a romantic liaison with her, but she blithely ignores his sexual overtures as well as his critique of her professional abilities. Soon, however, an amnesiac Gregory Peck arrives, and she immediately begins to demonstrate substantial competence in a variety of roles.

Dr. Peterson falls in love with the Peck character even though he quickly reveals himself to be an extremely troubled individual. Suspected of murder, he himself is unable to recall whether or not he killed Dr. Edwardes, the new director of the clinic whose identity he has assumed. Undaunted by these uncertainties, Bergman's character flees with her lover to Dr. Bruloff. Michael Chekhov, the eminent Russian actor and nephew of the playwright Anton Chekhov, plays Bruloff with occasional moments of irascibility and clownishness but presents both these qualities as necessary components of a wise and complex personality. When Dr. Bruloff scolds the Bergman character for succumbing to female emotionalism in her seemingly irrational conviction that Peck is innocent, he speaks with great authority. Yet Constance Peterson also speaks with authority, and it is with *her* that the film ultimately asks us to side, as should be clear from one of the film's production stills (plate 27). She tells Bruloff, "You know only science. You know his mind, but you don't know his heart." Later she adds, "The heart can see deeper. . . . I couldn't feel this pain for someone who is evil." Bruloff responds, "This is baby talk."

The scenes between Ingrid Bergman and Michael Chekhov contain the first detailed discussions of countertransference in the American cinema. As with *Private Worlds* in the previous decade, the producers of *Spellbound* enlisted a practicing psychiatrist for technical assistance: the credits list May E. Romm, M.D., as "psychiatric advisor." Nevertheless, the demands of Hitchcock's film necessitate the juxtaposition of a traditional female's nurturing instinct with the professional training of an experienced male. Constance Peterson can succeed only by exchanging her psychoanalyst's background for the emotional responses of a woman in love, and she herself says so. In this sense the film endorses the emerging ideology of the postwar years and implicitly supports the biological determinism of writers such as Lundberg and Farnham (1947). On the other hand, Constance's instincts turn out to be correct: she cures the psychological afflictions of the Peck character, and she personally solves the crime for which her lover has been convicted. The film says that women are ineffective as psychoanalysts unless they are fulfilled as women, but it also suggests that the efforts of an emotionally involved woman are vastly superior to those of male psychiatrists *and* male detectives. Dr. Peterson is even vindicated in her disputes with the wise old Dr. Bruloff. In reconciling contradictory myths about female psychiatrists, *Spellbound* provides an excellent illustration for the comparison between studio bosses (such as *Spellbound's* David O. Selznick) and "naive anthropologists" (Ray 1985, 13).

Spellbound also contains several conventions that were already established, or soon would be, in films about psychiatrists. In addition to the psychiatrist as lover and the psychiatrist as detective, the film also gives us the psychiatrist as criminal in the villain of the piece, Dr. Murchison (Leo G. Carroll). We also witness the conventional cathartic cure when Gregory Peck both regains his memory and recovers from a childhood trauma after a single skiing descent down a mountain slope. Miklos Rozsa's score for the film introduces the eerie sound of the theremin, an instrument that was often part of the melodramatic trappings that accompanied cinematic probings into the darker reaches of the human mind, although by 1948 the instrument was already being used for tongue-in-cheek purposes in *Let's Live a Little*. Although *Spellbound* is a long way from the free-flowing collection of Freudian dream images that made up the 1928 surrealist masterpiece *Un Chien andalou*, both films contain contributions from Salvador Dali. The brief montage of images appearing on the screen when Gregory Peck recounts his key dream was based on drawings by Dali and represents a further refinement in the rendering of dreams on the screen. No American film has matched the revolutionary mise-en-scène of the German expressionist classic *Cabinet of Dr. Caligari* (1919), but *Spellbound's* Daliesque dream sequence is a much more interesting representation of the dream work than the theatrical pageants of *Lady in the Dark* (1944) or the simple switch to negative stock in *Blind Alley* (1939).

In addition to listing the services of a psychiatric adviser, the opening credits for *Spellbound* conclude with a truncated quotation from Shakespeare, "The fault . . . is not in our stars, but in ourselves . . ." followed by these lines:

"Our story deals with psychoanalysis, the method by which modern *science* treats the emotional problems of the sane. The analyst seeks only to induce the patient to talk about his hidden problems, to open the locked doors of his mind. Once the complexes that have been disturbing the patient are uncovered and interpreted, the *illness* and confusion disappear . . . and the *evils* of *unreason* are driven from the human *soul*" (emphasis added). This is a fascinating statement with revealing contradictions and ambiguities: although psychoanalysis is at first named a science, it is later associated with both medicine and religion in the same sentence. But in spite of the broadly suggestive claims in its prologue, *Spellbound* does not take the practice of psychoanalysis much beyond the convention of the simple cathartic cure. When Gregory Peck arrives at the clinic, he is unaware that he is impersonating a dead man. Nevertheless, he is quite capable of functioning normally for the first few hours after his arrival, and he is even able to form a lasting romantic bond with the Bergman character. The film never questions the strength of a relationship initiated while one partner was not acting in an entirely rational manner. In fact, Peck's mental illness in *Spellbound* manifests itself entirely as an occasional lack of affect or as the sudden onslaught of panicky feelings. The "talking cure" suggested in the prologue appears only briefly, and ultimately, "the evils of unreason" that threaten the one disturbed character in the film are exorcised by detective work rather than psychoanalysis. Hitchcock himself called *Spellbound* "just another manhunt story wrapped up in pseudo-psychoanalysis" (Truffaut 1984, 165).

Two years after *Spellbound*, the talking cure was again subordinated to criminal matters in *Nightmare Alley* (1947). In fact, the patient in this film would have been much better off if he had kept his neurosis to himself. Stanton Carlisle (Tyrone Power), a "mentalist" who performs in a fashionable Chicago nightclub, visits "counseling psychologist" Lilith Ritter (Helen Walker) when he is driven into panic by the odor of rubbing alcohol. As the film shows us earlier, Stan accidentally gave wood alcohol to Pete (Ian Keith), a down-and-out alcoholic mind reader, when the two men were both working in a cheap carnival act. Stan's guilt over the old drunk's resulting death surfaces later when he has become a success by employing many of the techniques for phony mind-reading acts that Pete had taught him. Lilith Ritter terminates his guilt feelings in a very brief therapy session, but this is not the end of Stan's problems. The psychologist enlists the mentalist into her elaborate scheme for extorting money from wealthy patients who are obsessed with deceased loved ones. Armed with religious rhetoric, the psychologist's privileged information, and his own audacity, Stan convinces one Chicago plutocrat (Taylor Holmes) that he is in touch with the girl that the wealthy man loved long ago before her death. The man even donates $150,000 for the construction of a "tabernacle," but the mentalist entrusts the money to Lilith. The psychologist's name should have tipped Stan off, for when his project is exposed and he must flee Chicago, Lilith keeps the money for herself. When Stan threatens to expose her, she begins speaking in the patronizing tones of a therapist whose patient cannot remember the lessons of previous sessions. Just as she has done with the wealthy patients who have become her victims, Lilith has recorded Stan's confessions in their one session together, and she is prepared to use the information about Pete's death against him. The end of the film recalls its beginning, in which a young and naive Stan had expressed disbelief at the daily routine of the carnival geek whose act consisted of separating the heads from chickens by biting them in the neck. Unable to find work after fleeing from Chicago, Stan drifts into alcoholism and eventually to a traveling carnival where the job of geek seems to be awaiting him.

Nightmare Alley is still today an intriguing piece of filmmaking and one of the best examples of *film noir*. Literally "black film," movies of this type involve violent plots, often with a heavy dose of sexuality, and ruthless characters such as hard-boiled detectives, double-dealing women, and tough-talking criminals. Most of the films in this tradition were made just after World War II, and they reflect the less optimistic vision of America that was emerging in this period as well as the growing fascination with psychiatry that came with it. Just as psychiatrists were out of place in Frank Capra–land, they were welcome and even necessary in the more complex world of *film noir*. The darker corners of the mind that create irrational behavior were widely exposed and popularized in accounts of the psychiatric treatment for returning servicemen, and Hollywood had no trouble translating this knowledge into cinematic terms. The heavy emphasis on shadows and the "visual feel" in *film noir* were influenced by expressionist directors and cinematographers, especially those from Germany and, to a lesser degree, France, where there was a much greater interest in psychoanalysis. Fritz Lang, who made several classic *noir* films in the United States, had earlier used a number of expressionist techniques in Germany for his cycle of Mabuse films about a mad psychiatrist. On the other hand, much of what we now call *film noir* was only obliquely related to psychiatry: much of it grew naturally out of the wide range of techniques that American film-makers employed to render the bleak, urban vision of many novels of this period, particularly the detective fiction of Raymond Chandler and Dashiell Hammett. *Nightmare Alley* effectively exploits the techniques of this tradition and, like many other noirist films, creates a sinister world of victims and victimizers, populated by women of threatening, often ambiguous sexuality.

As plate 13 demonstrates, Helen Walker's Lilith Ritter dresses mannishly, and as the ultimate victimizer in *Nightmare Alley*, she provides one of the most complete examples of how *film noir* depicts women (Kaplan 1980). *Nightmare Alley* is another interesting example of how Hollywood has dealt with the troublesome image of a beautiful woman in an authoritative occupation. As we observed in chapter 1, female psychiatrists in the movies generally help their male patients only by falling in love with them. Lilith Ritter is an exception to test the rule. On the one hand, she does express some interest in forming a sexual relationship with Tyrone Power's character when she suggests a rendezvous in her cabin at the boat club. This overture is hardly consistent with the behavior of a sympathetic female therapist, especially since Stan (Power) is married. He refuses her offer, however, on the grounds that they cannot risk being seen together, and none of the conventional therapeutic romance we witness in *Spellbound* and many other films ever takes place. On the other hand, the psychologist's success with her patient is the work not of a competent professional but of a scheming and unscrupulous blackmailer with no "female" compassion whatever. She can help him recover from guilt feelings, but her real agenda is quite different from that of more honest therapists. The evil female psychiatrist in *Nightmare Alley*, who operates entirely without the nurturing spirit, is the obligatory complement to the more familiar female psychiatrist who can function successfully only by making sacrifices for the man she loves. Significantly, Lilith Ritter uses the term "transference," the magic word that women therapists in the movies often use in their first feeble efforts to cope with the sexual chemistry between themselves and their patients. In the mouth of Lilith Ritter, however, the word is part of a speech that has been carefully prepared both to convince the hero that he is mad and to keep him in place until police arrive.

Another intriguing speech in *Nightmare Alley* takes place during the first meeting between Stan and Lilith. At this point they are still circling each other, trying to determine what scheme the other is concocting. When Stan asks about her occupation, Lilith says, "Ever been psychoanalyzed?" Stan replies, "Saw it once in a murder movie. A good mentalist could have solved the whole thing in five minutes." This statement neatly captures the attitude toward psychiatry so often adopted in crime melodramas, or to use the genre suggested by Stan, "murder movies." Psychoanalysis is regularly confused with or relegated to detective work partially because its methodologies require gathering clues and following through on hypotheses, but also because crime detection provides a neatly simplified version of psychiatry—problems can be thoroughly solved

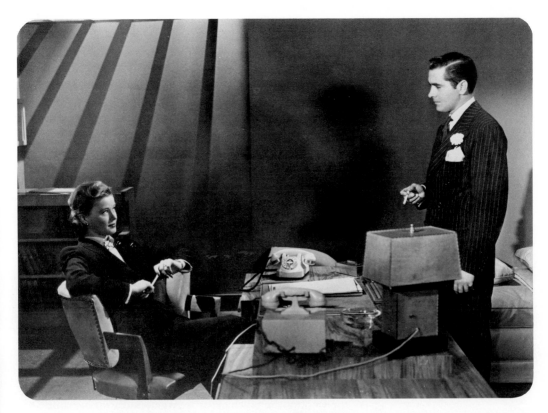

PLATE 13. The seductive and evil Lilith Ritter (Helen Walker) with Tyrone Power in *Nightmare Alley* (1947). Twentieth Century–Fox. The Museum of Modern Art/Film Stills Archive.

and forgotten once a culprit has been identified. This is one of the reasons why the easily identified parent is so often the cause of an individual's sufferings in psychiatrically oriented movies. Stories about people in trouble with their minds are often built upon the same foundations as stories about people in trouble with the law.

Other examples of films in which psychiatry appeared along with the conventions of *film noir* include *The Dark Past* (1948), which used noirist techniques to retell the same story as *Blind Alley* of 1939, and Steve Sekely's *Hollow Triumph* (1948, later released as *The Scar*), in which Paul Henreid plays a man who kills and then replaces his psychoanalyst double with a great deal of success, at least at first. In Curtis Bernhardt's *High Wall* (1947), Audrey Totter plays a psychiatrist who, like Ingrid Bergman in *Spellbound*, falls in love with an accused man (Robert Taylor) before she identifies the man who framed him.

Robert Siodmak's *The Dark Mirror* (1946) introduced a psychiatrist to the phenomenon of the "evil twin," a cliché which has surfaced in numerous films (such as Brian De Palma's *Sisters* and Paul Henreid's *Dead Ringer*), and which like many cinematic conventions has moved on to entrench itself thoroughly in television melodrama (most recently in made-for-television movies starring Jane Seymour and Ann Jillian). One of the twins in *The Dark Mirror*, both played by Olivia de Havilland, has committed a murder. The police know that one of the twins is guilty, but since they cannot discover which one, they are unable to indict either. Eventually they enlist the help of "psychologist" Scott Elliott (Lew Ayres), M.D., Ph.D., M.S., who has done research on the pathology of twins. (Actually, Ayres's character behaves much more like a psychologist than a psychiatrist, administering tests to the twins rather than working on a talking cure.) Dr. Elliott eventually identifies the guilty one (and falls in love with the other) largely through his findings with Rorschach, free association, and lie-detector tests, work that he does with the foreboding accompaniment of Dmitri Tiomkin's typically *noir* score.

Lew Ayres's performance as Scott Elliott in *The Dark Mirror* marks a further step in the acceptance and demystification of psychiatry in the movies of the 1940s. Although Dr. Elliott smokes a pipe, plays chess, listens to Brahms, and owns an office full of books, he also dotes on lemon drops and carries himself with the boyish charm that we expect from a leading man like Ayres (plate 14). Once again, the work of the psychiatrist is largely indistinguishable from detective work, and once again, the therapeutic relationship leads inevitably to romance, but the film also makes an effort to show how mental health professionals treat their patients. In several scenes we can compare the quite different reactions of the twins to the same Rorschach blots and free association series. Neither Freud nor medicine is invoked here, but in its attempts to make the mysteries of the unconscious accessible, the film suggests that by 1946 an audience that came to see a whodunnit could also appreciate the work of a psychotherapist.

The Snake Pit of 1948, also starring Olivia de Havilland, tries to present the dilemmas surrounding the treatment of mentally disturbed patients but, true to the Hollywood pattern, ultimately displaces them into melodrama. *The Snake Pit* fits most neatly into the genre of postwar social problem films best exemplified by *Gentleman's Agreement* (1947), *Crossfire* (1947), and *Pinky* (1949). The conclusion of *Snake Pit* resembles that of *Crossfire*, a murder mystery that takes anti-Semitism as its principal theme. Although the ugliness of anti-Semitism is plainly demonstrated in the near pathological behavior of the film's villain (Robert Ryan), his discovery and death at the end suddenly seem to suggest that the much more pervasive evils of Jew-hating have been completely eliminated. Similarly, the recovery of the heroine at the end of *Snake Pit* seems designed to make the audience forget the distress of the mental patients that are left behind.

In relation to the evolving history of psychiatry in the movies, *The Snake Pit* is important because it questions the profession's effectiveness from a more informed point of view. In films such as *Mr. Deeds Goes to Town*, psychiatrists are simply quacks, out of touch with the world in which human beings actually live. In *Snake Pit*, on the other hand, psychiatrists can heal the sick, but our society and the institutions it builds for troubled people do not always make psychiatric work easy. *The Snake Pit's* incipient notion that society may be at the root of people's problems would become fully developed in the 1960s.

Snake Pit dramatizes the chaos in state mental hospitals and replaces the gracious country manors of *Now Voyager* and *Spellbound* with a bedlam that can aid recovery only by giving the patient the desire to leave as soon as possible.

PLATE 14. Lew Ayres probes the mind of Olivia de Havilland and her "evil twin" in *The Dark Mirror* (1946). Universal Pictures. The Museum of Modern Art/Film Stills Archive.

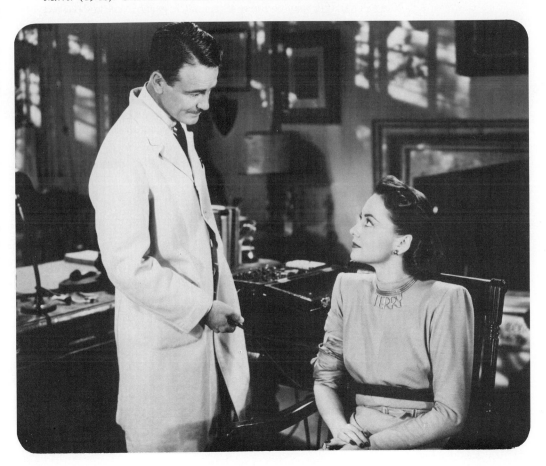

The film sends Virginia Cunningham (Olivia de Havilland) back and forth between the healing efforts of her psychiatrist (Leo Genn) and the disastrous effects of conditions at the "Juniper Hill" state mental hospital. Virginia first arrives at the hospital after a breakdown due to a crisis in her marriage. She is unable to accept love from a man because of guilt feelings stemming from the death of her father as well as from the subsequent death of a boyfriend who resembled him. We know this because Virginia tells part of the story while she is under the effects of narcosynthesis, a process which also appears in *Possessed* (1947) and *Home of the Brave* (1949), perhaps the first films in which psychiatrists use any kind of drug therapy. (The same process was used in the 1946 documentary, *Let There Be Light*.) We learn the rest of Virginia's story when her psychiatrist explains it to her while a portrait of Freud on the wall looms like an icon throughout the entire scene.

Virginia's psychiatrist in *Snake Pit* is played by the English actor Leo Genn, whose foreign accent is meant to be consistent with an unpronounceable last name, affectionately shortened by characters in the film to "Kik" (plate 15). He possesses a self-effacing but authoritative manner, and he frequently taps his pipe like Claude Rains in *Now Voyager*. In spite of his good intentions and sympathetic nature, Dr. Kik is up against more than just his patients' early traumas. Leo Genn's character may be the first cinematic psychiatrist to contend also with the inadequacies in state institutions, including overcrowding, arbitrarily authoritarian nurses, and incompetent administrators, which were widely publicized in the late 1940s. Even this knowledgeable practitioner must subordinate his treatments to decisions made in boardrooms. As a result, Dr. Kik tells Virginia's husband (Mark Stevens) that he must take "shortcuts" because of a lack of time. We also know that Kik's superiors have pressured him to release Virginia as soon as possible because there are already too many patients in her ward.

As we pointed out in chapter 1, *Snake Pit* simultaneously portrays ECT as barbaric and as helpful. The film also expresses ambivalence toward psychiatry in the immense difference between the analytic scenes, in which Virginia works out her own ambivalence toward her parents, and the more broadly played scenes involving other patients. The seriousness of her sessions with Dr. Kik could almost be part of an "educational" documentary about psychoanalysis. The scenes in the ward, on the other hand, exploit the horrifying as well as the farcical aspects of mental institutions. Virginia is clearly not helped by the flamboyant antics of the other patients or by the mindless regime enforced by the nurses. While other patients appear to be truly psychotic, Virginia's illness is almost charming, thanks especially to the affecting facial expressions and

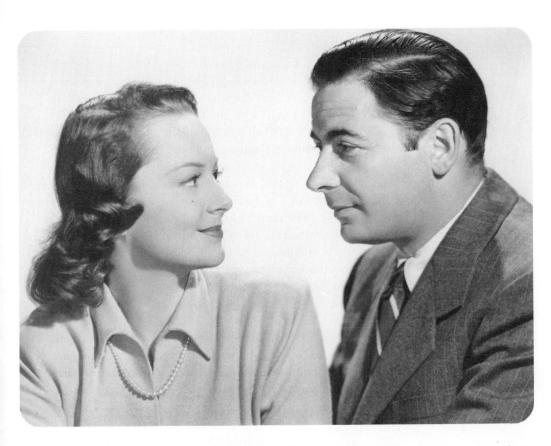

PLATE 15. Olivia de Havilland with caring, effective psychiatrist (Leo Genn) in *The Snake Pit* (1948). Twentieth Century–Fox. The Museum of Modern Art/Film Stills Archive.

gently humorous line-readings which won de Havilland an Academy Award nomination and made *The Snake Pit* one of the five top-grossing films of 1949. At one point, the film actually invites us to sympathize with Virginia when she bites the finger of a ridiculous psychiatrist who is badgering her with questions (plate 16). Since the occasion is a hearing to decide her readiness for release, Virginia's action is certainly counterproductive. Yet within the context of the scene, her defiance seems as reasonable as it is crowd-pleasing. De Havilland's performance itself may have been as important as any of many other elements in *Snake Pit* for fulfilling Hollywood's goal of presenting a serious problem and then deflecting it toward a single sympathetic character.

Films such as *Lady in the Dark, Spellbound, Nightmare Alley,* and *Snake Pit* clearly appropriate psychiatry for their own specialized purposes, but they do show a more sophisticated understanding of the subject than the films of the

1930s and before. Lest we give the impression that the 1940s were entirely characterized by this new sophistication, we should mention at least a few other films. Assorted quacks played highly conventionalized roles in *My Favorite Wife* (1940), *That Uncertain Feeling* (1941), *Murder, My Sweet* (1945), *Miracle on 34th Street* (1947), and *The Gay Intruders* (1948). In 1946 *Bedlam* appeared, featuring no less than Boris Karloff as the malevolent warden of an insane asylum in eighteenth-century London. *Shock* appeared in the same year with Vincent Price as a psychiatrist who kills his wife and then endeavors to dispose of the only witness (Anabel Shaw) to his crime. As if to demonstrate the potential menace of his professional skills, the psychiatrist first attempts to drive the witness crazy and then provides her with an overdose of insulin. Bosley Crowther of the *New York Times* was more indignant than usual about *Shock*, and his review expresses the sort of public response eventually responsible for the Golden Age of psychiatry in American film: "One is forced to challenge this picture as a social disservice at this time. Treatment of nervous disorders is being practiced today upon thousands of men who suffered shock of one sort or another in the war. A film which provokes fear of treatment, as this film plainly aims to do, is a cruel thing to put in the way of those patients or of their anxious relatives.

PLATE 16. Olivia de Havilland with incompetent quack (Howard Freeman) in *The Snake Pit* (1948). Twentieth Century–Fox. The Museum of Modern Art/Film Stills Archive.

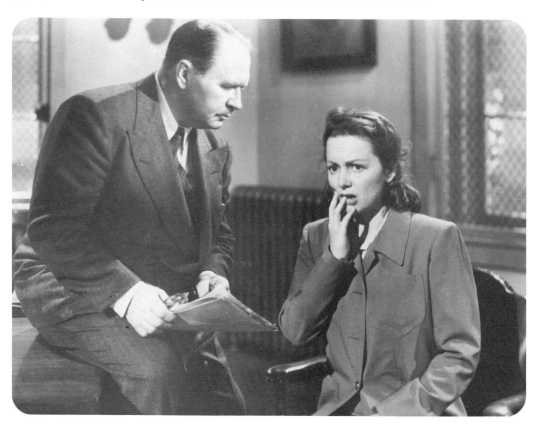

Aubrey Schenck, who produced this picture, and Twentieth Century-Fox, which is releasing it, have evidenced here a lack of public consideration that is most deplorable" (Crowther 1946, 10).

When he wrote these words, Crowther may have still been under the spell of *Let There Be Light* (1946), a documentary about the achievements of Army psychiatrists directed by John Huston before he filmed the biography of Freud in 1962. The film may be the most impressive piece of psychiatric propaganda ever made. The cameras follow several returning servicemen through eight weeks of therapy in a hospital on Long Island. All suffer initially from serious disorders related to their experiences during the war; their symptoms are presented quite graphically in a series of individual interviews. Early on, psychiatrists are shown using narcosynthesis and hypnotism on four male patients and achieving immediate results. Later, these same patients are shown learning to talk and even joke about their problems in group therapy sessions. And by the end of the film, all the men are filmed laughing, singing, and playing softball, apparently restored to emotional and physical well-being. According to the film's director, John Huston, the Army had wanted "a film to show industry that nervous and emotional casualties were not lunatics; because at that time these men weren't getting jobs" (Kaminsky 1978, 43). However, Huston also maintains that the Army decided not to release the film, citing the lack of signed consent forms from several of the patients who appear in the film. According to materials in a file on *Let There Be Light* compiled by Professor David Culbert for the Audio Visual Division of the National Archives, Huston claims the consent forms disappeared from a bank vault in Astoria, Queens. James Agee, one of a handful of critics who had the opportunity to see the film, offered a different explanation for the film's suppression: "The War Department has mumbled a number of reasons why it has been withheld; the glaring obvious reason has not been mentioned: that any sane human being who saw the film would join the armed services, if at all, with a straight face and a painfully maturing mind" (1958, 236). Agee may be correct, but a document in the clipping file at the National Archives quotes the legal officer of the Signal Corps as stating that the consent forms stipulated that the film could "only be used in furtherance of the war effort." He interpreted this to mean that it could only be shown to military personnel. The film was finally made available to the public in 1981. Even if allowed greater exposure at the time it was made, *Let There Be Light* would likely have done little to alter Hollywood's depiction of "the treatment of nervous disorders." With the exception of Mark Robson's *Home of the Brave* (1949), American films of that period seemed quite uninterested in psychiatry's efforts to heal psychological scars born by servicemen. *Shock* was typical of Hollywood's much greater fascination with the more sensational aspects of how doctors treat the mind.

THE FIFTIES: PRELUDE TO THE GOLDEN AGE

The American cinema continued to spin out its ambivalent mythology of psychiatry throughout most of the 1950s. While the profession was sometimes idealized, it was also shamelessly exploited in films such as *Glen or Glenda?* (1953), directed by the legendary Edward D. Wood, Jr. (best known for *Plan Nine from Outer Space*, a film that some hardened archivists have identified as the worst movie ever made). *Glen or Glenda?* subtitled *I Change My Sex*, features Bela Lugosi as a sort of occult philosopher surrounded by skulls, mysterious vapors, and other typical paraphernalia of the wizard's studio. Lugosi lectures the audience on the order of nature and then introduces a pompous psychiatrist who, in turn, narrates the story of a man haunted by the desire to dress in women's clothes. The film ends happily as the transvestite's understanding fiancée hands him her angora sweater in the final moments. The directorial ineptitude of Ed Wood makes unusually clear Hollywood's desire to "have it both ways," a tradition that goes back at least to Cecil B. DeMille. In *Glen or Glenda?* the psychiatrist articulates the dominant ideology's notion of normality while he simultaneously legitimizes the voyeuristic fascination with what is forbidden.

Another somewhat primitive film also reveals complex ways that psychiatry can function in the movies. *I Was a Teenage Werewolf* (1957) touches on a number of anxieties characteristic of the 1950s. The unleashing of the destructive forces in the atom is typical of metaphors that dominated the era's science fiction and horror films (most notably Gordon Douglas's *Them!* of 1954), and psychiatry had much in common with the scientific mystification of nuclear power: both were easily characterized as modern inventions for uncovering nature's forbidden forces. Just as Americans held mixed feelings about optimistic promises of "atoms for peace," they may also have harbored the unconscious concern that psychiatry derepresses powerful instinctual drives and leaves a patient in the throes of aggressive and sexual forces beyond his control. *I Was a Teenage Werewolf* expresses precisely this view. Whit Bissell plays a familiar B-movie mad scientist who works in a laboratory with an assistant named Hugo and dreams of saving the world from nuclear destruction by returning mankind to its primitive origins. The film seems to have identified the doctor as a "consulting psychologist" employed at an aircraft factory for the sole purpose of engineering his meeting with the young protagonist (Michael Landon), who comes to the doctor for help with his violent temper. The psychologist finds the teenager to be the perfect subject for his experiments and with the help of drugs and hypnosis transforms him into a lycanthropic monster. As the film ends with the police shooting the werewolf, they discover that the monster has killed his doctor. One of the more theologically inclined officers observes that "it's not for man to interfere in the ways of God."

Most of the films of this decade, however, merely perpetuate well-established traditions from the 1930s and 1940s. Ineffectual or oddball psychiatrists appear in *Fourteen Hours* (1951) and *The Seven Year Itch* (1955). The beautiful but unfulfilled psychiatrist who is "cured" by a male patient appears in both *Knock on Wood* (1954) and Blake Edwards's *The Perfect Furlough* (1958). In Frederick de Cordova's *Bedtime for Bonzo* (1951), Ronald Reagan plays an amiable professor of psychology who sets out to prove the ascendancy of nurture over nature by raising a chimp in his own house. Like the equally amiable Lew Ayres in *The Dark Mirror*, the professor succeeds in his experiment *and* wins himself a bride. In the tradition of *Nightmare Alley*'s Lilith Ritter, *I, the Jury* (1953) offers a seductive psychoanalyst who runs a decidedly more criminal operation than her prototype. Based on Mickey Spillane's novel, both the 1953 and 1982 versions of *I, the Jury* allow Mike Hammer to make love to therapist Charlotte Manning (Peggie Castle in 1953, Barbara Carrera in 1982) before he discovers that she is the murderer of his pal. Both films end with a deadly embrace in which Charlotte hopes she can distract Hammer with her kisses while she reaches for her gun. The shot we hear, however, comes from Hammer's gun. The films conclude with this memorable exchange:

CHARLOTTE: How could you?

HAMMER: It was easy.

Although it has little else in common with *Mr. Deeds Goes to Town*, the 1953 version of *I, the Jury* also relies on a nostalgic vision of stable individuals in stable communities to dismiss the unsettling claims that psychiatry makes for its legitimacy. Not only does the sex of the psychoanalyst in *I, the Jury* symbolize social disruption; when Hammer first arrives outside her office and sees the shiny plate near the door, we hear his omniscient voice on the sound track: " 'Charlotte Manning, Psychoanalysis.' Things have changed since I was a kid. Shingles were wood and carried a lot of weight. Now they were brass and could still weigh nothin'."

The vast majority of fifties films that included psychiatrists were still based on novels and plays. Henry Koster's *Harvey* (1950), for example, translated Mary Chase's popular stage play to the screen almost verbatim, including the conceit that Elwood P. Dowd (James Stewart), the good-natured drunk with the giant invisible rabbit, is less in need of help than the psychiatrists to whom his sister commits him. At one point he provides solace to the chief headshrinker, Dr. Chumley (Cecil Kellaway), whose one ambition is to escape to Akron, Ohio, where a sympathetic woman will continually say to him, "Oh, you poor thing. You poor, poor thing." Eventually, everyone comes to realize that the sanest person in the film is Elwood P. Dowd, whose vision of the world, except for the invisible rabbit, could have been borrowed from a Frank Capra film.

A few films from this period do however show a change in the image of psychiatry. Hollywood's drift toward the more positive view, one anchored in the unambiguous conviction that some people really do need help, is well illustrated by *The Shrike* (1955), a film based on the 1952 Pulitzer Prize–winning play by Joseph Kramm. Jose Ferrer was director and star of both Broadway play and film, but there are substantial differences between the works. In the New York production of Kramm's play, Ferrer played Jim Downs, a failed stage director who is committed to a New York psychiatric hospital after a suicide attempt. He soon learns that he is the captive not just of the unsympathetic corps of psychiatrists who examine him but also of his estranged wife, Ann, who has convinced the doctors to release him only into her custody. The wife even succeeds in severing any possibility of contact between her husband and Charlotte, the woman Downs fell in love with shortly before abandoning his marriage. In the play's disturbing conclusion, Downs realizes that he can leave the prison-like atmosphere of the institution only if he is willing to become the prisoner of his wife. He therefore capitulates, misrepresenting his true feelings toward her and telling the psychiatrists that he is prepared to reassume the traditional role of husband. When he finally walks out of the institution, he is a pathetically broken man (Kramm 1952).

By concentrating on the dark side of marriage, the play attacked what we have been calling "the dominant ideology." The 1955 film version of *The Shrike*, however, suggests that American movies were not yet prepared to make so drastic an appeal and that the pattern of reconciliation was still quite thoroughly entrenched. In the film, Jim Downs (Ferrer) again finds himself the victim of his wife (June Allyson) and her coconspirators in the psychiatric community, but screenwriter Ketti Frings has added a scene toward the end in which one of the psychiatrists, Dr. Bellman, uncharacteristically asks Ann (Allyson) if she has ever considered therapy. She reacts strongly in the negative, but at the end of the film, when Downs has been released into her custody, she reveals that she eventually went back to Dr. Bellman for treatment. Ann then tells her husband that she has seen the error of her ways and that she is prepared to let him go back to his lover Charlotte if he wishes. In an even more dramatic departure from the play, Downs tells his wife that he will stay with her and give their marriage another chance. The myth that any marriage can be transformed by two willing souls replaces Kramm's original vision of marriage as imprisonment. On one level, the film has simply added an upbeat "Hollywood ending" to a story that movie audiences might have found too depressing. On the other hand, *The Shrike* is a film that can be seen in the context of a gradual warming toward psychiatry in the years just before the Golden Age. *The Shrike* belongs to the genre of institution films in which psychiatrists are little more than jailers, but the part of Dr. Bellman (played in both film and original New York production by Kendall Clark) has been rewritten rather clumsily. In the new version Bellman suddenly becomes the oracular psychiatrist, capable of identifying and healing psychologically wounded people, that was about to become a staple of the American cinema.

Another film released in 1955, *The Cobweb*, not only echoes this tendency but presents the most elaborate treatment of the psychiatric profession in any Hollywood film to date. Produced by John Houseman and directed by Vincente Minnelli, the film employs an all-star cast and the wide-screen look of MGM CinemaScope. In fact, the film's lavish production values seem more appropriate to the musicals that Minnelli directed during the 1950s (*The Band Wagon, Brigadoon, Kismet, Gigi,* etc.) than to a serious drama about the daily operations of a mental institution. Ultimately, the plot in *Cobweb* turns around a set of drapes, and the disparity between subject and treatment may have been largely responsible for *The Cobweb's* failure to attract as large an audience as Minnelli's other dramatic films from the period (*The Bad and the Beautiful, Lust for Life,* and *Tea and Sympathy*) not to mention his musicals.

Based on William Gibson's novel of the same name, *The Cobweb* takes place at the "Castle House Clinic for Nervous Disorders" in Riverwood, Nebraska. The clinic and its fictional location were suggested by the Menninger Clinic of Topeka, Kansas, where Gibson lived while his wife, Margaret Brenman Gibson, was in psychoanalytic training. Like *Private Worlds* from twenty years earlier, *Cobweb* is much more about the personal lives and interactions of the staff members than about mental illness and its treatment. Yet unlike *The Snake Pit* of just seven years before, it makes a fairly coherent attempt to connect the private lives of psychiatrists with their work. Whereas Dr. Kik (Leo Genn) in *Snake Pit* is almost faceless, with no established family or personal problems and no apparent connection to the crazy patients and crazy nurses who surround the film's female protagonist, Dr. Stewart McIver (Richard Widmark) in *The Cobweb* has more difficulty dealing with the crises in his home than he does dealing with those of his patients. In fact, his most important clinical problem is one resulting from an action taken by his wife Karen (Gloria Grahame). And whereas *Snake Pit* gave us at least one godlike therapist surrounded by grotesquely disturbed patients in a chaotic institution, *Cobweb* presents several very human psychiatrists with only mildly troubled patients in an elegantly furnished institution. Of course, we must keep in mind that these two films concern, respectively, a state institution in an urban setting and an expensive private sanitarium in the cornfields of the Midwest. Still, compared to *Snake Pit, Cobweb* suggests that psychotherapy was rapidly losing the exotic, scientifically complex associations it had once held for the American mind.

The Cobweb begins with Gloria Grahame offering a ride in her car to a pleasant young man named Stevie (John Kerr). They joke about the nearby institution, at one point saying that it is difficult to tell the doctors from the patients. Minnelli surprises us early in his film by revealing that Stevie is an inmate with free access to the area around the sanitarium and that Karen (Grahame) is the wife of the head psychiatrist (Widmark) even though we might have suspected that Karen was the inmate. The interchangeability of "disturbed" and "normal" people is the central theme of the film, and a full half-hour goes by before all the doctors and staff have been distinguished from the patients.

One of the staff members is Victoria Inch (Lillian Gish), the ill-tempered business manager of the institution, who has little sympathy with Dr. McIver's (Widmark) new-fangled ideas such as self-governance for the inmates. She has already picked out the drapes she intends to put in the common room where the patients meet to discuss their problems, but at least two other parties become involved in the decision. One is Karen McIver, who has also chosen a pattern for the drapes; the second is Stevie (Kerr), whose paintings the other inmates feel should be printed onto curtains and placed in their meeting room.

The issue of the drapes creates a flare-up between Karen McIver and Vicky Inch, which then becomes an issue between Karen and her husband. Widmark plays Dr. Stewart McIver as a no-nonsense therapist and administrator who, despite his professional competence, is unable to devote enough time to his children and his scatterbrained wife. The film nevertheless portrays him as a loving father with equally understanding children, although his daughter claims to wish she were a patient so that she could see more of him. Because of the tension with his wife, Widmark drifts into a brief peccadillo with Meg Rinehart (Lauren Bacall), a sympathetic therapist at the clinic who lost her husband in the war and her only child to polio. McIver's wife (Grahame) is herself tempted by the institution's Don Juan, Dr. Douglas Devanal (Charles Boyer), an older analyst who turned to liquor and womanizing when his promising career became stalled. At one point he stares longingly at the faded cover of his own 1934 monograph entitled *The Theory and Practice of Milieu Therapy*. Presumably, he has written nothing in the twenty years since.

The most prominently featured patients in *The Cobweb* are played by Oscar Levant, John Kerr, and Susan Strasberg. Largely a comic character in the tradition of Shakespeare's Jaques, Levant enjoys his melancholy and cynicism but is often neglected by his therapist, Devanal (Boyer). Kerr and Strasberg, the juvenile and ingenue of the piece, are presented as beautiful losers who have been damaged by the outside world. Anticipating Keir Dullea and Janet Margolin in Frank and Eleanor Perry's *David and Lisa* (1962), Kerr and Strasberg's relationship becomes all the more appealing as they timidly help each other to conquer their fears. They both seem to make progress when they are able to go out together for a movie without suffering excessive anxiety.

At the film's climax, Karen (Grahame) learns that her husband has been seeing Meg (Bacall). She decides to punish him by putting up her own drapes in the patients' meeting room even though the group has decided to put up the set of drapes that bear the artworks of Stevie (Kerr). When he sees Karen's drapes in the room, Stevie flies into a violent rage and runs away from the institution. The doctors are so distracted by his disappearance that the inmates are left unsupervised. While the staff and police are busy searching for Stevie, even dragging the bottom of a nearby river, the patients quickly become involved in wild parties that just happen to take place before the clinic is to be visited by its board of directors. Dr. McIver's inspirational speech at the end convinces everyone that his unconventional methods of patient governance and freedom are working, and he is even reconciled with his wife after Stevie shows up at his house alive. The final moments of the film depict the happy home of husband, wife, and two children extended to include the much-improved Stevie, who sleeps peacefully on the couch.

The plot of *The Cobweb* is much more complex than this summary suggests, and it does afford the audience an extensive dramatization of life both inside and outside the clinic. As in *Now Voyager*, however, there is very little psychiatry practiced in the film, and its Hollywood ending is unfaithful to the novel, especially the film's suggestion that Stevie has undergone some kind of cathartic cure and is vastly improved after giving vent to his rage. Although the film does ultimately accept the necessity of psychiatric treatment for troubled individuals, it questions the administration of that treatment as strongly as did *Snake Pit*. It also introduces in Dr. McIver the soon-to-be-stereotyped image of the effective psychiatrist who can bring well-being to others but cannot establish harmony in his own life. (This same theme appeared in 1949 in Otto Preminger's *Whirlpool* as well as in the 1954 English film, *The Sleeping Tiger*.)

Although Charles Boyer's Dr. Devanal is more fleshed out than, say, the character played by Peter Sellers in *What's New Pussycat?*, Boyer plays the typical philandering psychiatrist, who disguises his lust with professional jargon. What is most significant about *Cobweb* is the humanization of psychiatrists: unlike the oracular or godlike therapists of *Snake Pit, Blind Alley,* or *Now Voyager,* Dr. McIver in *Cobweb* is a more complete individual, with recognizable problems and responses. Like many female therapists in the movies, the Lauren Bacall character is one more woman in need of a man to bring her fulfillment, but at least the film does allow her to continue practicing therapy after she has made the difficult decision to break off her affair with McIver. Moreover, she identifies herself as someone to whom psychoanalysis has given the courage to go on living after the loss of her family, so her character provides not only a slightly more positive image of a woman psychiatrist on film but a slightly more interesting one as well.

Another film from the 1950s that reflects the historical plan we have outlined is Edward Dmytryk's *The Caine Mutiny* (1954). The film was based on the novel by Herman Wouk and produced by Stanley Kramer, who also produced three other films involving psychiatry: *Home of the Brave* (1949), *Pressure Point* (1962), and *A Child Is Waiting* (1963). These films all present a thoroughly positive image of psychiatry, but *The Caine Mutiny* is a little more complex in how it handles the issue. In the film, three quite different officers aboard the USS *Caine* during World War II become concerned about the conduct of Captain Queeg (Humphrey Bogart), whose compulsive fondling of ball bearings convincingly reveals to the audience that something is wrong with the captain. Keefer (Fred MacMurray), a writer in civilian life, puts ideas into the head of Merrick (Van Johnson), a lifelong Navy man, who eventually agrees that Queeg's behavior is strange. The story is told primarily through the eyes of the third officer, an idealistic young student, Willie Keith (Robert Francis). When Queeg panics during a storm, Merrick submits to the urgings of Keefer and takes over control of the ship. A crucial witness against the defendants in the ensuing court martial is a psychiatrist, played by the ubiquitous Whit Bissell, one of the most faceless of actors, who played at least four psychiatrists during the 1950s and 1960s. (His other films are *Invasion of the Body Snatchers, Third of a Man* and *I Was a Teenage Werewolf.*) In *The Caine Mutiny*, Bissell portrays the psychiatrist as slightly pompous, and although his judgment is called into question by the defense attorney, he testifies that Queeg is quite sane and should not have been relieved of command. However, the defense attorney (Jose Ferrer) is able to win acquittal for the officers by reducing Queeg to a raving paranoid on the witness stand.

It is easy to forget that the opinions of the psychiatrist are largely vindicated in the final scene when the attorney arrives drunk at the mutineers' celebration and throws wine into the face of Keefer (MacMurray). He accuses the intellectual of sowing discord instead of supporting Queeg, holding Keefer responsible for the captain's breakdown during the storm. With drunken lucidity he argues that regular Navy men like Queeg and Merrick would have conducted the war quite well without troublemakers like Keefer and Keith. Students and intellectuals only come into the service during war, he asserts, and they should not interfere with the men who keep America safe in war *and* at peace. Even though the mutineers are acquitted, the film makes a strong argument in favor of Queeg, and the psychiatrist, though faceless and pompous, is shown indirectly to have been correct. Unlike the novel by Herman Wouk (1951), in which the psychiatrist is savaged, the film casts the psychiatrist and the attorney (Ferrer) as spokesmen for a society that, though it may have been unsettled by the trauma of World War II, can still preserve the values that made it great. In fact, the film's final credits go so far as to dedicate the film to the U.S. Navy. By encouraging the audience first to root for the mutineers and then to feel compassion for Queeg and pride for the military, a liberal filmmaker like Stanley Kramer could successfully negotiate the ideological minefields of the McCarthy era. Robert B. Ray sees *The Caine Mutiny* as an excellent example of how Hollywood's thematic paradigm could not hold up under postwar pressure to support the less glamorous official heroes such as Bogart's Queeg (Ray 1985, 174). The old pattern of reconciliation, which had characterized *Casablanca* and most of the films from classical Hollywood, was now breaking down, and even a psychiatrist could not conceal the absurdity in *The Caine Mutiny's* last-minute attempts to exalt an obviously neurotic hero. In many ways, the idealization of psychiatry that was about to become entrenched in American movies can be understood as a somewhat desperate means of preserving Hollywood's consoling paradigms for an American public that was increasingly unlikely to believe in them. This was surely the case for the awkward use of psychiatry to provide reconciliation at the end of *The Shrike* as well as *The Caine Mutiny*.

Whit Bissell appears as another psychiatrist in a film that also bears the mark of McCarthyism, Don Siegel's *The Invasion of the Body Snatchers* (1956). Actually there are two psychiatrists in this film: the local mind doctor in Santa Mira (Larry Gates), who turns out to be one of the "pod people," and the hospital psychiatrist (Bissell), who treats the protagonist (Kevin McCarthy) in the beginning and end of the film. Bissell's part was inserted late in production in an effort to tone down the film's disturbing conclusion. Like *The Cabinet of Dr. Caligari* (1919), the original version of the film was considered to be too unsettling for audiences, and a "frame" was added. *The Invasion of the Body Snatchers* was supposed to end with Miles Bennell (McCarthy) running up and down the highway screaming "They're here!" while cars whiz by unheeding. The final shot was to be a close-up in which he looks directly at the camera and warns the audience, "You're next!" Either the executives at Allied Artists or director Siegel decided to add scenes at the beginning and end suggesting that the invaders may not have entirely succeeded in taking over the world. The opening scenes show Dr. Hill (Bissell) being brought in to treat the raving Miles Bennell, who tells a story that turns the original film into one long flashback. When we return to the framing device at the end of the film, the psychiatrist and another doctor (Richard Deacon) assume the man is mad. However, when they overhear another patient talking about the curious pods that fell out when a truck was overturned, they realize that McCarthy is telling the truth. Dr. Hill jumps into action and confidently orders the police to call the FBI. In chapter 10 we will discuss how the premise of *Invasion of the Body Snatchers*—that our closest friends and relatives can suddenly be transformed into enemies—plays on early infantile anxieties as effectively as it does on 1950s anti-Communist hysteria.

The first few depictions of psychiatrists in the American cinema respond primarily to highly conventionalized plots about characters such as escaped lunatics. We have suggested that the almost complete absence of mental health professionals from movies throughout the first three decades of the century is a result of their incompatibility with the earliest scenarios for silent films as well as of the isolation of Hollywood from the psychoanalytic establishment. When producers began looking for scripts for the new talking pictures, they found a large library of books and plays that reflected the greater fascination with psychiatry existing in the eastern half of the country. And yet, when Hollywood made the plots of this literature their own, they recast them to accommodate the handful of cultural myths that kept Americans flocking to the cinema. Meanwhile, psychiatry was often found to be compatible with the needs of genres like the detective film, the women's film, and the screwball comedy, but only so long as the realities of the profession did not disrupt the illusions of escapist fantasy. Of course, the increasing acceptance of psychiatry as a part of American life in the 1930s, along with the profession's own willingness to give up its avant-garde image, resulted in the idealized portraits found in *Now Voyager, Since You Went Away, Spellbound,* and *The Dark Mirror.* But even in these cases, celluloid psychiatrists rarely practiced anything resembling true psychotherapy. So long as they were little more than glorified guidance counselors, doctors of the mind could help effect the consoling resolutions that characterized nearly all Hollywood films of the classic period. At the same time, however, the complexities of the profession presented genuine problems for the movies, and throughout the thirties, forties, and fifties, a bifurcated myth of psychiatry emerged. For every idealized healer there was a thick-accented, incompetent, and frequently malevolent quack. For every psycho-therapist who spoke the culture's inherent ideology, another confirmed it by embodying an unacceptable alternative.

The Golden Age

3

The Golden Age of psychiatry in the movies was over almost before it began. For a few years in the late 1950s and early 1960s, films reflected—however imperfectly—a growing conviction in American culture that psychiatrists were authoritative voices of reason, adjustment and well-being. Before this view became orthodoxy, however, the American cinema began responding heartily to the cultural upheavals of the 1960s, questioning the old ideas of sanity and conformity, and turning against the champions of these redefined concepts. Several historical forces played a role in making the Golden Age possible. Intrigued by successes with World War II casualties, young physicians had flocked into psychiatric residency training programs in the late 1940s, the same period during which *Life* magazine and other transmitters of popular ideology were making psychoanalysis fashionable for middle Americans. By the 1950s, Dr. Spock was advising mothers on the principles of psychoanalytically informed child rearing; psychoanalytic ideas were appropriated as cure-alls for a variety of social ills; and middle and upper-middle class professionals looked forward to the opportunity to lie down on The Couch.

During World War II, movie psychiatrists had been frequently idealized, most typically in *Since You Went Away*, a film that made a straightforward effort to contribute to the war effort by raising the morale of the women who kept the home fires burning. In the years immediately after the war, this shining image was considerably dimmed as a new disillusionment, pervasive in American society, began to set in. *Film noir* was one manifestation of this new malaise, but so was the inability of the social problem film to fit the old themes of reconciliation. The best example here may be the curiously ambiguous role of the psychiatrist played by Whit Bissell in *The Caine Mutiny:* audiences are asked first to reject his diagnosis and then to accept it some twenty minutes later. By the late 1950s, however, Hollywood was consistently producing idealized images of psychiatry: competent, compassionate, and/or lovable psychiatrists could be seen in at least twenty-two American films from 1957 through 1963.

One explanation for the new idealization of psychiatrists may lie in John Burnham's argument that the Golden Age of *medicine* in this country was coming to an end in the early 1950s (Burnham 1982). Perhaps the movies responded to this new disillusionment with medical doctors by shifting the sacerdotal mantle—which doctors had themselves appropriated from the clergy in the predominantly secular world of movie mythology—to the increasingly demedicalized psychiatrists. In fact, there are films extolling the virtues of psychiatrists at the expense of medical doctors. For example, the sexual anxiety that bedevils the two teenagers (Warren Beatty and Natalie Wood) in Elia Kazan's *Splendor in the Grass* (1961) produces shrugs and nervous laughter when Beatty asks the family physician for advice on how to deal with his desires. But when Natalie Wood's breakdown sends her into the care of an understanding and witty male psychiatrist, he is thoroughly knowledgeable about all aspects of her situation, and she emerges a wiser and healthier individual at the end of the film.

Burnham also provides a model for a more complex understanding of the Golden Age. We have already referred to his discussion of an important change in the role that analysts play in American culture. According to Burnham, the first doctors to practice psychoanalysis in the United States, such as A. A. Brill and Trigant Burrow, devoted themselves more to disseminating the revolutionary ideas of Freud than to actual practice and as a result were often associated with avant-garde movements in the arts such as "cubism, futurism, modernism . . . the problem play" (Burnham 1979, 128). The barrage of attacks upon Freud and his followers that were regularly published in periodicals such as *Current Opinion* during the teens and twenties allowed analysts like Brill, who took pleasure in shocking the sensibilities of mainstream Americans, to consider themselves in the vanguard of an intellectual revolution. In the 1930s and 1940s, however, as the emphasis in psychoanalytic circles shifted to practice, the field became one of many subspecialties in a bureaucratically organized medical establishment. Psychoanalysts could still see themselves as avant-gardists, but they were just as likely to consider themselves part of a pluralistic society that could tolerate a variety of points of view. The avant-garde role had more or less disappeared by the end of World War II, and analysts were by now regularly engaged in providing "a defense of traditional civilization" (Burnham 1979, 132).

Hollywood movies of the 1930s and 1940s absorbed only vaguely the roles described by Burnham, in particular by making little distinction between psychoanalysts and other psychiatrists or mental health professionals. Films of this period seldom acknowledged the iconoclasm of psychoanalysts, unless occasional oddballs such as the jargon-spouting quacks in *Free Love* (1930) or

Murder, My Sweet (1945) can be understood in these terms. We suggested in the previous chapter that the oracular creature played by Ralph Bellamy in *Blind Alley* (1939) may have embodied an idealized synthesis of both the avant-garde and tradition-defending roles that Burnham identifies. Within a few years, however, psychiatrists in films such as *Lady in the Dark* and *Now Voyager* spoke exclusively as advocates for a supposedly enlightened—but in fact highly conventional—view of the world even when the films portrayed their practice of psychotherapy simplistically or not at all. As psychiatry flourished in the postwar period, filmmaker Stanley Kramer showed this type of enlightened psychiatrist practicing a more dramatic, if not a more sophisticated, style of treatment in *Home of the Brave* (1949). Negative stereotypes of psychiatry were still very much alive, but in the 1950s the acceptance of psychotherapists in American life finally trickled down into the highly conventionalized world of movie myths. This process was in large part facilitated by a crisis in the Hollywood cinema, an industry which was beset by numerous forces, not the least of which was what Ray calls "the breakdown of the homogeneous audience" (1985, 129–52). As viewers began to drift away to television and European "art films," as audiences became more politically and aesthetically sophisticated, and as the film industry coped with assaults such as Communist witch hunts, desperate attempts were made to keep the old formulas alive. Ray lists the problem picture, the epic and the "inflated genre" film as examples of this trend: "These 'serious' movies revealed very little about postwar developments or about the concerns generated by them. Instead, they limited themselves to a few domestic issues (particularly race), dealt with along the safe, official lines encouraged by a studied ideological optimism. These movies almost never portrayed the central American anxiety of the time—the fear that World War II had permanently altered the conditions of American life on which so much of the culture's mythology depended" (Ray 1985, 154). This statement is especially true of the many problem pictures that featured psychiatrists during the Golden Age. The cinema's compassionate, effective healer of troubled minds, already perfected during the war years, was readily available to assist in Hollywood's project to revive its ailing formulas.

By the late 1960s, however, therapists who embraced the wisdom of "traditional civilization" had become easy targets for the increasing number of movies that absorbed a *new* set of "avant-garde" ideas and questioned outright the myths that had previously dominated American cinema. This chapter will focus primarily upon American films made during a seven-year period in which psychotherapists were most often characterized as competent healers and admirable human beings. We will divide the period into three shorter ones, examining the transitional films that led into the idealized portraits of psychiatry in the high Golden Age as well as those that heralded its rather definitive fall from the pedestal in the midsixties.

THE FIRST TRANSITIONAL PERIOD

The 1956 version of *Invasion of the Body Snatchers,* which we addressed in the final pages of the previous chapter, is one of the films anticipating the era of almost consistently positive images. The psychiatrist in the frame solves the mystery of Kevin McCarthy's story and immediately gives orders to begin the salvation of the world. Although he functions largely as a plot machine to set up the flashback, he anticipates the oracular character played by Simon Oakland at the end of *Psycho* (1960), who thoroughly explains the workings of Norman Bates's (Anthony Perkins) mind and then instructs the police on how Norman should be treated as well as on how they can find the bodies of three more murdered women. The 1956 version of *Invasion of the Body Snatchers* is transitional, however, because it contains the oracle (Whit Bissell), who is characteristic of the Golden Age, as well as the psychiatrist in the inner film (Larry Gates), who provides the stereotypically "rational" contrast to those who appreciate the powers of the unworldly. Much the same can be said of *The Shrike* (1955) with its good and bad asylum doctors as well as the more complex *Cobweb* from the same year, which offers an ambivalent view of the profession essentially by humanizing psychiatrists to the point of dwelling on their inadequacies.

Although it appeared a little late to fit perfectly into the transitional period before the Golden Age, Otto Preminger's *Anatomy of a Murder* (1959) may also be seen in this context. Orson Bean has a small part as the psychiatrist who testifies for the accused murderer (Ben Gazzara), defended by James Stewart. The attorney is attempting to prove that his client was temporarily insane when he committed the murder, and the psychiatrist testifies to that effect. What makes the film transitional is its self-conscious introduction of Orson Bean as a new breed of psychiatrist. When Stewart's sidekick (Arthur O'Connell) arrives at the train station to meet the psychiatrist, he apparently expects to see a Viennese gentleman with goatee and pince-nez or at least someone like Whit Bissell. He is not prepared for the youthful and friendly character played by Bean, and the psychiatrist's first speeches are aimed at countering the stereotypes of his profession. Although actors like Lew Ayres in *Dark Mirror* (1946) and Charles Drake in *Harvey* (1950) had played youthful, good-looking psychiatrists before, in *Anatomy of a Murder* Orson Bean seems to have been cast as a psychiatrist largely for the purpose of instructing audiences to dismiss the old stereotypes.

Anatomy of a Murder belongs more to the transitional period than to the Golden Age because the testimony of the youthful psychiatrist is undermined by the film's conclusion: it turns out that Stewart's client (Gazzara) was quite sane when he committed the murder. In a sense, this conclusion represents the complement to what happens at the end of *The Caine Mutiny* (1954). In the earlier film a rather unsympathetic psychiatrist is vindicated; in *Anatomy of a Murder* a fresh-faced psychiatrist is discredited. Unlike *The Caine Mutiny,* however, which exposes Hollywood's failure to adapt the old paradigms to postwar attitudes, *Anatomy of a Murder* undermines its psychiatrist's testimony primarily to set up a surprise ending. Much the same can be said of a more recent mystery film, *Jagged Edge* (1985), which also attempts to throw audiences off the track by briefly introducing a rumpled psychiatrist to attest to the sanity of the central male character (Jeff Bridges), who is later revealed to be a psychotic killer.

A true transitional film that fits more precisely into our historical pattern is Robert Mulligan's *Fear Strikes Out* (1957). This film tends to suggest that studio executives at Paramount were unsure whether audiences were ready to accept an entirely humanized psychiatrist who can do no wrong. Lawrence Alloway (1971) has described the dilemma facing movie producers, who must spend money on a venture that may no longer be to the taste of audiences when it is released months or even years later. As a result, movies speak to a "half known future" with images that are not easily datable as, for example, the clothes worn by women in forties films, poised "in a strange region of use, somewhere between negligee and ball gown" (Alloway 1971, 15). The tentativeness about audience acceptance of idealized psychiatrists at the beginning of the Golden Age may explain why *Fear Strikes Out* takes a supposedly true story for its text and casts the faceless Adam Williams as the psychiatrist (plate 17). Unlike Leo Genn's Dr. Kik in *Snake Pit* (1948) or Richard Widmark's Dr. McIver in *Cobweb* (1955), Adam Williams plays a sympathetic psychiatrist working effectively in an institution where *nothing* goes wrong. As we stressed in chapter 1, *Fear Strikes Out* even forgoes the opportunity to dramatize shock therapy. The treatment is portrayed as quite benign, with soothing music accompanying the shots of a bedridden Jim Piersall (Anthony Perkins) moving in and out of the door marked "electro therapy." We only see the room from the outside, and in each session, Piersall's psychiatrist stands by with a compassionate expression. The uncaricatured presence of a psychiatrist in such a

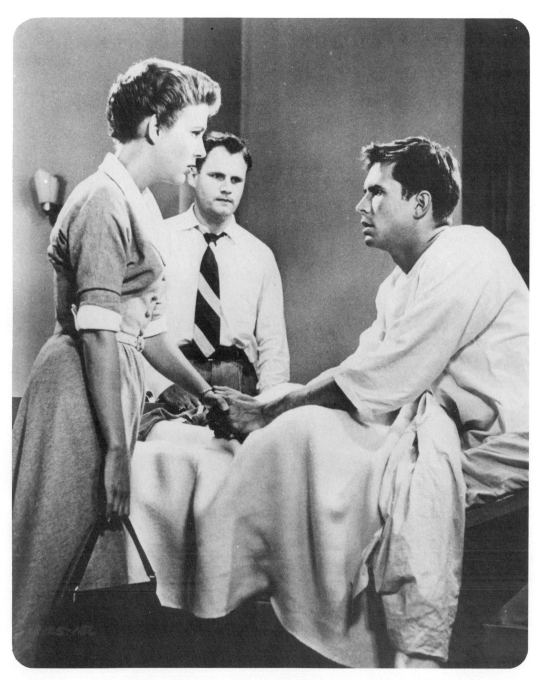

Plate 17. Like the audience for *Fear Strikes Out* (1957), Jimmy Piersall (Anthony Perkins) and his wife (Norma Moore) hardly notice the faceless psychiatrist (Adam Williams). Paramount Pictures. The Museum of Modern Art/Film Stills Archive.

film strongly suggests that the movie industry was granting new acceptance to the profession during this time.

The perfect complement for *Fear Strikes Out* is Nunnally Johnson's *The Three Faces of Eve,* also released in 1957 (plate 18). Both were problem pictures that grossly simplified actual case histories and gave no hints that the protagonists were not completely cured as the films concluded (Piersall and Hirshberg 1955; Sizemore 1977). In fact, Jim Piersall, like Chris Costner Sizemore ("Eve"), continued to suffer from mental illness for many years after the film was released. Both films also painted psychiatrists as competent healers with none of the personal or professional problems that had confronted many of their celluloid predecessors. However, just as the other transitional films seem tentative about presenting unabashedly positive images of psychiatry to the public, *Three Faces of Eve* actually harks back to the apologia for psychoanalysis that began *Spellbound* in 1945. While the earlier film ran a message explaining psychoanalysis in terms quite inconsistent with the romance and suspense film that Hitchcock actually made, *Three Faces of Eve* begins with an appearance by Alistair Cooke, behaving exactly as he had for several years on television's "Omnibus" and as he would later as the host of "Masterpiece Theatre." His function in *Three Faces*

PLATE 18. Joanne Woodward as Eve Black, one of *The Three Faces of Eve* (1957), confuses Lee J. Cobb and Edwin Jerome. Twentieth Century–Fox. The Museum of Modern Art/Film Stills Archive.

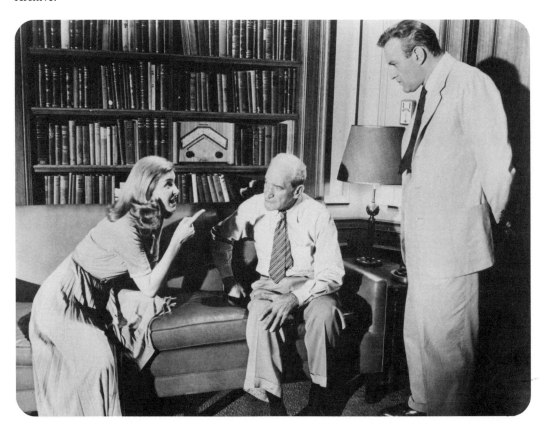

of Eve is to confirm the "truth" of what the audience is about to see, but even if he were to say that the entire film is a fabrication, his posturing legitimizes the film much more effectively than the prologues and "psychiatric advisers" of earlier films such as *Spellbound* and *Private Worlds.*

As much as anything else, *The Three Faces of Eve* is a star turn for Joanne Woodward, who won an Academy Award for her performance. Her Eve Black expresses as much sexuality as the waning Production Code was beginning to allow in 1957. In fact, this film was one of the first to use the pathology of mental illness to step beyond the usual limitations imposed on sex in the movies. In one scene, Eve's befuddled husband Ralph (David Wayne) realizes the common male fantasy of being married to two women, one for public acceptance and one for sexual adventure. Unfortunately for Ralph, Eve Black uses her sexual allure only to entice him into buying her clothes and does not provide anything in return. Eve Black also makes eyes at the principal psychiatrist in the film, Dr. Luther (Lee J. Cobb), telling him that he is "kinda cute." As Golden Age psychiatrists were wont to do, Dr. Luther parries her sexual overtures quite well, as much from personal as from professional ethics. Cobb even has some moments of gentle humor in his role as Eve's psychiatrist when he attempts to explain the phenomenon of multiple personality to her husband. As Ralph stares at him blankly, Cobb slips into jargon and then catches himself with a double take. The easy self-knowledge which Dr. Luther displays in this scene is definitely part of the humanizing process, which does not begin in American films until the 1950s. It would be difficult to imagine even Claude Rains in *Now Voyager* or Leo Genn in *Snake Pit* registering anything like Cobb's double take.

Although much less ambitious than *Three Faces of Eve,* another transitional film is *Oh Men! Oh Women!* These two films make a remarkable pair since they were both written, directed, and produced by Nunnally Johnson in 1957. (Johnson had earlier dealt with psychiatric subjects when he wrote the screenplay for *The Dark Mirror* in 1946.) But whereas *Three Faces of Eve* was hailed as something of a masterpiece, *Oh Men! Oh Women!* was dismissed as a mindless trifle. An English reviewer remarked: "CinemaScope discovers a solution for the problem of filling the wide screen; the characters spend most of their time full length on the psychoanalyst's couch" (Halliwell 1983, 602). Although this may not have been exactly true, the flashy use of new technology for the rather straightforward translation of a play to the screen does not hold up well today, especially in comparison with the almost documentary feel of *Three Faces of Eve.* (Ray would call *Oh Men! Oh Women!* "an inflated genre film," since it is basically a large-budget screwball comedy.) In fact, celluloid psychiatrists of the 1950s seem much more out of place in the Eastmancolor *Cobweb* and *Oh Men! Oh Women!* than in the black-and-white *Freud, Three Faces of Eve,* and *Fear Strikes Out.* This may have something to do with the fact that many people report that they dream in colorless images. (In *Whose Life Is It, Anyway?,* Richard Dreyfuss's dreams are in black and white.) On the other hand, the illusion of grainy realism offered by black-and-white cinematography captures the *ethos* of the social problem film much better than the fairy tale quality inherent in the gaudy palette of Technicolor and Eastmancolor.

Oh Men! Oh Women! fits squarely into the transitional period because of the ambivalence toward its central character, a psychoanalyst played by David Niven. The leading lady is a beautiful woman played by Barbara Rush, whose exasperating flightiness does not deter the analyst from asking her to marry him. Dr. Alan Coles (Niven) is shown to be an extraordinarily effective guidance counselor when it takes him a mere five minutes to put back together the marriage of two of his patients, Dan Dailey and that ubiquitous analysand, Ginger Rogers (plate 19). In his dealings with his fiancée, however, Dr. Coles has trouble handling his emotions, leading her to insist that he is too intellectual and detached to be a good lover even though she also disapproves when he deals violently with a meddling patient (Tony Randall) whose neurosis is co-incidentally related to his failed relationship with her. To paraphrase Freud, it is never exactly clear what this woman wants, but by the end she has told the analyst that their engagement is off. At this point Niven is visited by the man who appears to be his training analyst, Dr. Kraus (John Wengraf). Sporting the inevitable goatee and Viennese accent, the older analyst utters the phrase, "The distance from the library to the bedroom is astronomical, but it is worth the trip." Shortly after hearing this non sequitur, the Niven character unin-tentionally creates a situation that convinces his fiancée that he really loves her and that he desires to take charge of their relationship in a manner acceptable to her. All is well as the movie ends. As in Golden Age films, the analyst played by Niven is a swift and almost casually proficient mental health profes-sional even if the problems of the couple he treats have little to do with intrapsychic problems. But unlike the vast majority of Golden Age films, *Oh Men! Oh Women!* looks into the private life of the analyst and finds the same kind of trouble that beset Richard Widmark in *Cobweb:* the occupational hazards of a psychiatrist get in the way of personal relationships. The image of psychiatry in *Oh Men! Oh Women!* is actually quite positive—it would take a saint to endure the Barbara Rush character—but we have not yet encountered the psychiatrist who is a paragon in both his professional and private life.

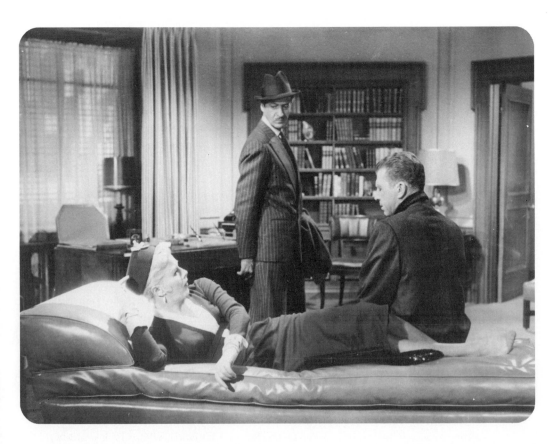

PLATE 19. Ginger Rogers (with David Niven and Dan Dailey) in her third decade as an analysand in *Oh Men! Oh Women!* (1957). Twentieth Century–Fox. The Museum of Modern Art/Film Stills Archive.

THE CANONIZATION

Fear Strikes Out (1957) was only one of many films from this period in which psychiatrists without personal lives were regularly portrayed as effective practitioners of healing arts. By 1958, these saintly doctors were already appearing in fictionalized stories as well as in pseudodocumentaries. In Mervyn LeRoy's *Home before Dark* (1958), Jean Simmons barely maintains her sanity while her husband (Dan O'Herlihy), a dispassionate philosophy professor, neglects her in favor of her stepsister (Rhonda Fleming). The Simmons character has just been released from an institution as the film begins, and a faceless psychiatrist specifically instructs the husband to do everything that we later see O'Herlihy not doing. By the end, the psychiatrist's admonitions have been thoroughly verified: Simmons reacts irrationally to the not-so-benign neglect of her husband, surviving her ordeal only because her husband's sympathetic but alienated colleague (Efram Zimbalist, Jr.) stands by her. (*Home before Dark* probably belongs most to the genre of women's film, but by identifying the character played by Zimbalist as Jewish, it also recalls the tendency of postwar problem films to confront racial issues.) When Simmons leaves her husband to join Zimbalist at the end, she vows that she will go to the big city and begin a life of her own that will include regular visits to a private psychiatrist.

We should mention a few other problem pictures from the Golden Age that present psychiatrists who are idealized but without a personal dimension. In an English/American production, Guy Green's *The Mark* (1961), Rod Steiger plays a heroic therapist who helps Stuart Whitman overcome the forces that drove him to commit sexual crimes against small children. Steiger then saves his patient again when the past comes back to haunt him. By the end, the Whitman character has established a healthy relationship with an attractive widow and her young daughter. Joseph Cates's *Girl of the Night* (1960) presents a very similar situation: Anne Francis plays a young woman who turns to prostitution because of a childhood rape trauma. She finds her way to the couch of a psychotherapist (Lloyd Nolan), who first cures her of the need to sell her body and then protects her when her pimp attempts to force her back into business. Whit Bissell appears as a psychiatrist once again in Robert Lewin's *Third of a Man* (1962), the story of how a small-town carpenter (James Drury) comes to accept his mute brother Doon (Simon Oakland), whom he has hidden away in a mental institution. The psychiatrist protects Doon from a posse after he escapes from the institution and eventually helps the Drury character to understand that people in sanitariums need love too. The film ends with the brother saying that he will visit Doon the next day. Doon then utters the first word he has spoken in years, "tomorrow."

There were other films from the early 1960s in which psychotherapists' private lives went completely unexplored. Simon Oakland appears again in Alfred Hitchcock's *Psycho* (1960), this time as a psychiatrist who is as successful a detective as he is a mind doctor. In Elia Kazan's *Splendor in the Grass* (1961), Natalie Wood's psychiatrist gracefully helps her put her life back together. Michael Callan in *The Interns* (1962) idealizes Dr. Bonny (J. Edward McKinley), a faceless psychiatrist whose stature is so august that intern Callan is prepared to lie and cheat in order to procure a residency with him. And as we have already suggested, Andrew Duggan in *The Chapman Report* (1962) brings the proper balance of science and humanism to his study of the sex lives of several beautiful women so that audiences can rationalize their voyeurism.

The Golden Age culminates in 1962 with, among others, *David and Lisa*. The fully integrated human being in psychiatrist's clothing emerges in this film as Dr. Swinford, played by Howard da Silva (plate 20). Significantly, da Silva was performing on the screen for the first time after a long period on the blacklist due to his outspoken pleading of the Fifth Amendment before the House Committee on Un-American Activities in 1951. The revolutionary character of da Silva's return to the screen complemented the film's breakthroughs not only in its treatment of psychiatry but also in its inauguration of an American tradition of low-budget "personal films." Made outside the studio system, such films attempted to abandon the old Hollywood myths and seriously examine themes of the family, love, and human communication. Although *David and Lisa* appropriates psychoanalysis in the same spirit as the old classic films, "as a doctrine of self-help" (Wood 1975, 38), it nevertheless brought a new, less sensationalized image of mental illness to the screen. In one scene, a group of young inmates on an outing are subjected to the abuse of a local man, who tells them that they do not belong in his town. Unlike several Laingian films yet to come in the 1960s (Philippe de Broca's *King of Hearts* of 1966 is the best example), *David and Lisa* does not quite suggest that the emotionally disturbed are superior to "normal" people, but it does confidently embrace psychiatry as the best hope for misunderstood and troubled individuals, associating the local man's hostility with blind conformity and intolerance. Furthermore, the film establishes its credentials as "art" by undermining familiar movie myths of America as a homogeneous culture exempt from unsettling ruptures such as mental illness.

David and Lisa also overturns myths of family in several scenes emphasizing the complete alienation of David (Keir Dullea) from his insensitive mother. American films of the classic period often created tension in their treatment of the cultural mythology, and as the editors of *Cahiers du cinéma* (Mast and Cohen 1985, 695–740) have written, even a filmmaker such as John Ford, who powerfully endorses the dominant ideology, contradicts that ideology through his personal style of filmmaking in *Young Mr. Lincoln* (1939). The much sharper critique of family in *David and Lisa* can be understood by comparing it with a somewhat similar situation in *Now Voyager:* Bette Davis's alienation from *her* unsympathetic mother in the earlier film also takes place in close proximity to psychiatric discourse, suggesting that both films strain at the same cultural myths. However, although the audience is allowed to cheer Bette Davis's rebellion against her mother's repressive regime, the heroine pays dearly for this rebellion when she feels responsible for her mother's death. The film also extols values associated with family in other ways, including Paul Henreid's unwill-

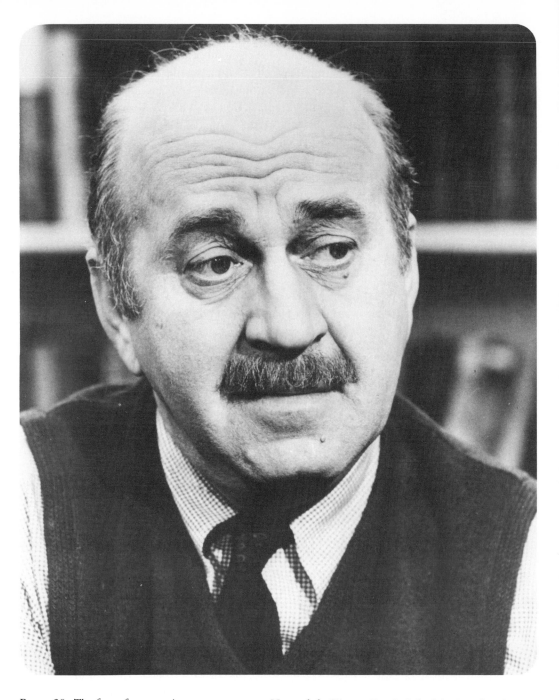

PLATE 20. The face of compassionate competence: Howard da Silva as Dr. Swinford in *David and Lisa* (1962). Continental. The Museum of Modern Art/Film Stills Archive.

ingness to leave his wife and Davis's mothering of Henreid's daughter. *Now Voyager,* following the Hollywood pattern of reconciliation, does not acknowledge that families can fail nearly so directly as does *David and Lisa,* in which David (Dullea) is effectively abandoned by his mother. Consequently, the later film has much greater need for the healing powers of psychiatry and the parent surrogate of da Silva's Dr. Swinford. Ideologically, *David and Lisa* no longer casts psychiatry as an agent for the project of verifying American myths; instead, the psychiatrist functions as the best hope in a fallen world without the consoling promise of eternally nurturing families. Even when the doctor performs the conventional function of telling David to forgive his parents, his quietly understated performance makes the statements seem fresh and even daring. Part of the film's success lies in da Silva's ability to communicate the compassion his character has for his patients without letting the trappings of the profession impede him. Swinford seldom uses jargon, and he occasionally reveals that the transference attacks of David affect him even though he tries not to show it. More than two decades after it was made, many psychiatrists still refer to *David and Lisa* as one of the most "realistic" depictions of psychiatric treatment.

The handling of countertransference feelings is actually the central issue in another film, Hubert Cornfield's *Pressure Point* (1962), certainly the best example of a racially oriented problem picture from the Golden Age. The film, however, has much more in common with *Home of the Brave* (1949) than with *David and Lisa,* especially since both were produced by Stanley Kramer. Furthermore, both *Home of the Brave* and *Pressure Point* substituted black characters for Jewish ones in the respective literary sources for the films. But unlike the earlier film, *Pressure Point* makes the psychiatrist the central character and casts a black actor as the psychiatrist rather than as the patient. Significantly, the first film appearance of a black psychiatrist takes place at the height of the Golden Age, and Sidney Poitier, the icon of the movement for black equality, endows psychiatry with his special aura during this period. *Pressure Point* begins when a psychiatrist in a state institution (Peter Falk) enters the office of the unnamed chief psychiatrist (Poitier) and asks to be taken off the case of a black youth who has suffered at the hands of white people and who has not responded to over seven months of Falk's treatment. The body of the film is a flashback illustrating why Poitier believes that Falk should continue to treat the boy. Twenty years earlier, Poitier had been a prison psychiatrist treating a disturbed bigot (Bobby Darin) who had been incarcerated for advocating Nazism (plate 21). In spite of Darin's constant taunting, Poitier eventually finds the root of his patient's problems, his hostility toward his father. (The film uses expressionist camera work in flashbacks to Darin's childhood.) The film does not hesitate to show us that Poitier is offended by many of Darin's remarks, but it also argues that Poitier's professionalism always subsumes his personal feelings and that his only goal is to treat the young man. On several occasions Darin tells Poitier that he is a fool to think that his white superiors will support a black man over a white man, even over a white convict who espouses Nazism. His prediction is borne out when Darin is paroled over the objections of Poitier, whose insistence that the bigot needs more treatment is interpreted by the warden as personal hostility. Poitier resigns from his job in the prison, and we learn that Darin is hanged for murder ten years after his release. Yet the black psychiatrist always believed that he could have helped the Darin character, and his insistence that Falk continue treating the black youth confirms this conviction. As in *Home of the Brave,* the real issues of racism that *Pressure Point* raises are finessed, and as in *The Caine Mutiny,* the solution offered at the film's conclusion does not ring true: the insuperable difficulties faced by Poitier in treating Darin contradict his optimistic belief that Falk can overcome the intractable resistance of a black patient. Obviously, the Poitier character himself should take over the case. Nevertheless, the heroism that the film finds in Poitier's struggle with himself is also invested in creating the portrait of a fully

PLATE 21. Sidney Poitier, as the movies' first black psychiatrist, overcomes the racism of Bobby Darin in *Pressure Point* (1962). United Artists. The Museum of Modern Art/Film Stills Archive.

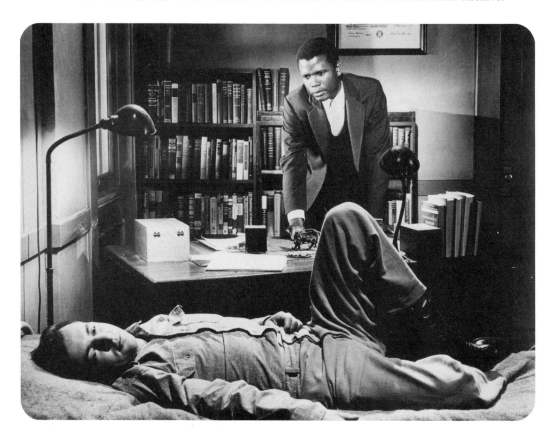

rounded, if idealized, human being whose expertise as a psychiatrist goes hand in hand with his nobility as a person.

One obscure film from the Golden Age is of interest primarily because of its title. Roger Kay's *The Cabinet of Caligari* (1962) hardly lives up to its name even though its script is by Robert Bloch, the same man who wrote the book on which Hitchcock's *Psycho* is based. In *The Cabinet of Caligari* (not *The Cabinet of Dr. Caligari* of 1919) Jane (Glynis Johns) is trapped in a strange house where everyone is dominated and sometimes even abused by a mysterious physician named Caligari. The one sympathetic character in the group is Paul (Dan O'Herlihy), a pipe-smoking, avuncular fellow who offers advice and comfort to Jane. But Paul is ultimately revealed to be Caligari in disguise, and the heroine feels more trapped and alone than ever. Only at the end does the film make clear why it has been named after a classic of the silent German cinema: all but the final moments of the action turn out to have taken place entirely within Jane's deranged mind. Paul (O'Herlihy) is actually Jane's psychiatrist, whose attempts to reach her have transformed him into a monster in her fantasies. The film ends with the revelation that in fact Paul has cured her, and as she leaves the sanitarium, we meet (much as in *The Wizard of Oz*) all the people from the sanitarium who inspired characters in her earlier dream. The expressionist mise-en-scène of the original *Cabinet of Dr. Caligari* is suggested only vaguely in one scene, and little else connects the film with the source for its title. Nevertheless, this "remake" is quite typical of the Golden Age, constituting a grand apologia for psychiatry: all the tricks with which Caligari seems to torment Jane are actually valid healing techniques that only a disturbed mind would regard as threats. When O'Herlihy appears at the end, he is the avuncular character from the dream, in other words, the typical film psychiatrist of the late 1950s and early 1960s.

We should call attention in this chapter to another minor film from the period, Philip Dunne's *Wild in the Country* (1961), one of the few Golden Age film that features a female psychiatrist. As we mentioned in chapter 1, Irene Sperry (Hope Lange) is perhaps the only female psychiatrist prominently featured in an American film who successfully treats a male patient without being transformed into his helpmate. (In 1935, when a young man thanks Claudette Colbert for curing him in *Private Worlds*, his total time on the screen is less than a minute.) Furthermore, *Wild in the Country* does not suggest at the outset that Dr. Sperry has chosen her profession because of her inadequacy as a woman. Nevertheless, she is sexually attracted to the Presley character and attempts suicide when their few chaste moments together in a hotel room are misinterpreted. This is, after all, an Elvis Presley film. On the other hand, Dr. Sperry is portrayed as a competent, compassionate therapist who transforms Presley from a juvenile delinquent into a promising young fiction writer and who at the end is capable of overcoming her feelings for him and returning to her practice. That all of this is accompanied by the obligatory fistfights and Presley's crooning should be sufficient proof that there was in fact a Golden Age of psychiatry in the American cinema.

We must also acknowledge that, even during the Golden Age, women were only occasionally allowed entry into the American cinema's psychiatric pantheon. In Blake Edwards's *The Perfect Furlough* (1958), Army psychologist Janet Leigh goes through the usual process of losing her heart to her leading man after he has thoroughly manipulated her for his own purposes. Leigh is, of course, a sympathetic character, but she is no different from female psychiatrists in movies from earlier decades who found their true calling in the arms of a male lover. Irwin Allen's *Voyage to the Bottom of the Sea* (1961) reserves an even harsher fate for its female doctor of the mind: Joan Fontaine plays a seemingly competent psychiatrist who has undertaken a study of men under stress on the futuristic submarine *Seaview,* the brainchild of a scientific genius played by Walter Pidgeon. The plot presents the scientist with a fire in the Van Allen Radiation Belt that is about to destroy the world. When Pidgeon sets out in his submarine to implement a controversial plan to extinguish the fire with a nuclear missile, Fontaine begins to spread doubts about his sanity among members of the crew. In this inflated genre picture, her function is a slight variation on that of psychiatrists in horror/science fiction films who deny the reality of supernatural forces. Rather than espousing a strictly rationalist unbelief in the supernatural, the Fontaine character in *Voyage to the Bottom of the Sea* fails to understand the unconventional but brilliantly effective plans of Walter Pidgeon. When Fontaine eventually resorts to sabotage to frustrate Pidgeon's plans, she receives a lethal dose of radiation for her troubles. Before she can expire from radiation sickness, however, she is eaten by a shark that another scientist (Peter Lorre) keeps aboard the submarine. Fontaine's sabotage attempts fail, and when Pidgeon finally launches his missile, he does in fact save the world. At the risk of overstating our thesis, we must point out that Fontaine, appearing in a film made during the Golden Age, is surely the least malevolent of all the negative female psychiatrists we have been able to locate in American movies. Unlike the villainesses in *Nightmare Alley, I, the Jury,* and *Shock Treatment,* Fontaine is motivated by concern for the safety of the ship's crew rather than by simple avarice.

We should also point out that a few films from the period 1957–63 take a skeptical view of psychiatry, even when the practitioner is male. In both

Pillow Talk (1959) and *Lover Come Back* (1961), Tony Randall presents an unmanly contrast to Rock Hudson as he pursues Doris Day. In the earlier film, when Randall discovers that Hudson has been wooing his girlfriend (Day), he says, "I should have listened to my psychiatrist. He told me never to trust anyone but him." Capitalizing on the success of *Pillow Talk*, Delbert Mann's *Lover Come Back* cast the same three actors in similar roles, this time allowing Randall's psychiatrist (Richard Deacon) to appear briefly and to dominate his neurotic patient as if Randall were a small child. In these two films as in *Oh Men! Oh Women!,* Tony Randall became stereotyped as an insecure male whose dependence on his therapist is a function of his unmanliness. The Rock Hudson of the movies would never require psychiatric treatment, even in the Golden Age. Twenty-five years later, revelations about Rock Hudson's sexual preference provide a thorough unmasking of this mythological conceit.

Delbert Mann again poked fun at psychiatry in still another Doris Day vehicle, *That Touch of Mink* (1962), and in William Castle's *Zotz!* (1962), a psychiatrist fulfilled the conventional role of the unenlightened rationalist who cannot appreciate the fact that the hero (Tom Poston) possesses magical powers. However, in these light comedies, psychiatry is hardly central, providing a few brief jokes as, for example, in *Call Me Bwana* (1963) when Bob Hope flies past the window of a psychiatrist, who immediately lies down on his own couch, begins talking about his childhood, and then is seen no more.

At least one film from the Golden Age poses special problems for our historical analysis of the psychiatrist in American films. Henry King's *Tender Is the Night* (1962), taken from the equally problematic novel of F. Scott Fitzgerald, can be seen as the straight version of a definitely post–Golden Age film, Marshall Brickman's *Lovesick* (1983). Dick Diver (Jason Robards, Jr.) is a handsome, well-liked, and promising young psychiatrist at a Swiss clinic who treats a wealthy young woman, Nicole (Jennifer Jones). Her mental illness gives her the same qualities possessed by Olivia de Havilland in *Snake Pit,* Susan Strasberg in *Cobweb,* and Janet Margolin in *David and Lisa*—a charming naiveté and vulnerability. Against the advice of his thick-accented supervising analyst, Dr. Dohmler (Paul Lukas), Diver falls in love with Nicole, and we hear this exchange:

DOHMLER: Love! How can a first class brain with a brilliant future fall in love so-called with a broken mind healing?

DIVER: There have been cases of good marriages between patients and psychiatrists.

DOHMLER: You cannot be both lover and psychiatrist to the same woman. You cannot be a guide, a doctor, a god, and a husband. For when she discovers that she married a human being, a fallible human being . . . crash, disaster, for one or the other or for the both.

Nevertheless, Dick marries Nicole and accepts the invitation of her manipulative sister, Baby (Joan Fontaine), to devote himself full-time to showing Nicole the good life. As Nicole's guardian, Baby can and will contribute unlimited financial resources toward her sister's happiness. But Dick and Nicole's marriage becomes one long binge during which Nicole has regular breakdowns. Returning to visit Dr. Dohmler some five years after leaving the clinic, Diver finds the old analyst on his deathbed. Dohmler repeats many of the remarks that he had made to Diver earlier, warning of the "tyranny of the weak" and of Dick's role as a "fallible human being, not a god." When Dohmler begins a sentence with the words, "And when the relapses end," Diver finishes it for him: "the love ends." Dohmler suggests, perhaps for the only time during the Golden Age, that the profession of psychiatry may actually attract people with personal problems. He even says that Nicole would get better without Dick and vice versa. Robards's performance suggests, however, that Dick Diver simply loves Nicole and wants to help her. The film also suggests that, almost until the end of their relationship, Nicole desperately needs Dick and that his love for her has forced him to succumb to the temptations offered by Baby.

Dick goes back to practicing psychiatry only when his little daughter becomes ill from drinking champagne, which constantly lies about in glasses during their extended and regular celebrations. Both Dick and Nicole, who has continued to improve, realize that they should get their lives back on track. But Dick returns to the clinic to discover that Dohmler has died and that Franz, the psychiatrist who has replaced him, is not fully prepared to accept Dick on his own terms. To complicate matters, Dick is no longer as effective a therapist as he was for Nicole, and in one scene he even attacks the father of one of his patients. During a later scene in which Dick uses terms like "anaclitic" and "countertransference," Franz suggests that Nicole has become the stronger member of their marriage. Their relationship continues to deteriorate until Dick decides to go back to upstate New York where he was born, presumably to start life over. Both Nicole and Dick realize they must separate for their own good, but the film, quite unlike the novel (Fitzgerald 1934), suggests that the love they still feel for each other might eventually have saved their marriage.

Tender Is the Night does not hold up well because of its soap opera treatment of what was already an overdrawn novel. The film follows Dick's degeneration and Nicole's improvement as if she were a vampire sucking the mental health out of him. A number of reasons are offered for Dick's succumbing so easily to this process, but none of them explain adequately why the physician cannot heal himself. Old doctor Dohmler was right to warn Diver not to fall in love with Nicole, but he speaks with a much better understanding of countertransference than the movie actually shows in its plot. Fitzgerald's novel is probably unfilmable, but it was especially so in 1962, the year in which the image of psychiatry had reached its apex in the American cinema. The picture of Dick Diver drowning in wasted love (Fitzgerald's onomastics are particularly bald in this story) clashes with the idealization of psychiatry that has seeped into the film from its historical context.

This idealization also comes to the movie directly from its source. *Tender Is the Night* is a largely autobiographical novel drawn from Fitzgerald's troubled marriage with the schizophrenic Zelda (Berman 1985, 60–86). Fitzgerald considered making his protagonist a film technician before deciding upon a psychiatrist. This choice was significant not just because Fitzgerald took psychiatry to be the best available equivalent for his own work as an artist. Dick Diver in *Tender Is the Night* also stands for "the decline of the supposedly solid, turn-of-the-century American morality, the disillusionment of the so-called Lost Generation, the ultimate futility of seeking material possessions, the emptiness of a purely sensual existence" (Guthmann 1969). Fitzgerald wanted to dramatize this vision by chronicling the destructive effect of these forces even upon a character who should be most equipped to withstand them. Even more so than in the film, the Dr. Dohmler of the novel represents the lofty traditions to which Diver's generation cannot measure up. It can be argued that the film version of *Tender Is the Night* does not possess the Golden Age qualities of, say, *Pressure Point* or *David and Lisa*. On the other hand, Dr. Dohmler is the most august and sympathetic elder statesman since Michael Chekhov in *Spellbound*. As played by Jason Robards, Jr., Dick Diver is a handsome, witty man who falls in love and then tries to pick up the pieces of his life (and his practice), leaving behind the woman he loves essentially for her own good. If the film had been made prior to 1955, there is little doubt that the portraits of the psychiatrists would have been much less positive. After 1963, the film simply would not have been produced at all unless as a made-for-television movie. In fact, a new version of *Tender Is the Night* appeared in 1985 as a miniseries on Showtime, a pay-cable television service.

The 1962 version of *Tender Is the Night* did not present the only dark cloud in the golden skies of cinematic psychiatry. A curious film from this period that deserves mention is Joseph L. Mankiewicz's *Suddenly, Last Summer* (1959), based on a short play by Tennessee Williams. Three years before he was to appear as Freud, Montgomery Clift plays a promising young brain surgeon who appears to be the only doctor in a mental institution, one that bears a great resemblance to the one in *The Snake Pit.* Strictly speaking, Clift does not belong in our study since his specialty is surgery, not verbal therapy. Yet there could be no more unlikely brain surgeon: Clift was just recovering from his disastrous automobile accident and was beginning the addiction to alcohol that would haunt him for the rest of his career. One scene in *Suddenly, Last Summer* shows his character about to perform a lobotomy even though Clift is apparently unable to stop his hands from shaking. Ultimately, however, Clift plays another idealized doctor of the mind, intervening in behalf of the institutionalized heroine (Elizabeth Taylor) and finally providing her with a complete cathartic cure and more than a suggestion of love interest. What makes the film problematic is its subtext: not only is Clift barely able to walk through several of his scenes, but the portrait of institutional care for the mentally ill falls back on the bedlam conventions of the 1940s, complete with wildly aroused male patients, arbitrarily repressive keepers, and a corrupt sanitarium director (Albert Dekker) willing to lobotomize a patient in return for the donations of a wealthy patron (Katharine Hepburn). According to Vito Russo (1981), Tennessee William's psychiatrist had recently convinced the playwright that he should renounce his homosexuality, and so Williams earnestly responded by writing a short play that portrayed Sebastian (the son of Katharine Hepburn's character in the subsequent film) as a homosexual monster. Mankiewicz's film expands this drama into a baroque horror film, featuring cannibalism, slightly displaced incest, and a conclusion that recalls the original *Frankenstein,* in which outraged villagers chase the monster to the top of a hill before destroying him. The spectacle of a barely functional Clift, however idealized his character, only contributes to the portrait of a moral universe that is profoundly askew and quite beyond the control of one benevolent therapist.

A similar situation exists with a number of films by Alfred Hitchcock. Interestingly, many of the director's most respected films were made during our Golden Age, and many of them feature a vision of psychiatry that seems on the surface to be rather positive. But the subtexts of almost all of these films undermine the grandiose claims by and for psychiatry during this time. Unlike *Suddenly, Last Summer,* in which the subtext seemed unintentionally at odds with the film's plot, Hitchcock's work reflects a carefully articulated vision that engaged psychiatry at several levels. The later films are much more interesting from a psychoanalytic view than is *Spellbound* (1945), which features psychiatrists much more prominently in its plot.

Perhaps the bleakest film of Hitchcock's career is *The Wrong Man* (1956), a semidocumentary account of a musician (Henry Fonda) who finds himself the victim of an astonishing array of coincidences that link him to a robbery he did not commit. During the long legal process to which the protagonist is subjected, his wife (Vera Miles) suffers a breakdown and is institutionalized. In his one brief scene, the wife's psychiatrist (Werner Klemperer) appears competent and concerned. Nevertheless, the profound pessimism of the film works against the hope offered by therapy. At film's end, although the hero has been vindicated, his wife is still deeply disturbed, and there is no suggestion that his Job-like sufferings will be requited.

Much the same can be said of a film that many critics consider to be Hitchcock's masterpiece, *Vertigo* (1958). When Scotty (James Stewart) collapses after what he assumes to be the death of Madeleine (Kim Novak), he is treated by an articulate psychiatrist whose diagnostic formulation and treatment recommendation are perfectly reasonable. Nevertheless, when he encounters Judy, the woman who had previously posed as Madeleine, the hero's obsession leads him on a necrophilic quest in which he finds himself hallucinating Madeleine over Judy's shoulder even as he is succeeding in transforming Judy into Madeleine. In his essential essay on *Vertigo*, Robin Wood has pointed out how well the film succeeds in its psychologically complex investigation of the human tendency "to form an idealized image of the other person and substitute it for the reality" (1977, 93). By the end, Scotty has been cured of his vertigo, but without the intervention of a therapist. More importantly, "his cure has destroyed at a blow both the reality and the illusion of Judy/Madeleine, has made the *illusion* of Madeleine's death real. He is cured, but empty, desolate. Triumph and tragedy are indistinguishably fused" (Wood 1977, 95). More important than the brief appearance of the therapist in this film is a subtext that finds madness in love, betrayal in friendship, and death in the displaced sexual climax when Scotty and Judy breathlessly arrive at the top of the church tower.

Even *Psycho* (1960), which we will discuss in more detail in both chapters 4 and 7, finds means for undermining the seemingly definitive statements of its psychiatrist, Dr. Richmond (Simon Oakland). Several critics have suggested that *Psycho's* psychiatric coda is actually a Hitchcockian joke or that the glib explanations of Dr. Richmond are inadequate to dispel the profoundly disturbing issues of matricide, voyeurism, and audience complicity that lie at the core of the film (Wood 1977; Braudy 1968). Harvey Greenberg argues persuasively that Hitchcock is a much better Freudian in his creation of *"Psycho's* authentic ambience of the dream"* than in the "inexact" pronouncements of the "officious" Dr. Richmond (1975, 134).

Robert Ray has identified Hitchcock's themes during this period: "His crowning achievements, *North by Northwest* and *Psycho,* specifically dealt with money, mothers, and movement. Of all his films' great sequences, the most memorable was the crop-dusting sequence in *North by Northwest,* an image that took the very basis of the American dream, open space, and revealed its hidden capacities for danger and claustrophobia" (1985, 158). In upsetting the old formulas so thoroughly, Hitchcock was hardly interested in the pat remedies that psychiatry so frequently offered in the social problem films of the Golden Age.

In spite of these few films that tarnished the psychiatric goldenness of the late fifties and early sixties, our period culminated in 1962 with John Huston's *Freud* (plates 22 and 23). The film is interesting if only for the role played by Jean-Paul Sartre in the genesis of its script. Huston had been planning a film about Freud ever since he had the opportunity to watch psychiatrists in action

PLATE 22. Young Sigmund Freud (Montgomery Clift) is about to come to terms with the problems of Cecily (Susannah York) as well as himself in John Huston's *Freud* (1962). Universal Pictures. The Museum of Modern Art/Film Stills Archive.

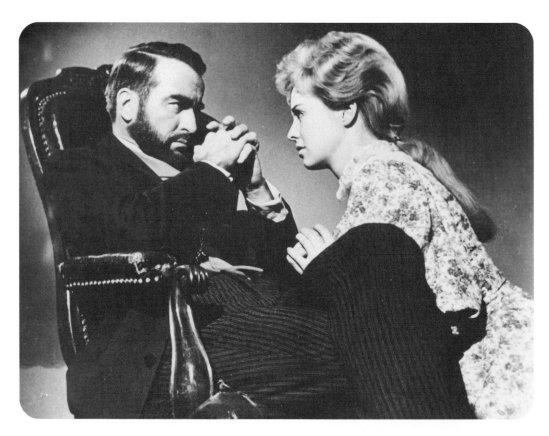

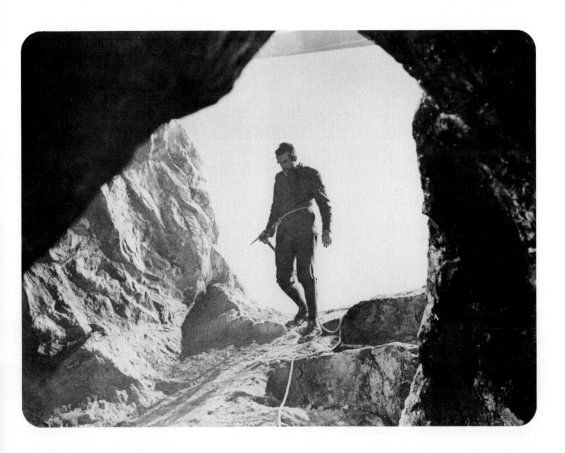

PLATE 23. Freud's dream is also a metaphor for his perilous journey into the unexplored regions of the mind: *Freud* (1962). Universal Pictures. The Museum of Modern Art/Film Stills Archive.

while filming *Let There Be Light* in 1946. Even though Huston refers to Sartre in his autobiography (1980) as an anti-Freudian, he says that he considered him to be the ideal writer for a script about Freud: "Sartre disagreed with Freud in a social sense rather than in a scientific sense. He regarded Freud's studies as valuable for what they discovered about the human mind, but of little social import because the role of the psychoanalyst was in fact so limited. I'm inclined to agree. Bored wives and problem children of the affluent make up the bulk of a top-ranking psychoanalyst's practice. Fees are exorbitant, and treatment is usually a matter of years. The movers and shakers have no time for it, and those who most need psychiatric counseling are precisely those who can't afford it" (Huston 1980, 294). Interestingly, the film that Huston eventually made carries none of the spirit of these remarks; in fact, it transforms Freud into a

Christ figure. Huston's statements in his autobiography reflect his (and typical Hollywood) ideas of 1980 much more than they do any ideas expressed in *Freud*.

According to Huston, Sartre wrote two drafts for a script, the first of which was long enough for a five-hour movie. After meeting with Huston for several days in order to make the script more manageable, and after being told not to worry about censorship, Sartre then produced a second draft, which was twice as long. (Sartre's *Freud* script was published in 1986 by the University of Chicago Press.) Some time later, Huston wrote a much shorter treatment with Wolfgang Reinhardt, son of the director Max Reinhardt. (Charles Kaufman also received credit though Huston says that his contribution was minimal.) Unlike Axel Corti's German film *Young Dr. Freud* (1977) or the six-hour miniseries made for British television in 1984, Huston's film takes a number of liberties with the chronology of events in Freud's life, and some characters, such as Susannah York's Cecily, are composites. The script relied on Sartre's work as its "backbone," particularly its focus on Freud's early career when he was developing the theory of the oedipus complex while confronting his own conflicts with his father. Yet Sartre denounced Huston when he eventually saw the script and demanded that his name not be associated with the film. Sartre never told Huston why he objected even though the director felt that the $25,000 Sartre received for his screenplay entitled Huston to an answer.

Still, the film is surprisingly frank about Freud's work, in particular his theories concerning infantile sexuality. On the other hand, the film attempts to romanticize and sensationalize Freud's work at the same time that it evokes a performance from the ailing Montgomery Clift so solemn as to obscure completely Freud's famous wit. The film is also the most claustrophobic of Huston's many works, employing a larger percentage of close-ups than does any other film by Huston or, for that matter, by almost any other Hollywood director (Kaminsky 1978, 140).

The film's credits first tell us that not one but two technical advisers were present during filming. We then hear John Huston's overripe narration behind obscure Rorschachesque images and Jerry Goldsmith's atonal score. After comparing Freud to Copernicus and Darwin for their "blows dealt us in our vanity," Huston introduces the Christ parallel by telling us we are about to see "the story of Freud's descent into a region almost as black as hell itself—man's unconscious—and how he let in the light." (The use of the word *light* in this context also recalls Huston's *Let There Be Light*.) The music of Jerry Goldsmith, whose effective score for Ridley Scott's *Alien* will be discussed in chapter 10, often telegraphs the psychosexual importance of what happens in the film. For example, when Freud learns through hypnosis that a troubled young man (David McCallum) has attacked his father because the son believed that his father raped a "young girl," a string crescendo and then a moment of pregnant silence precede McCallum's terse identification of the young girl as "my mother." Another musical flourish marks the oedipally charged moment when Freud unintentionally breaks the family heirloom pocket watch just after his father has given it to him.

In its cinematographic depiction of dreams and simple cures, *Freud* is in some ways no more sophisticated than a film as early as *Blind Alley* (1939). There is even a familiar cathartic cure for Cecily, the central patient in the film, played by Susannah York. (Both Huston and Sartre had wanted Marilyn Monroe to play the part, but according to Huston, Monroe's own analyst objected on the grounds that Anna Freud had not approved the project.) As Sartre had intended, the film unites Freud's progress toward defining the oedipus complex through the parallel analyses of Cecily and himself, arriving simultaneously at an understanding of why he and his patient both entertained troublesome feelings toward their parents. After a nocturnal moment of self-doubt when Freud's wife attempts to encourage him by reading to him from his diary, the truth of infantile sexuality suddenly becomes clear to him. As he realizes the importance of his discovery, his wife opens the drapes and the morning light pours in symbolically, recalling Huston's opening narration. The notion that Freud's discovery came from a stray remark by his wife is a little reminiscent of the joke about Beethoven hearing the opening motif of the Fifth Symphony in his wife's laugh. Like the author of the Beethoven joke, who capsuled a complex process into a single pregnant moment, Huston and his collaborators have attempted to find a cinematic means for presenting in concentrated form a discovery that was actually a series of processes within one person's mind. A film such as *Freud* provides an excellent example of the trivializing power of cinema, especially when, ironically, it attempts to impress us with the seriousness of what it has undertaken. Most film theorists agree that movies succeed more often when they put aside pretension and turn to material that is suited to a popular medium like the cinema. This is not to say that films cannot be serious or significant, but rather that they suffer when the complexity of the material lies outside the range of what cinema can dramatize effectively.

Ernest Callenbach, the editor of *Film Quarterly,* has said of *Freud,* "It is impossible, I would think, for any educated person to sit through *Freud* without bursting into laughter at least once" (Halliwell 1983, 303). This judgment may be a little harsh, especially of a film made during the unique moment when American films were most earnest in their romance with psychiatry, a moment that has been especially vulnerable to the changing attitudes and styles in the American cinema of the last two decades. In all fairness to Huston we should also point out that substantial portions of the film were excised under pressure from the heads of Universal-International studio, who nevertheless expected the film to be their most important release of the year. However, like most psychiatrically inclined films from the Golden Age, *Freud* was a box-office disappointment. Psychology was never as successful in attracting audiences as the singing and dancing and the biblical pageantry which usually characterized box-office hits in the late 1950s and early 1960s. When *Freud* was rereleased in 1963 with the subtitle, *The Secret Passion,* it was still unsuccessful. Huston is probably correct in his explanation of the film's failure to attract audiences: the film seemed too interested in education rather than in entertainment while its ability to produce titillation—or moral outrage—was greatly exaggerated. "Audiences didn't give a damn whether children thought about, were influenced by or practiced sex. They were, if anything, disappointed that there wasn't more sex in the picture, especially on an adult level. But what they wanted was 'healthy' sex—the Marilyn Monroe kind of sex" (1980, 304).

THE SECOND TRANSITIONAL PERIOD

Still, *Freud* is the ultimate example of a phenomenon toward which the American cinema had been moving since its inception: the portrayal of a sensitive human being dealing successfully with the interrelated problems of himself and others. It is no coincidence that in the single year of 1962 we meet this figure not only in *Freud* but also in the psychiatrists in *Pressure Point, David and Lisa,* and to a certain extent, *Tender Is the Night.* The Golden Age comes to an end very quickly, however, and like 1957, 1963 is a transitional year in which we can see a new, negative view of the profession emerging. Golden Age myths popped up briefly in 1963 films such as Daniel Mann's *Who's Been Sleeping in My Bed?,* in which Martin Balsam cures Dean Martin of compulsive woman chasing, or Norman Jewison's *The Thrill of It All,* in which James Garner wins back the attentions of his wife (Doris Day) thanks to the guidance counseling of a slightly eccentric psychiatrist. Yet both these movies are comedies, and like *Pillow Talk* and *That Touch of Mink,* they anticipate the irreverence toward psychiatry that was soon to become a regular feature of numerous satirical comedies in the sixties and seventies.

For our purposes, the most interesting transitional film of 1963 is David Miller's *Captain Newman, M.D.* Gregory Peck plays the title role of a psychiatrist during World War II who cares deeply about his patients but who must resist the efforts of his superiors to send men back into combat before he can finish curing them. Tony Curtis and Angie Dickinson appear in the film, largely for the purpose of showing the many ways in which Newman can be human and loving as well as effective and compassionate. However, he has mixed results with the three principal patients we actually see him treating. He never really succeeds in reaching an obsessed officer (Eddie Albert) who eventually jumps off a tower to his death. On the other hand, he wins a victory in his treatment of a nearly catatonic soldier played by Robert Duvall. The most effective element in the cure of Duvall comes when the doctor encourages Duvall's dispassionate wife (Bethel Leslie) to express more affection and to dress more alluringly. When his wife takes the advice and adopts a new approach to her marriage, the Duvall character has an outburst that turns out to be another cathartic cure. The most important patient, however, is played by Bobby Darin, just one year after his well-received performance in *Pressure Point.* After encountering more difficulty with him than with anyone else, Captain Newman turns the Darin character into a healthy individual and returns him to his unit a new man. In the final minutes of the film, however, the news comes back that Darin has been killed in action. Although the film's primary message has already been clearly stated, it ends with the psychiatrist bemoaning his fate of patching up the psyches of troubled soldiers only to send them off to be slaughtered. Psychiatry works, but it is no match, unfortunately, for the problems of the world. The suggestion that the diseases of society negate or mock the efforts of psychiatrists was present in earlier films such as *The Snake Pit,* but it becomes central to the view of psychiatry throughout the 1960s and 1970s. *Captain Newman, M.D.* is a transitional film because this theme appears alongside Peck's portrayal of one of the most idealized of all movie psychiatrists. Unlike *David and Lisa, Captain Newman, M.D.* is the big-budget product of a Hollywood studio that at this point appears to have abandoned the project of reconciliation and consolation. However sentimentalized its ending, the film does not blink at the terrible irony of Dr. Newman's career. The introduction of the idea that the world's problems render psychiatry ineffective also signals the end of the brief Golden Age of psychiatry in the American cinema.

The abrupt and unexpected end of the Golden Age coincided with an equally abrupt and unexpected decline in governmental support of psychiatric research and education (see chapter 6). In this context, we should mention one of the last Golden Age films, Hall Bartlett's *The Caretakers* (1963), in which Robert Stack plays an innovative young psychiatrist of idealized qualities who assumes command of a clinic and then overcomes the resistance of an authoritarian head nurse, appropriately named Lucrezia (Joan Crawford), in his efforts to help patients. The film, however, also exploits the sensational aspects of ECT and titillated the audience when a dazed but attractive female patient (Polly Bergen) wanders into a ward full of men, all of whom appear to be steely eyed rapists. *The Caretakers* was a strangely inappropriate film to ride the Golden Age wave and to garner the publicity benefits of being selected for a special preview screening before the United States Senate. The chairman of the Senate Committee on Labor and Public Welfare, Lister Hill, wrote to director Bartlett praising him for a film that "contributed to creating the very favorable climate and presenting the challenge that brought the victory in the passage of the Mental Health and Mental Retardation Act by an overwhelming vote" (Knight 1963). However, just as the movies were soon to begin projecting a much less flattering vision of psychiatry, the United States government was on the verge of reversing itself and cutting its expenditures for mental health: after two decades of dramatic increases, grant support from the National Institute of Mental Health for psychiatric research and education reached a peak and then began to decline in the mid-1960s (Pardes and Pincus 1983). The special attention afforded *The Caretakers* had little lasting effect upon the government or, for that matter, upon Hollywood itself.

THE MIGRATION OF A GENRE

We conclude this chapter both by departing from our exclusive concentration on theatrically released features and by pointing out that the idealized image of psychiatry does not disappear entirely from popular media after 1963. By the late 1970s, films such as *I Never Promised You a Rose Garden, An Unmarried Woman,* and, of course, *Ordinary People* project psychotherapists who would not have been out of place in the Golden Age. Nevertheless, the most positive images of psychiatry traveled from movie houses to television along with many other elements of the social problem film. The earnest realism of this genre quickly lost its allure for the increasingly youthful movie audiences of the 1960s, but its comforting view of souls being healed seemed ideally suited for the "cooler" medium of television. In 1962, the culminating year of the Golden Age of psychiatry, several therapeutically oriented films appeared that illustrate this point. Arthur Penn's *The Miracle Worker* from this year won Academy Awards for Patty Duke, who played the young Helen Keller, and Anne Bancroft, who played her teacher, Annie Sullivan. The story had originally appeared as an episode on television's high-art series, "Playhouse 90," before moving on to Broadway and then to the silver screen. Significantly, when *The Miracle Worker* was remade in 1979, it was not for theatrical release but for television once again, as a run-of-the-mill "movie of the week." (Scripts for all three versions of *The Miracle Worker* were by William Gibson, who also wrote the novel on which *The Cobweb* was based.) Similarly, in 1976 *The Three Faces of Eve* was more or less remade for television as "Sybil." The continuity between the originals and the remakes was established by casting Patty Duke as Annie Sullivan in the television version of *Miracle Worker* and Joanne Woodward (who had played the title role in *Three Faces of Eve*) as a psychiatrist treating a patient with multiple personality (Sally Field) in "Sybil." In 1981 Richard Sarafian directed an almost shot-for-shot television remake of *Splendor in the Grass* with the same Golden Age vision of psychiatry that had characterized the theatrically released original in 1961. As we will see in the next chapter, reassuring stories about people overcoming their problems were practically nonexistent in the movies made for theatrical release after the Golden Age.

The issue of alcoholism offers an even better illustration of how social problems move between media. In Billy Wilder's *Lost Weekend* (1945), Hollywood exploited alcoholism for its shock value and then tacked on a preposterous happy ending. In 1958, television's "Playhouse 90" presented a more disturbing look at the subject in "The Days of Wine and Roses." Blake Edwards made the film version of J. P. Miller's teleplay for "Days of Wine and Roses" in the crucial year of 1962, when audiences could also see *The Miracle Worker, David and Lisa, Pressure Point,* and *Freud.* In fact, in the film of *The Days of Wine and Roses* Jack Klugman plays a recovered alcoholic whose selfless devotion to helping the protagonist (Jack Lemmon) would have made him the perfect example of the Golden Age psychiatrist if only the film had decided to call him "doctor" instead of leaving his occupation unstated. *The Days of Wine and Roses* purposefully explores the dangers of alcoholism and then shows that at least some of its victims—including the Jack Lemmon character—can recover. Compared to *Lost Weekend,* we can hardly say that the film is optimistic, but the sadder-but-wiser ending for Jack Lemmon's character fits perfectly into an early sixties tradition that includes psychiatrically inclined films such as *Home before Dark, Splendor in the Grass,* and *Captain Newman, M.D.* Still, this view of alcoholism soon became the almost exclusive property of undistinguished television movies. "Sarah T.—Portrait of a Teenage Alcoholic," "Beatrice: Life of the Party," and "A Sensitive, Passionate Man" are three examples of made-for-television films that treat alcoholism with deadly seriousness, and although none are characterized by great dialogue and acting, they all emulate the tone established by *Days of Wine and Roses.* Theatrical films, meanwhile, have taken to portraying alcoholism through the lovable high jinks of Dudley Moore in Steve Gordon's

Arthur (1981) or the existential metaphors of John Huston's *Under the Volcano* (1984).

As for the Golden Age psychiatrist, he has been a regular feature of made-for-television movies for many years now, especially since the success of a Hollywood film that could almost have been a television movie, *Ordinary People.* Even when American movies were most consistently harsh in their portrayal of psychiatrists, two weekly (though short-lived) television programs, "The Psychiatrist" and "Matt Lincoln," presented heroic images of psychiatrists in 1970 and 1971. This is not to say that television does not occasionally cast psychiatrists in the same negative roles that Hollywood movies have found for them, but television psychiatrists are much more likely to solve those problems such as alcoholism, multiple personality, anorexia nervosa, and the sexual abuse of children that in the sixties moved off of the silver screen and onto the small screen. Large numbers of television viewers became well acquainted with a psychiatrist of Golden Age qualities during the years that Alan Arbus played Dr. Sidney Freedman on television's "M*A*S*H." In fact, when one of the largest audiences in television history watched the last episode of that program in February 1983, they saw the psychiatrist restore a deeply disturbed Hawkeye (Alan Alda) to his usual level of sitcom zaniness.

By 1957 psychiatry had become a fact of life for most Americans, at least as far as the movies were concerned. Consequently, psychiatrists were regularly appropriated for effects that they had only occasionally supplied in the previous fifty years of psychiatry in the American cinema. Psychiatrists were frequently on hand to confirm optimistic myths about how easy it is for troubled people to return to well-being, or they themselves become complex heroes, dramatically confronting issues quite unlike the stuff of crime plots that earlier psychiatric heroes had faced in *Blind Alley* or *The Dark Mirror*. The Golden Age may represent the culmination of several decades during which real-life psychiatrists had been steadily gaining acceptance, partially because of their willingness to undertake what Burnham (1979) has called the "defense of traditional civilization," a role especially accessible to cinematic myths of the late 1950s and early 1960s. The Golden Age also seems to be related to Hollywood's desperate attempt at preserving its familiar paradigm of reconciliation, an undertaking that made great demands on the healing powers of cinematic psychotherapists. Ironically, as reconcilers and defenders of tradition, psychiatrists were left wide open for the sustained attacks movies began to launch as soon as the brief Golden Age came to an end and the old formulas were revised to the detriment of psychiatry.

The Fall from Grace

4

Freud, the culminating film of the Golden Age of psychiatry in the American cinema, begins and ends with music and paintings designed to suggest the eerie world of the unconscious. At the close of the film, these sounds and images accompany words spoken off-camera by director John Huston: "'Know thyself.' Two thousand years ago these words were carved on the Temple at Delphi. 'Know thyself.' They're the beginning of wisdom. In them lies the single hope of victory over man's oldest enemy, his family. This knowledge is now within our grasp. Will we use it? Let us hope." The earnestness of this speech with its accompanying aura of the Great Unknown becomes especially ironic in light of John Huston's performance twenty years later as Dudley Moore's ridiculous supervising analyst in Marshall Brickman's *Lovesick* (1983). Although this film is a comedy, and although it's unlikely romantic hero (Dudley Moore) is a psychoanalyst, it is nevertheless one of the strongest attacks yet on Freud and his followers.

The swiftness and the vigor with which American movies turned against psychiatry is as remarkable as the staying power of the negative attitudes toward the profession, which have prevailed with few exceptions since the Golden Age. Only in the last few years has Hollywood ceased presenting psychiatrists almost exclusively as evil, incompetent, exploitative, or the agents of a repressive society. The success of *Ordinary People* in 1980 may mark the most dramatic reversal of this tradition after two decades of almost unrelentingly negative portrayals. However, 1980 was the same year that *Dressed to Kill* made its equally auspicious debut on the American screen. A comparison between *Dressed to Kill* and the film that most inspired it, Alfred Hitchcock's *Psycho* (1960), is a good way to introduce the striking differences between the Golden Age and what followed.

From *Psycho* to *Dressed to Kill*

Written and directed by Brian De Palma, *Dressed to Kill* is about Dr. Robert Elliott, a Manhattan psychiatrist played by Michael Caine. Throughout most of the film, he appears to be a respectable member of society, both likeable as a person and professional as a psychiatrist. He sternly reprimands an unscrupulous police detective (Dennis Franz) for referring to mental patients as "weirdos," and he steadfastly protects the confidentiality of his patients. Earlier in the film he is compassionate and wise with his patient Kate (Angie Dickinson), a sexually frustrated housewife. When she asks flirtatiously if he would like to sleep with her, the psychiatrist allows himself to be drawn into his personal reasons for refusing her, but he handles the matter gently, and few in the audience would reproach him for dealing a little awkwardly with a patient's transference wishes. At the film's conclusion, however, the psychiatrist is revealed to be a psychotic killer. He has taken a razor to Kate and is prepared to do the same to any other woman who arouses him sexually. The film asks us to believe that the doctor's personality is split into male and female halves: when the male half (Robert Elliott) is attracted to a woman, the female half (Bobbie) becomes threatened and, donning a wig and a dress, destroys the woman who has enticed the male half.

Like many of Brian De Palma's films, *Dressed to Kill* is clearly—and clumsily, some critics would say—modeled after a film of Alfred Hitchcock, in this case *Psycho.* Both films lead us to believe that a beautiful blonde woman (Janet Leigh in *Psycho,* Angie Dickinson in *Dressed to Kill*) is to be the principal character in the narrative. Hitchcock builds suspense as Marion Crane (Janet Leigh) flees across Arizona highways with stolen money. The director increases audience involvement with Marion by having a suspicious state policeman menacingly follow her through several scenes. But before the film is half over, Marion's perforated body has been dumped in the swamp, and the policeman is never seen again. Similarly, the afternoon dalliance of Kate (Dickinson) with the man she meets at the museum in *Dressed to Kill* promises to be central to the film, especially when she finds a note in her lover's desk announcing that he has venereal disease. Here too the assumed heroine is dispatched early, and the syphilitic lover is absent from the remainder of the film. Of course, the most obvious plot similarity between *Psycho* and *Dressed to Kill* is the eventual revelation that the supposedly female murderer of the blond woman is a man (Anthony Perkins in *Psycho,* Caine in *Dressed to Kill*), who ordinarily behaves in a fairly normal manner but who occasionally puts on women's clothes and kills people with a sharp instrument.

The plot similarities between the two films continue after the death of the woman who appeared to be the central character: in both films a young man who was close to the murdered woman goes off in search of clues. In *Psycho* John Gavin plays Marion's lover, Sam, and in *Dressed to Kill* Keith Gordon is

Peter, Kate's son. The young man is aided in his search by another attractive blonde who is in many ways the double of the murdered woman and who is nearly killed by the same murderer. In *Psycho* Vera Miles plays Marion's sister, Lila, who not only resembles the murdered woman but appears on the verge of inheriting her lover. The sisters have the same effect on Norman Bates (Anthony Perkins), and he tries to kill both of them. In *Dressed to Kill* Liz Blake (Nancy Allen) is a whore-with-a-heart-of-gold who takes the place of Kate, a woman the film goes to some lengths to characterize almost entirely in terms of her sex drive. Both women arouse the sexual passions of the killer, but both of them treat Keith Gordon with maternal gestures. By the end of *Dressed to Kill* Nancy Allen has taken Angie Dickinson's place in the house, just as at the end of *Psycho* Vera Miles appears to have replaced Janet Leigh.

Another similarity between the two films involves the shower scene in *Psycho*, the cinematic moment when Hitchcock perversely desecrated America's shrine to personal hygiene and transformed it into a place where no one has really felt safe ever since. De Palma playfully suggests this scene in both the beginning and end of *Dressed to Kill*. The actual slashing takes place in an elevator, but De Palma films the scene in a style that clearly recalls Hitchcock's famous shower murder. In addition, both films frustrate audience expectations not only with the early deaths of supposed heroines but also with early plot devices that go nowhere. For example, the $40,000 Marion steals in the beginning of *Psycho* appears to be the Hitchcockian "MacGuffin" (Truffaut 1984, 138) which will keep the plot going until the end but actually plays only a small role after she is murdered. Similarly, in *Dressed to Kill* Kate forgets her wedding ring in the apartment of her spur-of-the-moment lover. Since she is killed before she can retrieve it, we assume that sooner or later the ring will turn up as a clue. It never does.

The comparison between *Psycho* and *Dressed to Kill* becomes most compelling, however, when we turn to the images of psychiatry that each film presents. At the close of *Psycho*, Simon Oakland plays Dr. Richmond, a psychiatrist who thoroughly clears up any confusion that any member of the cast or audience may have had about Norman Bates's behavior. The part is both written and played for maximum effect: here is a man who speaks as an oracle of knowledge and who wears his authority without reluctance. When he begins to explain Norman Bates's split personality, the district attorney says, "Well now look, if you're trying to lay some psychiatric ground work for some sort of plea that this man intends to cop. . . ." The psychiatrist interrupts him and speaks with a kind of jocular humility, "A psychiatrist doesn't lay the ground work; he merely tries to explain it." Obviously, he can do much more than that, and before he has finished, he has also solved five murders besides that of the Janet Leigh character. When the sheriff asks about the location of the pseudo-MacGuffin $40,000, the psychiatrist delivers his line as if an afterthought: "The swamp. These were crimes of passion, not profit." Ordinary police work is a trivial business with which a psychiatrist has little patience. The scene ends with a policeman asking his superintendent if Norman should be allowed a blanket to keep him warm. Rather than answering the policeman immediately, the superintendent defers to the psychiatrist, who nonchalantly nods his approval while lighting a cigarette. Although Hitchcock may have purposefully undermined the psychiatrist's formulation in the film's subtext (see chapters 3 and 7), his Dr. Richmond is quite consistent with other cinematic portrayals during the years we have called the Golden Age of psychiatry in the cinema.

Of course the dominant image of the psychiatrist that appears in *Dressed to Kill* is the psychotic Dr. Elliott (Caine). But as in *Psycho* a psychiatrist also appears in the police station at the end of *Dressed to Kill* to explain the mind of the murderer. Here, however, the resemblance ends. In *Psycho,* Hitchcock had Simon Oakland standing before a seated group of spectators who look up at him and hang on his every word. In *Dressed to Kill* the psychiatrist, Dr. Levy (David Margulies), is seated during his speech; his gestures are a little effete; and he speaks without conviction. Furthermore, his explanation of Elliott's behavior is only a subsidiary factor in the solution of the crime. The streetwise police detective (Dennis Franz) is the focal figure in the scene, giving only minimal attention to Levy and leering at the prostitute (Nancy Allen) during the psychiatrist's gratuitously graphic explanation: "Elliott's penis became erect and Bobbie took control, trying to kill anyone that made Elliott masculinely sexual." Both *Psycho* and *Dressed to Kill* present unlikely interpretations of unlikely characters in their psychiatrically informed conclusions, but the more recent film offers the uniquely absurd proposition that the female component of a psychotic multiple personality was being favorably considered for transsexual surgery while the male side of the character was able to function competently as a psychiatrist.

In fairness to Brian De Palma, we must point out that he knows how to make the most of familiar film genres, both as a reverent student and as an irreverent satirist. He has learned from his idol Hitchcock—with whom he has carried on a kind of dialogue in *Hi! Mom, Sisters, Obsession, Blow Out,* and *Body Double,* as well as *Dressed to Kill*—that mock seriousness is often the most effective means of telling a far-fetched tale. De Palma's often perverse sense of humor can best be appreciated by the more devoted film buffs who can recognize how he toys with famous and not-so-famous conventions. This explains on the one hand why his films have seldom found a large audience and on the other why his *Phantom of the Paradise* and *Carrie* have cult followings.

De Palma's handling of psychiatrists, however, is entirely consistent with the mainstream of popular American films, and it may even be remembered as a culminating film after two decades of reaction against psychiatrists. The oracular character played by Simon Oakland in Hitchcock's 1960 *Psycho* fits as perfectly into the Golden Age as Michael Caine's Robert Elliott into the years of negative characterizations of psychiatrists: completely different images emerge from two quite similar films. Hitchcock may have subverted the psychiatrist's formulations on a subtextual level, and De Palma probably did not care how seriously his audience took the psychiatric elements in *Dressed to Kill*. But the images of psychiatry in the works of the two directors powerfully date these two films to specific moments in cinema history.

Another comparison between a Golden Age film and one from the more recent period demonstrates how the trend against psychiatry can transform the work of a single writer-director team. Frank and Eleanor Perry created the supremely sympathetic and competent Dr. Swinford (Howard da Silva) in *David and Lisa* (1962), one of the most prominent films of the Golden Age. A mere eight years later, however, they made *Diary of a Mad Housewife* (1970), in which a psychiatrist is one of several extremely unpleasant male figures inflicted upon the long-suffering heroine. Based on a novel by Sue Kaufman, *Diary of a Mad Housewife* chronicles several days in the life of Tina Balzer (Carrie Snodgress), a Manhattan housewife whose egotistical, domineering husband (Richard Benjamin) has as little to offer as her violent, mean-spirited lover (Frank Langella). In addition, her children emulate all the worst aspects of their father, and she finds absolutely no compassionate souls in the domain to which she has been confined. Nevertheless, her psychiatrist, whose dour visage usually appears upside down in the frame (as she might see him from the couch but also as the film asks us to understand his upside-down values), regularly tells her that she ought to be able to fulfill herself as a wife and mother. (Tina's psychiatrist appears in the version of the film shown on television, not in the theatrical print. The psychiatrist scenes and other footage were cut from the film just prior to its release and then added to the television version to fill up time left by the excision of several minutes of nudity and sex.) Her psychiatrist even discourages her from expressing her creative impulses through painting, urging her instead to engage in more conventionally healthful activities such as jogging and scrubbing floors. After her lover throws her bodily out of his apartment, Tina returns to her husband only to discover that he is about to lose his job, that he has squandered all their savings on a failed investment in a French vineyard, and that he is having an affair. At the film's memorable conclusion, Tina presents her story to a collection of misfits at a group therapy session and endures a chorus of loudly unsympathetic responses as the final credits roll.

After breaking ground with a "personal" film like *David and Lisa,* the Perrys may have realized that the age of earnest realism and reconciliation was over, and that a more satiric, socially critical vision was appropriate for the late 1960s. It is difficult to determine if Frank and Eleanor Perry had a change of heart about psychiatry between the time of *David and Lisa* (1962) and *Diary of a Mad Housewife* (1970) or if they merely accommodated the new wave in serious commercial filmmaking with the required character types. According to Roy Huss (1986, 111), Eleanor Perry earned a degree in psychiatric social work before becoming a writer. Regardless of motives, however, comparison of the two films suggests that the motion picture industry's reaction against psychiatry was so overwhelming that even filmmakers who once created the most sympathetic of all movie psychiatrists were caught up in it.

The psychiatrist in *Diary of a Mad Housewife* is a feminist cartoon with roots in the "you need a man to dominate you" psychiatrist of *Lady in the Dark,* but films of more recent vintage do not always present the psychiatrist-as-society's-agent only in terms of the oppression of women. In 1971, just one year after the release of *Diary of a Mad Housewife,* Lawrence Turman's *The Marriage of a Young Stockbroker* appeared, providing an interesting comparison with the Perrys' film and illustrating the extent to which psychiatry was under assault from both sexual camps simultaneously. Both films center around troubled marriages; both adopt sixties myths about the corrupt values of the affluent professional class; in both the husband is played by Richard Benjamin; and both films suggest that a psychiatrist intervenes to change the behavior of the character who is least in need of help. Yet, whereas in the feminist *Diary of a Mad Housewife* the female spouse (Carrie Snodgress) is asked by a male psychiatrist to sacrifice her individuality, in *Marriage of a Young Stockbroker* the husband (Benjamin) is asked by a female psychiatrist (Patricia Barry) to do the same thing. In the earlier film, Benjamin plays Tina's husband as a domineering monster who blithely makes wildly unreasonable demands of his wife. In *Marriage of a Young Stockbroker* Benjamin plays Bill, a perfectly likeable young professional who takes pleasure in looking at nude or seminude women either in pornographic movies or on beaches. Falling back on the truisms of the sexual revolution, *The Marriage of a Young Stockbroker* presents these activities as the natural and completely understandable result of Bill's boring job and his difficulty in communicating with his pretty wife Lisa (Joanna Shimkus). The villain of the piece is the wife's sister, Nan (Elizabeth Ashley), who encourages

Lisa to leave Bill because of his voyeurism but who is also quite willing and even eager for him to gaze at her own body.

The antifeminist ideology of *Marriage of a Young Stockbroker* argues that women are prepared to give up normal sexuality for the sake of controlling men, and Nan's husband, Chester (Adam West), is a thoroughly controlled male. We learn that Chester has been brainwashed by the psychiatrist, Dr. Sadler (Barry), a friend of Nan (Ashley) whose psychobabble includes words like "insight" and "productive" but who clearly seeks to turn healthy, normal men into docile breadwinners for their domineering wives. Dr. Sadler sets to work on Bill as well, but he is immediately able to see through her manipulative and acquisitive motives: after learning that she charges fifty dollars per half hour for her time, he pays her in cash and sends her away after ten minutes. The film ends when Bill quits his stifling job as a stockbroker and seduces Lisa in the women's locker room of a country club. As they are about to drive away together in renewed connubial bliss, Nan tries to stop them by demanding that Chester "do something." Chester, however, has had enough, and he pushes his wife to the ground. Now both men have overcome the efforts of the emasculating female therapist.

Another pair of filmmakers whose portrayal of psychiatry and its practitioners appears to have changed with the times is the producer/director team of Alan J. Pakula and Robert Mulligan. In 1957 they made one of the first Golden Age films, *Fear Strikes Out*. In 1966, however, they made *Inside Daisy Clover*, the story of a 1930s child star (Natalie Wood) reminiscent of Judy Garland who is crassly manipulated by a studio mogul (Christopher Plummer). When Daisy breaks down from the strain of being a star, a pipe-smoking psychiatrist is brought in to achieve one of two goals that Plummer offers him: either she is certifiable, and the studio can collect insurance money; or she is sane, and the doctor must give her a quick fix so that she can get back to work. The psychiatrist demurs slightly, but he is definitely prepared to do whatever work the money men request.

The calmly reassuring image of ECT appearing in Pakula and Mulligan's *Fear Strikes Out* provides the basis for still another contrast between Golden Age films and those that followed. As soon as the Golden Age began to wane, mental institutions were made out to be something akin to torture chambers in both Samuel Fuller's *Shock Corridor* (1963) and Denis Sanders's *Shock Treatment* (1964). The notion that ECT is used as punishment subsequently occurs most memorably in *One Flew over the Cuckoo's Nest* (1975) but also in Michael Winner's *Death Wish II* (1982). In this grim glorification of vigilante justice, Charles Bronson masquerades as a psychologist in order to kill the man who raped and murdered his daughter. Although the film portrays the villain as simply vicious rather than "insane," he escapes prosecution because a judge consigns him to a mental hospital. When Bronson gains entry to the killer's quarters, an orderly tells him that he will meet with the patient in a room full of unused electronic equipment. The orderly says that "you guys," meaning the new breed of talking therapists to which he assumes Bronson belongs, no longer use shock treatment. "Now it's all done with kindness," he says. Appropriately, Bronson dispatches the killer by jolting him with electricity after the villain's fist misses Bronson's jaw and catches in the inner workings of the ECT apparatus.

PSYCHIATRY IN THE SIXTIES: POLITICS AND THE HERO

The drastic changes in the representation of psychiatry after the Golden Age are undoubtedly related to the cultural revolutions of the 1960s. The swiftness of the changes may not, however, reflect correspondingly dramatic changes in American attitudes toward mental health professionals. Winick (1963) has reported data from a number of studies conducted in about 1960, in the middle of what we have called the Golden Age of psychiatry in the movies. One study found that only 1 percent of the subjects polled expressed active support for the psychiatric profession but that only 7 percent expressed active opposition. Another study found that although psychiatrists themselves were regarded quite favorably, their techniques were held in very low esteem.

This "softness" in American attitudes apparently provided a wide range of tolerance for the wildly inconsistent images that characterized movie psychiatrists in the early as opposed to late 1960s. Popular films of the decade continued to activate myths of freedom and the primacy of the self, somewhat revised from the patterns of classic Hollywood films but still grounded in fundamental American mythology. Just as American movies had always exploited psychiatry, American psychiatry had in some ways exploited these movie myths, largely by presenting itself as a means of removing obstacles to happiness. The French psychiatrist Henri Ellenberger (1955) visited the United States in 1952 and subsequently wrote, "In Europe, people go to the psychiatrist because of a symptom, in America because of a problem." Burnham (1978) has demonstrated how psychiatry in America allowed itself to become associated with an individual's pursuit of happiness through its claims of problem-solving, especially after the therapeutic successes with veterans of World War II. Consequently, psychiatry was especially vulnerable in the sixties when disillusionment accompanied the profound questioning of postwar ideas of happiness.

Although few Americans appear to have had strong feelings about psychiatrists during this period, the movies pounced upon the profession's new vulnerability.

Burnham has also stressed the ease with which the profession's focus on solving "personal problems" was appropriated by the "managers of the increasingly bureaucratic American society" as "a tactic to head off, indeed, deny, the existence of social discontent" (1978, 65). Even the teachings of Erik Erikson, one of the great post-Freudians and hardly a conservative, were nevertheless "easily corrupted into the conservative assumption that any changes that needed to be made were on a one-by-one, individual basis—as in psychoanalytic psychotherapy—and in that individual, not in the culture" (1978, 65). In the climate of 1960s social protest, psychiatry could easily be tied to the conformity and repressiveness of the 1950s, and psychiatrists were regularly portrayed as part of the establishment forces perpetuating the false values of old America. An excellent example of how films used psychiatry for this purpose is Jack O'Connell's *Revolution* (1968), a crude documentary that extolled the virtues of the hippies and invited their sympathizers in the audience to ridicule pious and often hyperbolic warnings by doctors, police, and psychiatrists about the physical and mental dangers of hippie culture. In a more familiar genre film, John Guillermin's *House of Cards* (1969), Inger Stevens refers to her psychiatrist as "the man who polices my psyche."

The social problem film, which had afforded psychiatry the most amenable surroundings in the early 1960s, was as good as dead by 1965. Many of the most successful films of the 1960s adopted a more overtly irreverent and satiric vision of America and its values, especially in comparison to the dominant genres of film comedy in the late fifties. Compare, for example, *Pillow Talk* (1959) with *The Graduate* (1967). Compare also the Swiftian view of world leaders and the military in Stanley Kubrick's breakthrough masterpiece, *Dr. Strangelove, or How I Learned to Stop Worrying and Love the Bomb* (1964), with Sidney Lumet's mirthless and didactic *Fail-Safe,* which addressed the same questions of nuclear defense in the same year as *Dr. Strangelove. Fail-Safe* must now be regarded as one of the final films of the 1950s while *Dr. Strangelove* is one of the first in a long series of 1960s films that took a satirical and apocalyptic view of the world and its institutions (Cagin and Dray 1984). The gravity and solemnity with which Hollywood had handled psychiatrists in the Golden Age made them easy targets for the youth-oriented filmmakers of the sixties, who often strove to shake up bourgeois audiences as much as to confront what they considered to be the tired old conventions of earlier movies.

As we begin now a year-by-year survey of Hollywood's reaction against psychiatry just after the Golden Age, we should point out that, as in every decade, psychiatrists were still introduced for the sake of plot mechanics but that after 1964 they were knocked off their pedestals even when their functions were most trivial. A classic example of the psychiatrist-as-plot-machine from 1964 is J. Lee Thompson's *What a Way to Go!* In this vehicle for Shirley MacLaine, a psychiatrist (Robert Cummings), whose office includes a hydraulic couch controlled by a button on his desk, listens to the story of the heroine's several marriages so that the film can cut to flashbacks. Each of MacLaine's husbands was hugely successful at earning money but quite unsuccessful at remaining alive. When MacLaine tells Cummings early in the film that she wants to give her $200 million inheritance to the IRS in the form of a check, he naturally assumes that it is all part of her fantasy and settles back to hear her story. The film ends with the psychiatrist's secretary entering to announce that MacLaine's check is genuine. Cummings then falls to the floor in a faint. A Golden Age psychiatrist might have done a quick double take at this information, but even if he functioned as a mere plot expediter, he would not have lost consciousness. *What a Way to Go!* has little of the emerging sixties ambience, but its irreverence toward psychiatry is portentous.

The year 1964 was also the release date for *Shock Treatment,* in which Lauren Bacall plays another evil female psychiatrist. She runs an institution as a front for illegal financial gain, but at the conclusion she herself becomes psychotic. The same year marked the appearance of a low-budget exploitation film, William Castle's *Strait Jacket.* This film suggests that Joan Crawford has been cured after twenty years of confinement in an institution. Yet when her ineffectual psychiatrist comes out to check up on her, he is decapitated by an axmurderer. *Sex and the Single Girl* presents a lecherous male psychiatrist (Mel Ferrer) as well as an easily manipulated female therapist (Natalie Wood), and in *Lilith,* Warren Beatty plays a therapist trainee who falls in love with, and is eventually driven mad by, a schizophrenic patient (Jean Seberg).

By 1965, the reaction is complete. Psychiatrists are thoroughly devalued in at least four films from that one year: Peter Sellers plays a libidinous Viennese quack named Dr. Fritz Fassbender in *What's New, Pussycat?* (plate 24); "Mrs. Koogleman" (Hermione Gingold) in *Harvey Middleman, Fireman* is a female shrink too involved with her own extramarital affairs to be of any help to the eponymous hero; an amnesiac Gregory Peck, this time with no Ingrid Bergman to save him, has to make do with a pompous and thoroughly unhelpful psychiatrist (Robert H. Harris) in *Mirage;* and the familiar female psychiatrist who is "cured" by a male patient reappears as Leslie Caron in *A Very Special Favor.* Negative stereotypes of psychiatrists adorned even more American screens in 1966. That year introduced the "Dr. Bluebeard" (Rock Hudson) of *Blindfold;*

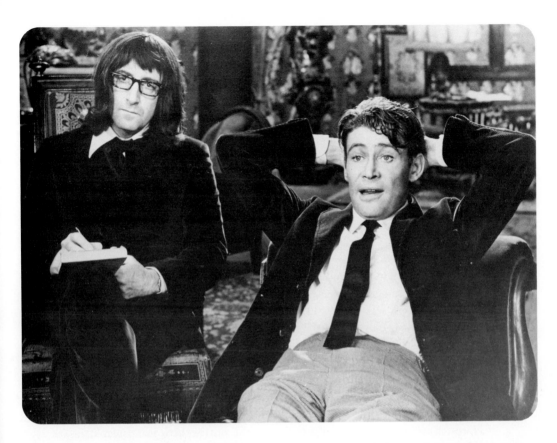

PLATE 24. Peter O'Toole details his sex life for Dr. Fritz Fassbender (Peter Sellers) in *What's New, Pussycat?* (1965). United Artists/Famous Artists. The Museum of Modern Art/Film Stills Archive.

the beautiful but unnecessary psychiatrist played by Janet Leigh in *Three on a Couch;* an easily seduced prison psychologist in *Dead Heat on a Merry-Go-Round;* Natalie Wood's mentally unbalanced analyst (Dick Shawn) in *Penelope;* a female therapist (Sarah Marshall) who is driven to hysterics by Roddy McDowall's refusal to find her Rorschach blots "dirty" in *Lord Love a Duck;* a dispassionate analyst (Arthur Hill) who so neglects his wife (Jean Seberg) that she becomes involved in a sordid love affair in *Moment to Moment;* the willing agent of a corrupt studio boss in *Inside Daisy Clover;* and even the LSD-dispensing director of a sanitarium in a bizarre film called *Movie Star, American Style or LSD, I Hate You.* In Sidney Lumet's *The Group,* a rare distinction is made between medical psychiatry and psychoanalysis, reserving special scorn for the latter. *The Group* suggests that the inadequacies of Shirley Knight's married lover (Hal Holbrook) are a function of his dependence on his analyst. Although the film presents Knight as the solution to Holbrook's problems, he eventually drifts away, offering specious reasons supplied by his psychoanalyst. Knight finds happiness, however, when she falls in love with a hospital psychiatrist (James Broderick), outspokenly anti-Freud and anti-couch, who expresses the desire to give up his practice and devote all his efforts to "research."

The year 1966 was also the release date for Irvin Kershner's *A Fine Madness,* one of the first films that clearly casts the institution of psychiatry against the prototypical hero for the 1960s and 1970s: an eccentric but vital loner, often doomed, who rejects the obsolete values of the Establishment even when he has not thought about them very much. Ray argues that films of the 1960s and 1970s appealed to a politically bifurcated audience, generating "left and right cycles" (1985, 296–325): the mythology of classical Hollywood never died, but the 1960s marked the end of a thematic paradigm that never forced the audience to choose between an outlaw hero and an official hero. The strength of this paradigm was waning in the 1950s: the ending of *The Caine Mutiny* is incoherent because the classical formula had been strained to justify the actions of a neurotic official hero. Ray cites Howard Hawks's *Red River* (1948) as an example of a parallel phenomenon: the film's ending struggles unsuccessfully to provide the reconciliation between the official hero (Montgomery Clift) and an obviously disturbed outlaw hero (John Wayne). In the 1960s and 1970s, the official hero became the exclusive property of films of the right cycle (*Dirty Harry, Walking Tall, Death Wish*), while the outlaw hero was isolated in the left cycle (*Easy Rider, Cool Hand Luke, Little Big Man*). The choice between which hero the audience should favor was made even before the film began. In effect, Humphrey Bogart's Rick no longer played against Paul Henreid's Victor Laszlo. Although many of these films seemed radical at the time, they were still firmly rooted in American myths. Ray points out that Bobby Dupea (Jack Nicholson), the outlaw antihero of *Five Easy Pieces* (1970), is based on American heroes such as Huck Finn and Holden Caulfield: surrounded by phonies, he lights out for the territory at the end (1985, 297). Furthermore, Nicholson's character recalls the "roughneck classical musician" heroes of *Golden Boy* (1939) and *Humoresque* (1946).

Since the right and left films had abandoned the reconciliatory pattern, they no longer needed psychiatric healers. Rather they created straw men to reinforce the validity of the hero's cause. In a right-cycle film such as *Death Wish II,* psychiatry represents a feeble, unmanly attempt to solve problems that are more effectively addressed by vigilante violence. In one scene, the ineffectual psychologist who gives directions to Bronson cannot immediately distinguish between his left and his right. The filmmakers had no such difficulty. In left films such as *One Flew over the Cuckoo's Nest,* the power of psychiatry was more ominous than in films made for right-wing audiences. In general, the heroes of the right cycle always seemed to survive the climactic violence at the end of the film, while in left films the heroes were no match for the destructive power of the Establishment and were usually destroyed in an apocalyptic ending. This was the case in *Cool Hand Luke, Easy Rider, Bonnie and Clyde,* and even the glibly fatalistic *Butch Cassidy and the Sundance Kid.* The sixties image of the doomed antihero was tied to perceptions of the Kennedy assassination and the Vietnam War, but the character type had earlier appeared in one of the most influential films for American filmmakers of the 1960s, Jean-Luc Godard's *Breathless* (1961).

A *Fine Madness,* an obscure film of the left cycle, finds its outlaw hero in Samson Shillitoe (Sean Connery), a brawling, womanizing New York poet who is eventually institutionalized and put at the mercy of a team of psychiatrists. The most stereotypical of the group is Dr. Menken (Clive Revill), who speaks in a thick accent about his plan to appropriate Connery for his behavioristic and dehumanizing experiments in lobotomy. A female psychiatrist, Vera Kropotkin (Colleen Dewhurst), opposes Revill's plans because, predictably, she has succumbed to the hero's sexual appeal. Although the third participant, the strict Freudian Dr. Vorbeck (Werner Peters), is broadly caricatured, he opposes Dr. Menken's lobotomy proposal on largely humanitarian grounds. The final decision must be made by the fourth psychiatrist, the no-nonsense director of the clinic, Dr. West (Patrick O'Neal), who sees through Menken's crackpot schemes. Yet when he learns that Shillitoe (Connery) has been carrying on an affair with his wife (Jean Seberg), Dr. West grimly votes to allow the lobotomy to take place. The operation turns out to be a failure, at least for the psychiatrists, and Shillitoe emerges from the experience as feisty as ever. Future victims of psychiatric intervention in left-cycle films would prove less resilient.

A *Fine Madness* has much in common with *One Flew over the Cuckoo's Nest* (1975). Both are adapted from novels written in the early 1960s: Elliot Baker published *A Fine Madness* in 1964, and Ken Kesey's *One Flew over the Cuckoo's Nest* appeared in 1962. As Jeffrey Berman (1985) has demonstrated in his thorough and psychoanalytically sophisticated study of psychiatry's image in literature, these novels were part of a literary attack upon psychoanalysis that goes back at least to 1892 with Charlotte Perkin Gilman's "The Yellow Wallpaper." Like Gilman's work, Virginia Woolf's *Mrs. Dalloway* (1925) also presents an unsympathetic psychiatrist, but negative portrayals of psychiatry became most common in the 1950s with the appearance of T. S. Eliot's *The Cocktail*

Party (1950), Joseph Heller's *Catch-22* (1955), Saul Bellow's *Seize the Day* (1956), Vladimir Nabokov's *Pnin* (1957), John Barth's *End of the Road* (1958), and Iris Murdoch's *A Severed Head* (1961). All of these books present the same arguments informing the attacks on psychiatry in films after 1964: doctors of the mind are repressive, often self-deceiving egomaniacs. These novels predate the antipsychiatry movement of the 1960s, and most interestingly, coexisted with many of the most sympathetic treatments of psychiatrists in the movies. The messages in these novels, however, were readily available when American films sought a new vision of psychiatry in the 1960s.

Like their literary sources, *A Fine Madness* and *One Flew over the Cuckoo's Nest* share the more specific view of psychiatry as an emasculating activity that promotes social harmony at any cost, and both suggest that psychiatrists are quite willing to act out their own hang-ups to the detriment of their unsuspecting patients. *A Fine Madness* delivered this message with none of the sentimental panache of *One Flew over the Cuckoo's Nest* and was consequently much less of a critical and commercial success. Nevertheless, *A Fine Madness* paved the way for numerous films, including *Cuckoo's Nest,* that presented psychiatry as the nemesis of those sensitive and usually victimized loners who so often emerge as the protagonists of left-cycle films. We have already mentioned *Diary of a Mad Housewife* and *The Marriage of a Young Stockbroker* as films that present psychiatrists as the natural agents of a society that seeks to dehumanize its most sensitive citizens whenever they attempt to break out of the stifling lives that have been inflicted upon them. The mental health professions fill this victimizing role even in Larry Peerce's *The Bell Jar* (1979), in which the female psychiatrist played by Anne Jackson is usually caring and compassionate. But this screen adaptation of Sylvia Plath's autobiographical novel presents the soothing words of the psychiatrist as a poor anodyne for the malevolent and overpowering forces in society that drive the feminist heroine (Marilyn Hassett) to psychosis. The film makes the protagonist into still another lone antihero as it catalogs all the characters—mother, employer, fiancé, lover, friends—who would force her to become anything but her own woman. The psychiatrist must be devalued because she would prepare the heroine to accept a world that the film baldly characterizes as crazier than anyone in an institution. This conceit was taken to its most absurd extreme by "underground" director Robert Downey in his 1967 film *Chafed Elbows.* Downey's hero ignores the stern advice of his psychiatrist and fulfills his desire to marry his mother, an event which the film portrays as a joyous and fortuitous occasion for all. *Titicut Follies* and *Marat/Sade* were also released in 1967, as was Theodore J. Flicker's *The President's Analyst,* which actually turns a psychiatrist into the lone antihero.

As the credits for *The President's Analyst* roll, we see Dr. Sidney Shafer (James Coburn) on the couch, talking presumably to his training analyst (Will Geer, made up to look like Mark Twain). We then see Dr. Shafer in the analyst's chair while a number of different patients appear on the couch, including an attractive woman with whom he exchanges meaningful glances. Meanwhile, Don Masters (Godfrey Cambridge), wearing a curly wig and a "Dizzy Gillespie for President" sweatshirt, very professionally assassinates a suspicious man who has just accepted information from another suspicious man. The film then cuts to Dr. Shafer sitting on the floor of his office practicing on a large oriental gong. When his next patient enters, it is Masters (Cambridge), now dressed in a business suit. Within a few minutes, Masters has confessed to being a secret agent for a CIA-like organization as well as a killer. Assuming that the spy is there for help, Shafer begins philosophizing about hostility, morality, society, and a paper he might write on the subject. But Masters interrupts him with the information that he has been attending the analytic sessions only because his agency is running a security check on him. Now that the check is complete, Masters invites him to proceed to a more private place since Shafer's office might be bugged. When the doctor responds indignantly, "The sanctity of a psychiatrist's office is like a confessional," Masters replies, "Oh, really. I put this one here myself," and he picks a bugging device off the diploma on the psychiatrist's wall.

Shafer is eventually told that he has been selected to be the analyst for the president of the United States, because, as we are told in this pre-Watergate film, the chief executive is not neurotic, just overworked and overtired. He needs to talk with someone who "does not want something from him." Honored, Shafer takes the job and is at first fascinated with his proximity to so august a presence. Yet Dr. Shafer soon discovers that he has become a major security risk, that he is not allowed any private life, and that he is constantly being followed by men in dark glasses. Unable to bear the strain, the hero "drops out," even joining a group of hippies for a brief journey through American subculture. The film's level of irreverent sixties satire rises substantially at this point, soon degenerating into an exploration of political paranoia in which agents for numerous countries attempt to kidnap the psychiatrist. The film concludes with an escapist happy ending for the principals but also with the revelation that the *telephone company* and not the various intelligence agencies of American and foreign governments is the most powerful force in the world.

The President's Analyst has more in common with the light-weight psychedelic satire of television's "Laugh-In" than it does with *The Graduate* (the two films and the television program all appeared in 1967), but it does offer an interesting synthesis of psychiatric myths since the 1930s. Like Ralph Bellamy in *Blind Alley* (1939)—our touchstone for the American cinema's idealized image of the "avant-garde" psychiatrist—Dr. Shafer appreciates exotic cultures from the East, even having joined a presumably ancient cult of the gong sometime before he takes up with hippies. The film also addresses myths of oracularity by having the psychiatrist early on engage in self-aggrandizing illusions of omniscience only to discover later that he is being controlled by a government agent. Analysands commonly fantasize that they control and manipulate their therapists rather than the other way around: Katherine Hepburn realizes this fantasy in 1938 when she outsmarts Fritz Feld in *Bringing up Baby.* The situation becomes much more common in the 1960s, specifically in *The President's Analyst* as well as in another James Coburn vehicle, *Dead Heat on a Merry-Go-Round* (1966), in which the hero makes love to a prison psychologist (Marian Moses) only in order to win a quick parole. *The President's Analyst* is perhaps the only film in which the myth of the manipulable psychiatrist coexists with an attempt to cast the same psychiatrist as a lone antihero.

Of course, not all films with psychiatrists from the 1960s were characterized by irreverence and satire. Richard Fleischer's *The Boston Strangler* (1968), for instance, took the allegedly true story of Albert De Salvo quite seriously even though the film indulged in some graphic violence that was very much of the sixties. The film probably belongs more to the right cycle, but *The Boston Strangler* can be considered radical for being the first commercial film to use the potential of CinemaScope for split-screen editing, offering the audience multiple views of an action on the same wide canvas. Dr. Nagy (Austin Willis), the faceless psychiatrist in this docudrama, functions somewhat like Simon Oakland in *Psycho,* a film Director Fleischer surely had in mind when he made *The Boston Strangler.* Dr. Nagy often steps forth to explain the multiple personality of Albert De Salvo (Tony Curtis), a real-life character who was charged with but never tried for the strangulation deaths of eight women in Boston during the early 1960s. As in *Psycho,* the killer has a "normal" self that has no knowledge of the murderous self. De Salvo's normal personality even lives a quiet life with his wife and children. The film reveals its right-cycle orientation when Dr. Nagy becomes involved in a professional argument with police officer Bottomley (Henry Fonda), who has been put in charge of a special task force to apprehend the strangler. The psychiatrist is convinced that De Salvo will lapse into permanent catatonia if his normal side is ever forced to confront his murderous side. Bottomley (Fonda) realizes that he will have to bring about such a confrontation if he is to get a confession but that any confession will be useless if the strangler becomes legally insane. Eventually, the policeman decides that "cracking" De Salvo may be just as effective as a conviction. Over the objections of Dr. Nagy, Bottomley proceeds with an interrogation of the strangler that brings him to the brink of integrating the two sides of his personality. The psychiatrist tries to put De Salvo under sedation when he sees that the prisoner is about to break down. Bottomley, however, stops him.

PSYCHIATRIST: You're looking at a sick animal.
POLICEMAN: So were the women he strangled. I want him now!

In the last moments of the film, De Salvo is clearly on the verge of a complete breakdown. The final credits tell us that De Salvo has never been tried and that he is still institutionalized. We then read the following: "This film has ended, but the responsibility of society for the early recognition and treatment of the violent among us has yet to begin." The earnestness is reminiscent of the Golden Age, but the sentiment is a little different. What is to be the "treatment" for violent people such as De Salvo if the prognosis is permanent catatonia? Unlike *Psycho,* in which psychiatry was superior to police work, *The Boston Strangler* clearly endorses the policeman's point of view over the psychiatrist's. Not only does Bottomley win the arguments with the psychiatrist, but Austin Willis (Dr. Nagy) cannot compete with Henry Fonda's star presence. As is frequently the case in Hollywood films, the casting director is as responsible as anyone for the ideology of the film.

THE ARTIST/ANALYSAND COMES OF AGE: WOODY ALLEN AND PAUL MAZURSKY

Our year-by-year survey could be continued into the mid-1970s with little change in the negative images of psychiatry. Nevertheless, we will abandon our chronological approach at this point and consider two directors, Woody Allen and Paul Mazursky, who deserve special attention as we move from the 1960s to the 1970s. In his own films, Woody Allen has consistently played the disenchanted analysand, a phenomenon increasingly common during this period as more and more people sought respite from the complexities of their lives on the analyst's couch. For Allen, as well as for many of his college-educated and affluent admirers, psychoanalysis has not fulfilled its old promise of bringing happiness through the elimination of "personal problems" even though the narcissistic indulgence it provides makes it hopelessly addicting. More specifically, for Manhattanites like Allen, psychiatry is another troublesome fact of life, comparable to brown tap water or pseudointellectuals who pontificate in movie waiting lines.

In *Annie Hall* (1977), Alvy Singer (Allen) delivers several one-liners about psychiatry that have been widely quoted. In the context of the critical and commercial success of *Annie Hall,* they represent the culmination of a tradition of psychoanalytic humor that goes back at least to the couch-and-notepad cartoons that first appeared in popular magazines in the 1940s (Plank 1956). Alvy/Allen says that he has been in analysis for fifteen years, but that if he has not made progress after one more year, he will go to Lourdes. Later, when Annie's family inquires about his prolonged analysis, he says, "I'm making excellent progress. Pretty soon, when I lie down on his couch, I won't have to wear the lobster bib." Alvy also delivers the following speech during a standup monologue before a college audience: "I was suicidal, as a matter of fact, and would have killed myself, but I was in analysis with a strict Freudian, and if you kill yourself, they make you pay for the sessions you miss."

Yet, Woody Allen has brought an irony to his characterization of psychiatry that sets his films apart from the vast majority of American movies with their stereotypical psychiatrists perfunctorily fitted to generic formulas. For example, in *Stardust Memories* (1980), the filmmaker hero played by Allen is showing clips at a retrospective of his films. In a fantasy sketch from one film, "Sidney Finkelstein's hostility" is portrayed as a tall hirsute monster in the process of destroying everyone against whom Sidney bears a grudge. One of the characters who attempts to stop the beast is a man in a dark raincoat (Victor Truro) who approaches the monster and, holding up a pipe, calls out sheepishly, "Please, uh, we don't want to hurt you. We . . . we want to reason with you. I'm a psychoanalyst. This is my pipe." Allen is of course poking fun at psychiatry, but he is also ridiculing the B-movie idea that scientists are rationalist fools who approach violent beasts with talk instead of force. Moreover, Allen is sending up the stale Hollywood convention of the pipe as icon of the psychiatrist's pensive intellectualism, a cliché that goes back at least as far as *Blind Alley* (1939).

In *Annie Hall* Allen uses split-screen technique to show Annie (Diane Keaton) and Alvy (Allen) simultaneously discussing their troubled sex life with their respective psychiatrists. Each analyst asks how often Annie and Alvy have sex. Alvy says, "Hardly ever, maybe three times a week." Annie says, "Constantly, I'd say three times a week." Here Woody Allen is using psychiatry as the traditional plot device for establishing character, but the joke can be understood in several other contexts, including Alvy's Pygmalion-like attempts to transform Annie, even by paying for her analysis. Naturally, she will feel guilty if she leaves him, but any progress in her analysis would almost necessarily make her less dependent upon him and thus more likely to leave him. Psychiatry then becomes one of several forces making their relationship impossible, a reality that Alvy acknowledges in the joke that closes the film: a man tells a psychiatrist that his brother thinks that he is a chicken, but when asked why he does not have his brother committed, the man says, "I would, but I need the eggs." Alvy uses the joke as a focus for his feelings about relationships: they are painful and perhaps not worth the trouble, but he needs the eggs. Much the same can be said for his feelings about his analyst. Like the split-screen presentation of parallel analytic sessions, this juxtaposition of Borscht Belt humor with the troubling complexities of romantic love is one of several "modernist" devices Allen uses in *Annie Hall*, both to comment upon earlier romantic comedies and to separate his film from this tradition (Schatz 1982). Although the psychiatrists in Allen's films often appear ineffectual or pompous, his purpose is not simply to condemn them or to exploit them for conventional generic purposes. If anything, Allen is more interested in poking fun at their *patients*. Allen also uses psychiatry, along with a wide range of cinematic techniques, to explore the ambivalences in human relationships.

Since his 1977 breakthrough with *Annie Hall*, Allen has continued to find new ways of integrating his eccentric humor, as well as his fascination with diverse traditions of filmmaking, with affecting observations about complex relationships. In *Hannah and Her Sisters* (1986) he has created the most artistically successful synthesis yet of his many obsessions, and he appears to have made his most commercially viable film since *Annie Hall*. Once again, Allen has appropriated psychiatry as an important element in the lives of the witty, beautiful, and delicately flawed characters who interact in *Hannah and Her Sisters*. Playing Mickey Sachs—Hannah's ex-husband and an almost peripheral character—Allen has an introspective monologue just after he discovers that he does not have the fatal brain tumor he thought was about to end his life. Reflecting on the inadequacy of philosophers such as Socrates or Nietzsche to make sense of life's absurdities, Allen's character then expresses his disillusionment with Freud: "I was in analysis for years. Nothing happened. My analyst got so frustrated, the poor guy, that he put in a salad bar." As usual, this is not the only time that the issue of psychiatry is raised. Later on we see Elliot (Michael Caine), Hannah's husband, talking through his midlife crisis with a psychotherapist. Elliot is unsure whether to leave his well-adjusted and supportive wife (Mia Farrow) for her heart-breakingly beautiful sister, Lee (Barbara Hershey). Although the briefly glimpsed therapist never speaks, Elliot eventually overcomes his infatuation with Lee and by the end appears to have reestablished a strong loving relationship with Hannah. Meanwhile, Mickey Sachs (Allen) has found the reason for living while watching the Marx Brothers in *Duck Soup*. Allen has never been a propagandist for psychiatry, and he is much too subtle a filmmaker to suggest a direct relationship between therapy and "cure." But in *Hannah and Her Sisters,* at least one character appears to have benefited from treatment. We will have more to say about Woody Allen in chapters 8 and 9 of this study.

Paul Mazursky's films also use psychiatry to deal with the inevitability of ambivalence in human relationships, but his work is particularly interesting because he has regularly cast real-life psychiatrists in his films. Donald F. Muhich, for many years a Beverly Hills psychiatrist, has appeared in four of Mazursky's films and has advised the director on virtually every film he has made since 1969. Muhich gives low-key performances as a psychotherapist in both *Bob and Carol and Ted and Alice* (1969) and *Blume in Love* (1973). He also appears briefly in *Willie and Phil* (1980) and *Down and Out in Beverly Hills* (1986). In the most recent (and most broadly satirical) film, Muhich plays a solemnly earnest psychiatrist for a wealthy family's dog, at one point announcing that the pet suffers from "nipple anxiety."

On one level, the character played by Muhich in *Bob and Carol and Ted and Alice* fits into the historical pattern of reaction against the profession that in 1969 was still powerfully active in American films. For example, when Muhich is consulted by Alice (Dyan Cannon), the more traditional of the film's two eponymous women, she is appalled to learn that the analyst encourages his young daughter to refer to the female genitals as "vagina." Alice's befuddlement is handled comically, but so is the studiously detached pose of the psychiatrist: Mazursky's camera presents both Cannon and Muhich in uncomfortably tight close-ups and invites us to laugh at the therapist's habit of idly tugging at his cheek, a mannerism that Muhich himself created in order to achieve "the fine line between realism and satire," on which most of Mazursky's films take place (Muhich, personal communication, 1985). The session nevertheless begins to bring Alice to a better understanding of her situation, but just as she seems to be on the verge of a major insight, the analyst informs her that her time is up. Even though she protests that she needs more time, he steadfastly refuses to continue. The analyst may be acting professionally, but the audience is not asked to applaud his behavior.

In a certain sense, the psychiatrist in *Bob and Carol and Ted and Alice* is equated with the range of alternative therapies such as encounter groups, which are sampled by the "hip" couple played by Robert Culp and Natalie Wood: neither psychoanalysis nor the more contemporary experiences offered by the human potential movement seem to be of any real help to the characters. (The most popular among the alternative therapies of the 1970s was probably est, an institution subjected to devastating parody in both *Semi-Tough* [1977] and *The Big Fix* [1978].) Mazursky's film begins with Bob and Carol (Culp and Wood) visiting "the institute," where participants in a twenty-four hour marathon are invited to wallow in their problems *ad nauseam;* Muhich's arbitrarily terminated session with Alice (Cannon) may be intended as representative of the opposite extreme. On the other hand, the exchange between Alice and the therapist has some relevance to the inner lives of the four protagonists, whose failure to follow their convictions into group sex is never fully explained. The film ends with the two couples strolling out of their Las Vegas hotel room and into the world to the tune of Burt Bachrach's "What the World Needs Now (Is Love, Sweet Love)." It is unclear what kind of love the song is meant to endorse in the long dialogueless conclusion to the film, but it is not likely that the film's huge audience believed that the song referred to that love which, according to psychoanalysis, is inevitably tempered by unconscious hatred and aggression. Yet these forces clearly play a part in the loving relationships cultivated by the couples. Mazursky is one of several directors such as Martin Scorsese, Francis Coppola, and, to a certain extent, Robert Altman who attempted in the 1970s to strike a balance between commercialism and social criticism. Consequently, there is an unstable irony in *Bob and Carol and Ted and Alice* that allows some viewers to identify with the couples' leisure-time explorations of cultural revolutions at the same time that it allows others to condemn their superficiality. Mazursky has not made clear just who is making the highly generalized call for love at the end of the film and how it should be interpreted: the plea for love could come from the film, from the couples, or from the crowds that they walk past, and the audience can accept the plea as genuine or satiric. Similarly, the audience is offered a number of alternatives for evaluating the experience of Alice with the psychiatrist played by Muhich. This kind of complexity has led Schneider to refer to the scene in the psychiatrist's office as "the best and most realistic therapy session ever portrayed on film" (1977, 618).

In Mazursky's *Blume in Love* (1973), Dr. Muhich plays the psychiatrist for both Blume (George Segal) and his wife, Nina (Susan Anspach). Like Bob and Carol and Ted and Alice, Blume and his wife are upwardly mobile adults trying to cope with the new sexual/cultural mores, which they may not be young enough to manage successfully. Nina has caught Blume in the midst of a peccadillo with his secretary and has taken up with a docile drifter named Elmo (Kris Kristofferson) after which Blume drifts into an unsatisfying affair with Arlene (Marsha Mason). Blume, however, is still in love with his wife, and like Proust's Swann in a story with a similar title, he frequently stands outside Nina's quarters and stares into her windows with longing and jealousy. In a session with his psychiatrist (Muhich), Blume speaks of his spells of impotence just after he sees his wife with Elmo. The analyst, wearing an extremely wide and garish tie, inquires innocently—but to the great surprise of Blume—if he has been engaging in "sport-fucking." Although the psychiatrist insists that he is not recommending the activity as a cure for impotence or depression, the next scene shows Blume with a sexually adventurous young woman whom he has met in a bar but who does little to cheer him up. In a subsequent scene, Blume questions the effectiveness of his analytic hours:

> BLUME: Sometimes I think this is a waste of time. That it doesn't really do any good.
> ANALYST: Sometimes it doesn't.
> BLUME: Then why do you do it?
> ANALYST: Sometimes it does. And until we find something better, what else is there to do?

Immediately after this scene, Blume goes home and rapes his wife.

In another crucial scene, *Blume in Love* flashes back to an earlier time when Blume and Nina were still living together and Nina was working for the California Department of Welfare. Coming home from her yoga meditation class, Nina starts to cry but cannot say why she is unhappy.

> BLUME: Maybe you should go back to the shrink.
> NINA: (after a pause for composing herself) A woman came into my office today . . . to talk to me about her son. He's a junkie; she's already on welfare; and she wants more money. Do you know why?
> BLUME: So the son can buy dope.
> NINA: It's getting very depressing there.

Not only does the film imply that an analyst is of little help to Blume and Nina, but in her deflection of Blume's suggestion that she return to therapy, Nina expresses a sixties and early seventies notion that reverses the vulgarized ego psychology of the 1950s identified by Burnham (1978). Rather than locating the cause of problems in the individual and not in society, Nina implies that the real problems are in the culture as a whole and that psychiatry can do little to help. This kind of glib social criticism is typical of most of the films of this era, but like Woody Allen, Mazursky is less inclined to oversimplifications of this sort. As in *Bob and Carol and Ted and Alice,* the irony in *Blume in Love* is difficult to locate precisely. When Nina refuses to return to her psychiatrist by complaining that her job is "depressing," are we being asked to agree that psychiatry can be of no help, or are we to suppose that Nina is unwilling to face her own problems? Similarly, the scene in which Blume forces his estranged wife to have sex can be interpreted in a variety of ways. Rape is not something that a filmmaker as sensitive as Mazursky is likely to endorse, but on the other hand, Nina appears to be sharing Blume's passion during the scene, and the couple *is* reunited by the end of the film. Also, the fact that Blume has committed rape just after a frustrating session with his analyst cannot be blamed entirely on the analyst. Muhich articulates most completely the unpleasant realities that Blume faces, yet it is Blume himself who ultimately must decide how he will respond to the new sexual roles for which he is not prepared. He must decide this, just as he must decide whether to continue courting his wife and whether to continue therapy. Until recently, few American films offered their protagonists such ambiguous choices.

Blume in Love does have a Hollywood happy ending of sorts, although we should point out that the dramatic reunion of Blume and Nina in Venice to strains of Wagner's music could be Blume's fantasy. But if it does not take place in the hero's imagination, the film's conclusion can be understood as the fortuitous result of Blume and Nina's coming to terms with problems that were at least identified in therapy. The analyst's wide tie and his salty language can be regarded as a function of his humanity (and of the film's wry humor) as much as they can be seen as evidence of ineffectuality. Since Mazursky has used a real-life psychiatrist, chances are that his intentions toward psychiatry are at least somewhat honorable, even if he does not return to the myths of the Golden Age. In fact, Mazursky and Woody Allen have expressed an ambivalence toward psychiatry that may nevertheless represent a new and sophisticated appropriation of the profession for gently humorous explorations of complexity in loving relationships. The Golden Age psychiatrist of heroic stature never appears in Mazursky's films, but neither do the grotesque shrinks from the years immediately following the Golden Age. Furthermore, Mazursky rejects the sixties and seventies mystique of the lone antihero. James Monaco's statement is quite relevant here: "Almost alone among his contemporaries, Mazursky takes it for granted that the natural state is marriage, and that single people are anomalies" (Monaco 1979, 380). He is not as likely then to be hostile to psychiatrists when they fulfill their usual cinematic function of reconciling patients to their social roles.

In this sense, Mazursky's *An Unmarried Woman* (1978) is quite similar to his earlier work. The film stars Jill Clayburgh as Erica, the unmarried woman attempting to find herself after her husband Martin (Michael Murphy) announces that he has fallen in love with a woman he has met in Bloomingdales. Like most of Mazursky's characters, Erica and Martin inhabit the world of sophisticated, affluent professionals who are just close enough to the audience (and Mazursky) to win affection and understanding in spite of the satirical treatment to which they are often subjected. Mazursky, who also wrote the script for *An*

Unmarried Woman, had projected a scene in which Erica (Clayburgh) seeks help from a therapist who is a short, fortyish woman with a European accent. However, at the suggestion of Director Claudia Weill (who later used Clayburgh in her 1980 film, *It's My Turn*), Mazursky cast the six-foot-two-inch, sixtyish American psychologist Penelope Russianoff as Erica's therapist. In fact, Russianoff is the real-life author of a book, *Why Do I Think I'm Nothing without a Man?,* which addresses many of the same problems Erica faces in the film. According to Russianoff (personal communication, 1984), Mazursky did several takes of the scene between Erica and her therapist in which Clayburgh read lines that Mazursky had scripted while Russianoff ad-libbed a number of different responses. The take that Mazursky eventually used presents one of the most sympathetic images of psychotherapy in American film since 1963 and clearly anticipates the return of the Golden Age psychiatrist in *Ordinary People,* a film that was released two years after *Unmarried Woman.* Nevertheless, Erica later encounters the therapist at a party, and the film raises the question of the doctor's sexual orientation when she introduces Erica to her female companion. Mazursky had filmed a subsequent scene in the therapist's office in which Erica confronts her about her sexuality. Russianoff, a married heterosexual in real life, explains in the scene that she is bisexual and that Erica must accept the fact that sexual fulfillment can be found in a variety of contexts. Erica is so upset by this revelation, however, that she decides to break off therapy. After an emotional confrontation, patient and therapist embrace. According to Dr. Russianoff (personal communication, 1984), Mazursky says that he cut this scene from the final print because it made the therapist too important a character and deflected the film's focus from Erica.

Of course, the issue of the therapist's lesbianism is still present in *An Unmarried Woman,* especially in Erica's facial expression when the doctor introduces her female friend. For even after excising the discussion of bisexuality, Mazursky has introduced one of his favorite themes into the film: the fact that Erica receives good advice from a practicing homosexual underlines the morally and culturally ambiguous sphere in which she must operate now that she, like Blume, is deprived of the clearly defined role that married life offers. The doctor's unconventional sexuality may also be the same kind of off-beat humanizing touch Mazursky gave to the analyst played by Muhich in *Blume in Love.*

PSYCHIATRY IN THE SEVENTIES: MCMURPHY AND NURSE RATCHED

A real-life psychiatrist also appears in Milos Forman's *One Flew over the Cuckoo's Nest* (1975), but there the similarity between Mazursky's and Forman's films ends. Dr. Dean Brooks appears as Dr. Spivey, the director of the institution to which McMurphy (Jack Nicholson) has been confined, but he seems to be little more than an administrator. The most potent figure in the film—and the one who seems most active in seeking psychiatric solutions to the problem that McMurphy presents—is Nurse Ratched (Louise Fletcher). We have already mentioned how *One Flew over the Cuckoo's Nest* presents psychiatry as the accomplice of a culture that does not hesitate to use electroshock and lobotomy to punish its transgressors. In addition, we have identified the film's protagonist (Nicholson) as another of the era's inspirational but doomed outlaw heroes. At this point, we should also call attention to how the film transforms the treatment of mental illness into a metaphor for emasculation (plate 25). The great majority of the inmates in the institution with McMurphy are not really crazy. They are simply weak. Most have voluntarily committed themselves and are unwilling to face the real world. They are, however, quite content to submit to Nurse Ratched's fantasies of omnipotence. Only when McMurphy arrives in their midst do any of them begin behaving like "real men." He shows them that sitting about like women and discussing their personal feelings is not nearly

PLATE 25. McMurphy (Jack Nicholson) looks for help in his efforts to overcome the regime of Nurse Ratched (Louise Fletcher) in *One Flew over the Cuckoo's Nest* (1975). United Artists. The Museum of Modern Art/Film Stills Archive.

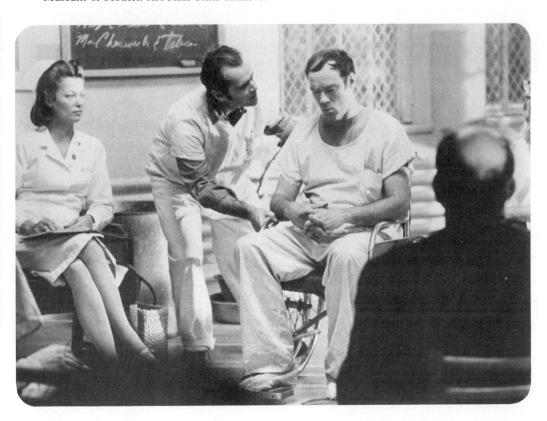

so fulfilling as more masculine and competitive activities such as poker, fishing, and basketball.

The sexual politics of *One Flew over the Cuckoo's Nest* separates women into two groups: emasculating martinets like Nurse Ratched and submissive floozies like McMurphy's girlfriends. The inmates seem to prefer the former to the latter, even allowing themselves to be fed saltpeter tablets to repress their sexual appetites. McMurphy, who would be their sexual liberator, is especially committed to masculinizing Billy Bibbit (Brad Dourif), a stuttering mama's boy who nevertheless develops a special affinity for McMurphy. Because Billy has expressed what the film suggests is a healthy interest in McMurphy's girlfriend, the hero is quite willing to carry out his program of men's liberation by loaning her to Billy for the night. When Nurse Ratched arrives the next morning, she confronts Billy with his transgression, but now that he has partaken of the right kind of woman, Billy can talk back to the nurse, even with a marked reduction in his stuttering. He has not reckoned on all the weapons in Nurse Ratched's arsenal, however, and he loses his confidence when she threatens to report his behavior to his mother. In his panic, Billy takes his own life, and in a play upon the film's sexual themes, McMurphy dives on top of the nurse in an attempt to strangle her.

At the conclusion of *One Flew over the Cuckoo's Nest*, lobotomy is portrayed as psychiatric vengeance against an almost Christlike savior, whose inspirational force is confirmed in Chief Bromden's eventual escape. Still, in terms of the film's sexual metaphors, the lobotomy inflicted upon McMurphy is an upward displacement of the castration performed upon those who would express their masculinity. The misogynist ideology of *One Flew over the Cuckoo's Nest* did not prevent the film from garnering four major Academy Awards. The film also confirmed Nicholson's status as a superstar and established Director Forman, who would later win his second Oscar for *Amadeus*, as a director to be reckoned with. Nevertheless, its casting of psychiatry in the role of assistant to the repressors was nothing new.

A few films from the 1970s deserve special attention for the extent to which they have extended this formula of psychiatry-as-repression. In Hal Ashby's *Harold and Maude* (1971), Harold (Bud Cort) is a quietly appealing young man whose wealthy mother (Vivian Pickles) refuses to acknowledge his fascination with death and suicide, a trait the film presents as a healthy alternative to any other activities available to him. When he decides to marry Maude (Ruth Gordon), an exceedingly eccentric and elderly woman who is, again, vastly preferable to any available alternative in the film, Director Ashby sets up three complementary scenes in which representatives of establishment authority voice their opposition. In each of the three scenes a man sitting behind a desk speaks directly into the camera, presumably to the unseen Harold, while a single photograph is visible on the wall behind him. In the first scene Harold's uncle, a hawkish Army general, expresses befuddlement while an official portrait of Richard Nixon looks on. In the third scene, a sexually obsessed priest gives vent to his disgust beneath a picture of the pope. The middle scene places Harold's pompous and transparently foolish shrink (G. Wood) beneath a photograph of Freud as he exposes his inability to understand the boy even with the help of psychoanalytic clichés: "A very common neurosis, particularly in this society, whereby the male child wishes to sleep with his mother. Of course, what puzzles me, Harold, is that you want to sleep with your grandmother." Sandwiched between Nixon and Pope Paul VI, Freud has become another icon for a system that demands blind conformity to a sterile and obsolete set of norms.

The idea that psychiatry colludes in society's efforts to destroy its vital but unconventional individuals is spelled out by a psychiatrist himself in Sidney Lumet's 1977 film of Peter Shaffer's play *Equus*. The audience here is asked to believe that the competent therapist Dysart (Richard Burton) envies young Alan Strang (Peter Firth), a psychotic teenager whose only passion is an occasional night ride during which he masturbates on the back of a horse. Eventually this activity issues in Alan's blinding of several horses with a metal spike. However, since Alan's relationship with horses has a strong religious component, and since Dysart sees himself as the sterile practitioner of a science that robs people of worship, the psychiatrist regrets that he must be the one to prepare Alan to lead a "normal" life. Critics and audiences shunned the movie largely because of its inability to translate the striking theatricality of the play into film, but the overstated portrayal of a psychiatrist's despair at his own success was seldom questioned. Dysart ends the film with a long speech about the damage he has done to Alan Strang as well as to himself: "I'll heal the rash on his body. I'll erase the welts cut into his mind by flying manes. And when that's done, I'll set him on a metal scooter and send him puttering off into the concrete world, and he'll never touch hide again. Hopefully, he'll feel nothing at his fork but approved flesh. I doubt, however, with much passion. Passion, you see, can be destroyed by a doctor. It cannot be created. You won't gallop anymore, Alan. Horses will be quite safe. . . . You will, however, be without pain, almost completely without pain. But now, for me, it never stops, the voice of Equus, out of the cave. Why me?"

For the most part, the seventies continued to offer the same stereotypes of psychiatry that were introduced or refined in the late 1960s: in contrast to the heroic black psychiatrist from the Golden Age's *Pressure Point,* James Earl Jones in Aram Avakian's *End of the Road* (1970) runs a clinic in which patients are encouraged to have sex with chickens, a particularly grotesque variation on the "avant-gardist" psychiatrist played by James Coburn in *The President's Analyst.* Like many out-of-touch shrinks in the sixties, a young psychologist in Jack Lemmon's *Kotch* (1971) is entirely incapable of appreciating the problems of the elderly widower played by Walter Matthau. Joanne Woodward plays another neurotic psychiatrist who is cured by a male patient in *They Might Be Giants* (1971), and Patricia Barry attempts to emasculate Richard Benjamin in *The Marriage of a Young Stockbroker* (1971). Ernest Lehman's *Portnoy's Complaint* (1972) sends its characters to analysts who are completely wordless, even depriving the protagonist's psychiatrist of the one sentence that is the "punch line" in Philip Roth's novel, "So. Now vee may perhaps to begin. Yes?" In a tepidly feminist film, Bryan Forbes's *The Stepford Wives* (1975), a female psychiatrist appears to be part of a plot to replace the wives of wealthy suburbanites with automatons. A pompous psychologist in Richard Donner's *The Omen* (1976) is the conventional rationalist who has plausible but completely wrong explanations for the "fantasies" of Lee Remick, who is correct in believing that her son is the Devil. Similarly the female psychiatrists in John Boorman's *Exorcist II: The Heretic* (1977) and Jack Gold's *The Medusa Touch* (1978) are powerless in the face of supernatural forces. An army psychiatrist asks inane and insensitive questions of a deeply troubled Christopher Walken in Michael Cimino's *The Deer Hunter* (1978); Richard Benjamin indulges in the grossest kind of countertransference as the analyst for his girlfriend in Stan Dragoti's *Love at First Bite* (1979); and in Blake Edwards's *10* (1980), Dudley Moore, in the midst of a midlife crisis, is about to call his dour black psychiatrist but thinks better of it and hangs up.

There are dozens of post–Golden Age films that we have not mentioned in this chapter although the interested reader can find them listed in the filmography. If only because the negative portrayal of psychiatrists may have become overly familiar, a few films began to appear in the midseventies that were less hostile to the profession. We have already mentioned *I Never Promised You a Rose Garden* (1977) (plate 26), *An Unmarried Woman* (1978), and *Starting Over* (1979), all of which take much more sympathetic views of therapists. We should also point out that Alan Arkin played a somewhat idealized version of Sigmund Freud in Herbert Ross's *The Seven-Per-Cent Solution* (1976), a portrait that was all the more remarkable since it coexisted with a deromanticized revision of the Sherlock Holmes myth.

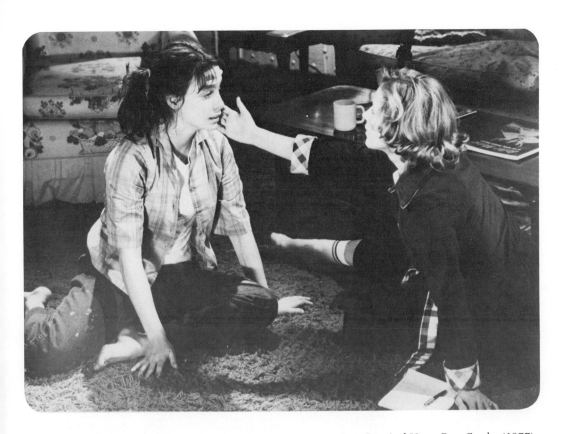

PLATE 26. Bibi Andersson heals Kathleen Quinlan in *I Never Promised You a Rose Garden* (1977). New World Pictures. The Museum of Modern Art/Film Stills Archive.

Still, the most successful film to reverse the antipsychiatrist tradition, and in a sense to bring back the old pattern of reconciliation, was the Academy Award—winning *Ordinary People* of 1980. Hollywood almost always attempts to follow up on its successes, and in the next few years even more films appeared that were much less aggressive in their attacks upon psychiatry. Jack Hofsiss's *I'm Dancing as Fast as I Can* (1981) begins with the revelation that a faceless male psychiatrist (Joseph Maher) and a violent, jealous lover (Nicol Williamson) have turned filmmaker Barbara Gordon (Jill Clayburgh) into a Valium addict. Yet the second half of the film introduces the therapist Julie (Dianne Wiest), a fully rounded human being in the tradition of *David and Lisa*'s Dr. Swinford (Howard da Silva), who swallows her pain at Barbara's transference attacks and stays with the case until her patient has thrown off her addiction. Although the psychiatrist played by Kathryn Harrold in *The Sender* (1982) is the typical rationalist foil for superior supernatural powers, she is nevertheless portrayed as concerned and devoted to her possessed patient. In Bryan Forbes's *The Naked Face* (1984), Roger Moore was cast against type as a pensive, nonviolent analyst pursued by both the Mafia and a vindictive police lieutenant (Rod Steiger). The chain-smoking psychiatrist played by Jane Fonda in Norman Jewison's *Agnes of God* (1985) is quite similar to Harrold's character in *The Sender:* she strives mightily to help her patient (Meg Tilly), but she is completely unwilling to entertain the possibility—suggested by the film with leaden ambiguity— that Agnes (Tilly) has been impregnated by an angel. Dr. Sam Rice (Roy Scheider) in Robert Benton's *Still of the Night* (1982) is another intrepid detective in the mold of Ingrid Bergman's Constance Peterson in *Spellbound,* and Dudley Moore is the lovable psychiatrist hero in Marshall Brickman's *Lovesick* (1983), but we will have more to say about these two films in the next chapter.

After the midsixties, movies dramatically abandoned the Golden Age psychiatrist and most often associated psychotherapists with society's false values and malevolent ideologies. Psychiatry had been an essential part of a fifties fantasy— created by psychiatry itself as well as by the movies—which failed to deliver on its promise of social harmony and individual fulfillment. The 1960s found new movie myths—most notably that of the inspirational antihero—which perfectly accommodated the new vision of psychiatry although many of the older myths were revived with only minor revisions. More sympathetic portraits of psychiatrists may have emerged in the past decade simply because the unrelieved vehemence of the attacks made a character such as Dr. Berger (Judd Hirsch) in *Ordinary People* (1980) seem fresh and original. Golden Age visions of psychiatry may now be returning as American culture in the 1980s appears to be longing once again for myths of reconciliation. The movies have already begun to move away from left- and right-cycle heroes and to return to films in which outlaw heroes are again balanced against official heroes. *Star Wars* (1977), perhaps the most influential film of the last ten years, is clearly "a disguised western" with an old-fashioned outlaw hero (Han Solo) eventually coming to the aid of an old-fashioned official hero (Luke Skywalker). As this yearning for reconciliation continues, psychiatrists may once again be called upon to help troubled individuals make the necessary adjustments. The best films may continue to present the profession with the ironic ambivalence tempered by reality that characterizes the films of Paul Mazursky and Woody Allen. Nevertheless, the vast majority of American movies are not likely to depart substantially from the conventions that have characterized Hollywood's approach to psychiatry during the last eighty years.

Countertransference in the Movies

5

■ The glut of movies with highly conventionalized portraits of bad psychiatrists may have inspired a parody of the tradition in *St. Ives* (1975), an unlikely film starring Charles Bronson. Directed by J. Lee Thompson, *St. Ives* contains a moment that ought to be included in "Great Moments in the Countertransference." Dr. John Constable (Maximillian Schell) is the live-in psychiatrist for millionaire Abner Procane (played with unusual understatement by John Houseman), whose treatment of his one patient includes showing movies, especially old ones, which, he tells St. Ives (Bronson), are like dreams. Although Schell plays the psychiatrist as obsequious and a little effeminate, he eventually reveals that he has been scheming to deprive Procane of his fortune. When Dr. Constable produces a gun and prepares to shoot Procane, he delivers the following speech:

> DR. CONSTABLE: What have I been paid all these years to listen to your mewling little troubles? Your mewling little troubles drove me mad! For nights, for hours. And what did you pay me? Compared to the millions you stack in your Swiss bank accounts, I have been paid in pennies.
>
> PROCANE (innocently): I had no idea. I . . . thought, John, I really believed . . .
>
> DR. CONSTABLE: That we were friends? It was a Freudian relation, Abner. God knows I loved you, but God knows I hate you now.

With these words, the psychiatrist shoots and kills his patient. This perversely sophisticated exploitation of psychiatry may represent a point at which the motion picture industry's attack upon the profession became self-conscious to the point of parody. At any rate, it provides the most extreme example of countertransference in the movies, crystallizing the worst fears an analysand could harbor.

The present chapter is devoted to how the movies have dealt with countertransference, specifically with how the phenomenon has been appropriated to conform to well-established myths and generic patterns. In the three recent films to which we will devote most of our attention, countertransference seems to be primarily a vehicle for reviving older genres. The regular presence of the countertransference theme in American movies reflects the long-standing controversy and misunderstanding surrounding Freud's suggestion that the psychoanalyst should maintain the dispassionate objectivity of the surgeon while striving to be as opaque as a mirror that simply reflects back the patient's own image. Freud's proscription against emotional involvement with patients has resulted in stereotypical portraits of aloof and unresponsive psychoanalysts as in the joke about the analyst who is dead for three days before his patients realize it. The public also reacts skeptically to the notion that psychotherapists are able to avoid acting on their feelings toward patients. Filmmakers have amply demonstrated that skepticism, as we have illustrated in the preceding chapters. It is no wonder that the movies' most negative images of psychiatry involve the mishandling of countertransference feelings: psychiatrists fall in love with patients, exploit them sexually, sadistically manipulate them, punish them with ECT and psychosurgery, even murder them as in *Dressed to Kill, I, the Jury,* and, of course, *St. Ives.*

Countertransference, narrowly defined, refers to the therapist's unconscious reaction to the patient's transference. More broadly defined, it is the total emotional reaction of the therapist to the patient (Kernberg 1965). It is true that all practicing psychiatrists experience countertransference feelings to varying degrees every day. Consequently, years of training and supervision are hopefully devoted to the goal of ensuring that each psychiatrist properly manages these feelings. Nevertheless, filmmakers have grossly simplified psychiatrists' susceptibility to forces outside therapeutic objectivity and have consistently portrayed psychiatrists—good and bad—as the prisoners of countertransference fantasies. Seldom does the professionally appropriate handling of these feelings appear in American films, and only on rare occasions do movie audiences see a psychiatrist in supervision, in a training analysis, or in other personal therapy where the meaning of countertransference reactions can be addressed.

Even when countertransference is actually discussed in films, the audience is usually asked to side with the guilty party, especially when romance is involved. Everything that Dr. Bruloff (Michael Chekhov) in Hitchcock's *Spellbound* (1945) tells Dr. Constance Peterson (Ingrid Bergman) about her reckless love for John (Gregory Peck) is perfectly valid from a professional point of view. Yet the film clearly sides with the dewy-eyed heroine (plate 27). On the one hand, Dr. Peterson renounces her profession and appears at the film's conclusion to be headed for the traditional wifely role, thus pushing the issues of countertransference into the background as far as the film is concerned. On the other hand, the kind of work that she does to save her lover from his mental distress as well as from the clutches of the law is closely related to psychotherapy (especially as it is portrayed in the movies), and her ultimate victory is entirely the result of her emotional commitment to her patient/lover, in other words, of countertransference.

In general, movies ask us to sympathize with female psychiatrists when they fall in love. When the smitten psychiatrist is male, however, the audience is not as likely to congratulate him. For all its flaws, *Tender Is the Night* (1962) intelligently invites an ambivalent reaction to the marriage of Dr. Dick Diver (Jason Robards, Jr.) and Nicole (Jennifer Jones) as well as to the psychiatrist's willingness to reject his profession. When his supervising analyst, Dr. Dohmler (Paul Lukas), warns him about "the tyranny of the sick," the film does not ask us to reject the advice as strongly as *Spellbound* asks us to dismiss the warnings of Dr. Bruloff to the Ingrid Bergman character. When we move out of the Golden Age, and the tone of psychiatrically inclined films becomes less grave, we are regularly invited to ridicule libidinous quacks such as Peter Sellers in

PLATE 27. Countertransference observed. Ingrid Bergman nurtures Gregory Peck while her training analyst (Michael Chekhov) looks on disapprovingly in *Spellbound* (1945). David O. Selznick. The Museum of Modern Art/Film Stills Archive.

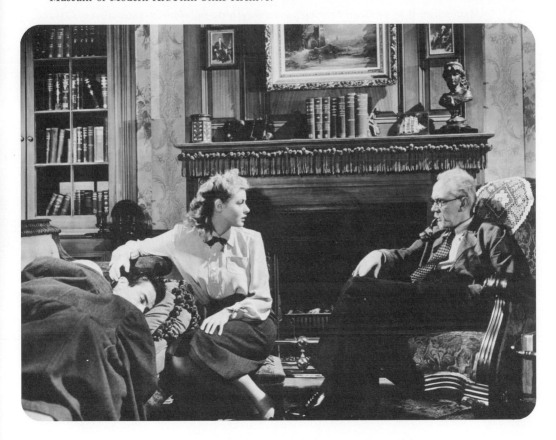

What's New, Pussycat? (1965) (plate 24) or Richard Benjamin in *Love at First Bite* (1979).

In this chapter we will focus on three recent films that at first glance seem to go beyond the familiar stereotypes of the psychiatrist in love. Although Marshall Brickman's *Lovesick* (1983), Graeme Clifford's *Frances* (1982), and Robert Benton's *Still of the Night* (1982) would seem to have little else in common, all three involve psychiatrists acting on countertransference feelings, and as we shall demonstrate, they can all be understood in terms of the well-established cinematic genres to which they belong. In fact, we maintain that the films present *necessary* images of the psychiatrist in order to fulfill the conventions of their genres.

Lovesick

The most psychiatrically sophisticated of these three films is probably Marshall Brickman's *Lovesick* (plate 28). Brickman, who shared screenwriting credit with Woody Allen on *Annie Hall* and *Manhattan* before directing his first film, *Simon* (1980), seeks to present a sympathetic psychoanalyst hero named Saul Benjamin (Dudley Moore). Early in the film, Benjamin is sought out by a distraught colleague, Otto (Wallace Shawn). This fellow analyst consults with him about a young female patient with whom he is madly infatuated. When Benjamin advises him that he cannot throw away everything for countertransference, Otto objects, saying he cannot possibly give her up. Foreboding trouble for Saul, the psychiatrist played by Shawn soon succumbs to a heart attack, and Benjamin finds himself contacted by the patient, a young playwright named Chloe (Elizabeth McGovern). The psychiatrist falls in love with Chloe at first sight, engaging in romantic fantasies about her only minutes after she sits down in his office.

Enter the ghost of Sigmund Freud (played by Alec Guinness), who serves as the protagonist's conscience, admonishing him that he is not in control of his countertransference and that he should refer the patient to another therapist. Benjamin ignores his warning and proceeds to fall madly in love with Chloe. He even sneaks into her apartment and hides in her shower. Chloe, who has already revealed strong romantic feelings for the analyst, discovers him in the shower, and they promptly go to bed after he professes that he is in love with her and that he can no longer treat her. Realizing that he is treading on dangerous ground, Benjamin seeks help from a mentor (John Huston) who, along with other members of the psychoanalytic society, meets with him to advise him further about the perils of a love affair with a patient. Benjamin protests that

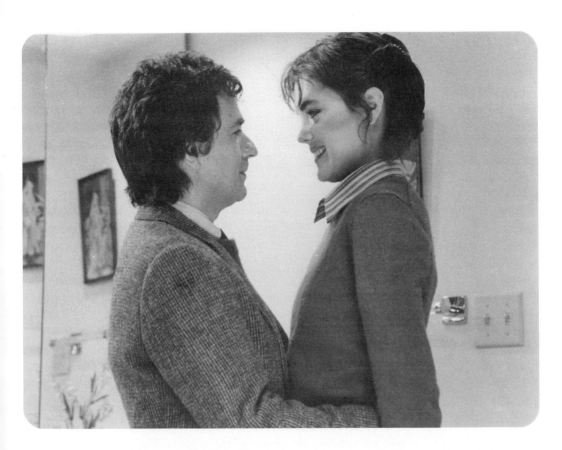

PLATE 28. Saul Benjamin (Dudley Moore) succumbs to the transference wishes of his patient (Elizabeth McGovern) in *Lovesick* (1983). Warner Brothers. The Museum of Modern Art/Film Stills Archive.

he is not experiencing countertransference but "real feelings," and he eventually rejects his colleagues and quite likely his profession. At the end, despite an intense argument with Chloe in which she asserts that he is crazy, the lovers reunite and romantically stroll off together in the moonlight.

Although *Lovesick* was not a success at the box office, *Newsweek* critic David Ansen called it "as airy and charming a movie as is likely to be made about countertransference" (1983). The film may have a certain charm, but to be truly inoffensive and benign, the film would need to be much *less* sophisticated about the psychiatric profession. It can be argued that *Lovesick* is the most insidious depiction of a psychiatrist acting on erotic countertransference feelings that has ever appeared on film. The treatment of the sexually obsessed psychiatrists in *What's New, Pussycat?* and *Love at First Bite* is so broadly farcical that no reasonable person would take their actions seriously. Movies such as the made-for-television "Betrayal" (1978), based on an actual case of a patient's seduction and manipulation by her psychiatrist, portray the psychiatrist as a clearly sick man rather than a typical member of his profession. *Lovesick,* by contrast, portrays Saul Benjamin (Dudley Moore) in a very sympathetic fashion—he is not an outrageous caricature but rather an ordinary man in love.

On closer scrutiny, however, the movie reveals an inherent destructiveness toward the principles of psychoanalytic treatment since Brickman's knowledge of psychoanalysis is sufficient to offer a pretense of the proper management of such feelings. Benjamin's reaction is correctly labeled countertransference by Sigmund Freud himself, and Benjamin does in fact seek consultation with a colleague. In a rare instance in American film, the audience is privy to a scene showing a psychiatrist in the throes of countertransference seeking help from a colleague. The only other instances of supervision that we have located are handled much more scrupulously. Although we side with Ingrid Bergman over Michael Chekhov in *Spellbound,* the training analyst is endowed with a great deal of authority and effectively represents the ideals of his profession. In the Golden Age, the supervisors of psychiatrists are even more august. The eminent Dr. Dohmler in *Tender Is the Night* is largely vindicated in his statements, and in the framing plot of *Pressure Point* (1962), the infallible Sidney Poitier tells Peter Falk how he himself was able to overcome his own hostility and that of the racist patient played by Bobby Darin.

But in *Lovesick,* when Benjamin comes to the office of Larry Geller (John Huston) and lies down on the couch, the older analyst offers him a cookie and tells Benjamin that countertransference "comes from the bottom. It's the muck." He further advises him to relax and take a tranquilizer. He reassures Benjamin that everything will be all right since he trained him. Then Dr. Geller (Huston) promptly falls asleep as Saul continues to ramble on the couch. One cannot infer from this ambiguous scene whether Geller is the hero's former training analyst, his current analyst, his former supervisor, or simply a consultant. It is certainly highly unusual for a colleague to lie down on the couch of a supervisor or consultant. It would be even more unusual for the training analyst to offer his analysand a cookie. Moreover, Geller's shallow advice and his lapse into somnolence make a mockery of the entire consultative or supervisory process. Hence, even Benjamin's apparent attempt to get help for his problem is depicted as farce.

In a subsequent scene, Geller advises Benjamin to go back into analysis. He further suggests that he wait a while and take up with Chloe at a later point, after the dust settles. The suggestion here is that a good facade must be maintained—it is the analyst's reputation that must be guarded, not the patient's health. This view is further reinforced in a dinner meeting with senior analysts composing the membership committee of the psychoanalytic society. Benjamin is told that he has been a "bad boy" although his superiors seem most concerned about what his actions will do to the reputation of the profession and to Benjamin's future as a psychoanalyst. They warn him that he will be practicing in North Dakota if he continues. Again, no concern is expressed for the patient. How, for example, will Benjamin's action affect the patient's anxiety attacks, the symptom for which she sought out psychiatric help?

Earlier, when Benjamin explains to Chloe over lunch that he can no longer have an affair with her because she will eventually feel betrayed and angry, she stands up indignantly and asks, "Eventually?" She then proceeds to stomp out of the restaurant. The movie would indicate that the real betrayal, the real cruelty of the analyst, would be to dump his heartbroken patient rather than to continue their romantic involvement.

Meanwhile, Benjamin deteriorates in his ability to function as a psychiatrist. He falls asleep while listening to one patient. He tells another that he really cannot help her at all and that she would be better off to take a walk or a jog. He abuses diazepam and methaqualone and begins drinking heavily. He responds to a patient's emergency call by showing up at his office intoxicated, forcing the patient to arrange for his transport by ambulance to the local emergency room. Benjamin apologetically explains to his patient that psychiatry is a young science. He then returns over six thousand dollars to one patient because he feels he has not helped this patient adequately. He compares himself to a plumber who would not charge if he failed to fix his customer's sink.

Despite this obvious decompensation, Benjamin is portrayed as a positive character, a man in love who is misunderstood by his colleagues. In a sense he is a well-heeled 1980s version of the outlaw hero. The members of the analytic society are seen as stuffy, repressive, authoritarian types who subscribe to outmoded and archaic principles of ethics. If there is any question of their absurdity, Brickman's camera further distorts their visages with a fish-eye lens. When Benjamin finally throws off the shackles of these reactionaries who would destroy his love for Chloe, Freud informs him that it is time to terminate the relationship. Freud is going to Mexico to study how hallucinogenic mushrooms and group dreaming are being used therapeutically. He comments that this mixture of psychology, religion, and chemistry is the wave of the future. In his exit line, Freud comments, "Psychoanalysis is an interesting method. I never intended it to become an industry." Even Sigmund himself is disillusioned by the principles of the science he founded. The audience is asked to feel exhilarated when Benjamin and Chloe walk off together at the end of the movie. This psychiatrist has had the courage to buck the establishment, to follow his instincts, to be his own man, to listen to his heart. Problems such as the patient's anxiety attacks will now go away: all she needed was a man to take care of her. The film also neatly disposes of the analyst's wife by showing her in the midst of an affair with a Bohemian painter (Larry Rivers). Furthermore, there is no suggestion that the age difference between the lovers may pose difficulties or that Benjamin's behavior is part of a midlife crisis. After all, as the psychiatrist himself says, these are "real feelings," not countertransference.

The comments of the *real* Sigmund Freud on this outcome are germane in this context: "If the patient's advances were returned, it would be a great triumph for her, but a complete defeat for the treatment. She would have succeeded in what all patients strive for in analysis—she would have succeeded in acting out, in repeating in real life, what she ought only to have remembered, to have reproduced as psychical material and to have kept within the sphere of psychical events. In the further course of the love relationship, she would bring out all the inhibitions and pathological reactions of her erotic life, without there being any possibility of correcting them; and the distressing episode would end in remorse and a great strengthening of her propensity to regression. The love relationship, in fact, destroys the patient's susceptibility to influence from analytic treatment" (1915, 156).

In spite of its hostility to the psychoanalytic profession, *Lovesick* belongs to a familiar style of romantic comedy in which the hero rejects what society considers to be success for the love of a sympathetic partner. We can find films of this kind in the 1930s, (*It Happened One Night, Bringing up Baby, Holiday*) and in the 1950s (*Born Yesterday, The Apartment,*) in which the protagonists find that their lovers have more to offer than any rewards their societies might hold out. Northrop Frye (1957) sees this archetypal situation as "the mythos of spring" or "new comedy," in which a negative society is supplanted by a more spontaneous, positive world built around the lovers. In the 1960s, the conviction that society is hopelessly corrupt became so strong that the lovers often run away with no new world in mind, only a rejection of the one they live in. The best example of this version of the genre is Mike Nichols's *The Graduate* (1967), in which the "plastic" world can be escaped only by a definitive break. At the film's end, Dustin Hoffman wields a crucifix against a culture that has perverted such symbols and then takes a bus to nowhere with his true love. We have already discussed *The Marriage of a Young Stockbroker* (based on a novel by Charles Webb, who also wrote the source novel for *The Graduate*), in which a female psychiatrist fails to deter the hero and his wife from a similar act of dropping out. Although it hedges on the extent to which its hero actually escapes his society, Dudley Moore has already appeared in one film like *The Graduate,* Steve Gordon's *Arthur* (1981). His final acceptance of Liza Minnelli as his mate must be perceived as vastly preferable to the company of those who would otherwise run his life. Similarly, in *Lovesick,* Chloe must make us believe that her charms outweigh any benefit that Saul Benjamin could possibly derive from the grotesque collection of colleagues who sustain him in his extremely lucrative career.

On the other hand, both *Arthur* and *Lovesick* represent a 1980s revision of *The Graduate*'s formula. Although all three films belong to the left cycle, in which an outlaw hero is opposed exclusively by caricatured representations of official ideology, the two characters played by Dudley Moore do not perform anything like Dustin Hoffman's ritualized renunciation of his parents' culture. Arthur is promised a large portion of his inheritance from the family matriarch (Geraldine Fitzgerald), and Saul Benjamin in *Lovesick* has reconciling encounters with his estranged wife, with Freud's ghost, and even with his older colleague (Huston), who lustily applauds Benjamin's table cloth maneuver at the dinner table. *Lovesick* has more in common with films of the 1950s that strained unsuccessfully at extending the old formulas into a different era. *Lovesick* seems to strain in several directions, recapturing the formulaic magic of neither classical Hollywood nor *The Graduate.* The film's inability to succeed in either direction may be primarily responsible for its failure at the box office.

Nevertheless, *Lovesick* belongs to a time-honored genre, and like all good escaping and escapist heroes, the psychiatrist must be likeable, and he must be portrayed as misused by society. Benjamin's five patients, whom we meet in the opening scenes of *Lovesick,* are treated as contemptible fools who are wasting their analyst's time. The only patient that Benjamin seems to enjoy treating is a down-and-out paranoid schizophrenic. Although a colleague warns him that schizophrenics are incurable, Benjamin achieves breakthroughs with this patient, and by the film's end he appears to have devoted himself to the treatment of impoverished chronic patients on the street instead of the much more affluent group of narcissists he is treating in the opening scenes. The genre to which *Lovesick* belongs also demands that we see love—especially the love for a dewy fresh heroine—as the only alternative to a comically demented world of foolish analysands and their equally foolish analysts. The dramatic conflict is strengthened when Benjamin's peers explicitly demand that he choose between them and her. Benjamin will live in less regal surroundings, but he will undertake the more meaningful work of treating the street people who really need him. We hardly need to know this fact, however, because the most important issue is Benjamin's relationship with Chloe, one that can only be arrived at through the phenomenon of countertransference. As a result, those who oppose Benjamin's acting out on countertransference must be devalued, including Freud's ghost. This is the kind of ending we have learned to expect from watching Jack Lemmon reject the executive suite for Shirley MacLaine in Billy Wilder's *The Apartment* (1960), Cary Grant reject big time banking for Katharine Hepburn in George Cukor's *Holiday* (1938), Ryan O'Neal reject musicological acclaim for Barbra Streisand in Peter Bogdanovich's *What's up, Doc?* (1972), and, of course, Dustin Hoffman reject suburban affluence and Mrs. Robinson for Katharine Ross in *The Graduate*. We may wish to view *Lovesick* not as a carefully conceived frontal attack on the American psychoanalytic establishment but rather as an unambitious romantic comedy, which must not disturb its audience by straying from its generic conventions and portraying its psychiatric hero as anything but a sympathetic fellow who *must* act on his erotic countertransference feelings for the heroine.

Nevertheless, audiences for *Lovesick* leave the theater having entertained, if only for a few minutes, the following assumptions: (1) a married, middle-aged analyst's instant infatuation with a patient young enough to be his daughter is not a countertransference reaction but real love; (2) sexual relations between analysts and patients are not damaging to the patient; (3) it is more cruel for the analyst who is in love with his patient to abandon her than to continue a sexual affair with her; (4) supervision is totally ineffectual in helping an analyst with his countertransference feelings, as is the analyst's personal treatment experience; (5) the main reason that psychoanalysts prohibit their own kind from having affairs with patients is that it would look bad for the profession; (6) psychoanalytic principles of ethics are outmoded and repressive restrictions that prohibit the analyst from emotional spontaneity with his patients.

Frances

Frances, directed by Graeme Clifford (who edited Robert Altman's 1972 film *Images*) and written by Eric Bergren, Christopher Devore, and Nicolas Kazan, presents quite a different picture of countertransference. This biographical account of the tragic life of Frances Farmer (played by Jessica Lange) is reportedly based on the actual experiences of Farmer in psychiatric treatment settings. The protagonist first comes to a psychiatrist halfway through the film after being dominated by a narcissistic mother, jilted by a lover, and abused by Hollywood moguls. Frances's mother (Kim Stanley) brings her to an asylum, where a psychiatrist named Dr. Symington (Lane Smith) greets her. He informs her with a smile that he has followed her career and finds her to be a "fascinating case." Furthermore, he tells her that he looks forward to "solving her predicament." As is the case with many borderline patients that psychiatrists deal with every day, Farmer is uncooperative and contemptuous of his efforts to help her. She avows that she will not tell him anything about her personal life and does not want to talk with him about her "predicament." However, Dr. Symington seems incapable of handling this negative transference reaction on the part of his patient, and we see beads of sweat develop on his upper lip, which he seeks to hide with his hands. An increasingly menacing look appears on the doctor's face as Farmer continues to devalue him and his attempt to help her. He is portrayed as so narcissistically injured and humiliated at her refusal to be helped that he becomes punitive. When it is time to order her out of his office, he intones the following inanity: "Symington says." As she leaves the office, the film flashes to the next scene, in which Farmer is being administered insulin shock, inducing a grand mal seizure.

The audience is led to believe that Dr. Symington's countertransference anger at being humiliated by his patient is punitively acted out by administering a cruel and inhumane treatment to his patient. In a subsequent scene, he interviews her in his office and is portrayed as an almost crazed sadist who aggressively sharpens a pencil while he talks with her and then obsessively puts the shavings into a container. He clearly looks more disturbed than Farmer and is portrayed as forcing her to stay in the hospital when she really does not need it. He is depicted as victimizing her, as though she is a misunderstood innocent mislabeled as mentally ill. Hence, unlike *Lovesick, Frances* portrays the lone patient, not the psychiatrist, as the sympathetic figure. Dr. Symington is not only a buffoon but a sadistic buffoon who punishes patients when they do not conform to his expectations.

The countertransference portrayed in *Frances* can also be understood in terms of the generic demands of the film. The genre to which *Frances* belongs is the familiar story of a real character who takes a rocky emotional road to stardom. The rise and fall of female celebrities was a genre unto itself in the 1950s, but more recent forerunners for *Frances* are *Lady Sings the Blues, Funny Girl,* and *The Rose. Frances* also resembles films in which a free-spirited or individualistic hero is victimized by a repressive society and its agents in the psychiatric community. The best example of this type of film is of course Milos Forman's sentimental *One Flew over the Cuckoo's Nest,* but we have also found the same conventions in sixties films such as *A Fine Madness* and *Harold and Maude.* In the seventies, the oppressed protagonist is often female, especially in feminist films such as *Diary of a Mad Housewife, A Woman under the Influence,* and *The Bell Jar.* In a sense, these films recall Golden Age movies such as *Three Faces of Eve* and *Splendor in the Grass.* However, the successful therapies that the women undergo in these earlier films become punitive, repressive, and ineffective in the later ones.

Although *Lovesick* uses comic means to deliver a fairly definitive condemnation of psychoanalysis, *Frances* is even bolder in its attack on the profession. Although we are never sure exactly what Jessica Lange's Frances wants, we know it is not what her mother undertakes to inflict upon her. Proceeding from the seemingly logical premise that any woman who does not want to become a successful movie star must be mad, Mrs. Farmer (Kim Stanley) enlists the aid of psychiatrists to employ the most grotesque means to restore her daughter to "sanity." Like *Cuckoo's Nest, Frances* suggests that society is upside down and that the true crazies remain outside the institutions while a few nonconforming but vital souls become inmates. Again, the movies have taught us that such thoughts are legitimate, and as we pointed out in chapter 1, the genre of the institution film relies upon the conventions of the old prisoner-of-war camp films to show that those inside should be outside and vice versa. Recent left-cycle prison films such as *Cool Hand Luke, Papillon, Midnight Express,* and even *Escape from Alcatraz* (with the same star and director as the right cycle's *Dirty Harry*) have given almost Christ-like qualities to inmates in contrast to the demonic goons who keep them there. We should not be surprised then that the psychiatrists encountered by Frances are weak, neurotic, and prone to grandiose fantasies. They cannot deal with her claims that they have no right to tamper with her life, so they resort to insulin shock, ECT, and, ultimately, lobotomy. As in *Cuckoo's Nest,* we are asked to grieve over the affectless protagonist who appears at the film's end.

In order to validate the claims of left-cycle heroes such as Frances Farmer, psychiatrists within this genre are caricatured as willing and malevolent agents of a repressive society, one which cannot tolerate nonconformity and punishes those who attempt to be creative and different. In a later scene in *Frances,* Farmer appears before a board of four psychiatrists who will determine whether or not she can be discharged. These psychiatrists look more like a gang of mobsters than a group of concerned physicians, and they scrutinize Farmer carefully as she tries to say exactly the right things to effect her discharge. They are then easily duped by her performance and decide to discharge her. Their reactions as she talks would indicate that Farmer can deceive them because of their narcissistic fantasies about being able to cure patients. When Farmer returns home, her mother tries to force her back to Hollywood against her will, and Farmer shouts at her mother, "You are breaking my spirit." Indeed, the movie would have us believe that psychiatrists also break a patient's spirit.

The real Frances Farmer was certainly not helped by psychiatry. According to Carrie Rickey (1982), Farmer first suffered a breakdown due to a combination of stress and the mixing of alcohol with Benzedrine, the drug which studio doctors regularly prescribed to actresses in order to keep their weight down. Although there are conflicting accounts of what actually happened to her during her several periods of confinement in institutions, Farmer was the kind of celebrity upon whom at least one psychiatrist relished the opportunity of experimenting, and she may actually have been lobotomized. As the film suggests, it is also possible that patients in one of the asylums to which she was committed were raped repeatedly by whomever the night orderlies allowed into the institution. However, Rickey also writes that Frances was an extremely complex individual whose story allows widely divergent interpretations. In Graeme Clifford's film, Frances is simply the victim of Hollywood, men, her own mother, and psychiatrists, and there is little suggestion that she herself might be at least partially responsible for her own unhappiness. In *Frances,* psychiatry is an extension of the protagonist's mother, and regardless of their own needs, patients are punished by psychiatrists for not performing according to their parents' expectations. Near the end of the film, we see a psychiatrist lecturing to a group of his colleagues about a primitive form of lobotomy. He explains to them that the imagination and the emotions are disturbed in mental illness and that lobotomy cures the problem. Hence, psychiatry is also seen as opposed to free expression of emotions, creativity, and imagination. Movies in this genre can offer us a limited number of story patterns, and audiences can only accept a limited number of conventions. Thus, the manner in which Frances Farmer contributed to her own difficulties and the possibility of effective treatment for such problems go unexamined in the film.

As with *Lovesick,* audiences are not invited to take the conventions of *Frances* very far, but if they do extend the film's assumptions into the real world, they will arrive at the following conclusions: (1) a patient dare not express anger and contempt toward a psychiatrist, because it is likely to make the psychiatrist angry; (2) psychiatrists react punitively to patients who do not cooperate with them; (3) psychiatrists have a narcissistic need to cure patients and can be conned by flattery; (4) psychiatrists are likely to be as disturbed as or more disturbed than their patients; (5) psychiatrists are likely to collude with parents in committing patients who do not conform to parental expectation; (6) psychiatrists react negatively to people who express creativity, imagination, and spontaneity.

Still of the Night

A third recent example of cinematic countertransference can be found in Robert Benton's *Still of the Night.* Benton first won acclaim when he cowrote Arthur Penn's *Bonnie and Clyde* (1967). Like Graeme Clifford, Benton was given early support by Robert Altman, who produced one of the director's first efforts, *The Late Show* (1977). Benton eventually won an Academy Award for his *Kramer vs. Kramer* and has since received acclaim for *Places in the Heart. Still of the Night* is a mystery-thriller that belongs to a genre created almost entirely by Alfred Hitchcock: as in *The Thirty-nine Steps* (1935), *The Lady Vanishes* (1938), *Notorious* (1946), *Rear Window* (1954), *The Man Who Knew Too Much* (1934 and 1956), *North by Northwest* (1959), and even his last film, *Family Plot* (1976), Hitchcock builds stories around mostly innocent but resourceful protagonists who become entangled in desperate situations and must use their wits to solve mysteries and, frequently, to exonerate themselves. Hitchcock often delves into the psychology of his characters, and in *Spellbound*—the most obvious antecedent for *Still of the Night*—a psychiatrist relies on dream analysis as well as her somewhat unprofessional intuitions in order to identify the real villain and save her client/lover. *Spellbound*'s conclusion with its happy-ever-after for the lovers is not atypical Hitchcock. Some of his films, such as *Shadow of a Doubt* and *The Wrong Man,* belong to the *film noir* tradition, in which romance seldom flowers, and other aspects of his work can be traced back to cinematic influences from Fritz Lang and Carl Dreyer, hardly masters of the light comedy. At least on the surface, however, the basic Hitchcock ending allows some kind of romantic resolution for a sympathetic and romantic couple. Hitchcock once directed a more or less conventional romantic comedy, *Mr. and Mrs. Smith,* and as Cavell (1981a) has pointed out, even Hitchcock's *North by Northwest* can be thought of as a "comedy of remarriage," a subgenre of what is usually considered to be "screwball comedy." In spite of Hitchcock's acclaimed obsession with evil and sin, his films usually end with justice done and the lovers united. Although critics have correctly identified undercurrents of disorder profoundly disturbing the seemingly happy endings to certain of his films, Hitchcock was just as likely to unite his lovers unambiguously at the conclusion. This is certainly the case with *Spellbound.*

Because Robert Benton has appropriated Hitchcock's conventions in *Still of the Night,* the depiction of psychoanalyst Sam Rice (Roy Scheider) becomes paradoxical, much in the same way that the Ingrid Bergman character in *Spellbound* can be seen as both a good and a bad practitioner of her profession. The movie depicts Rice as an old-fashioned hero who rescues his lover (and himself) from a desperate situation, but his heroism is in many ways the acting out of self-destructive and irrational countertransference. The audience is meant to see Rice in a sympathetic light from the very beginning of the film when we see him reassure an analytic patient that he need not stop treatment just because he cannot afford it. Rice is struggling with a bout of depression in reaction to his divorce, which has just been finalized at the beginning of the movie. He is also suffering from a grief reaction over a recently murdered patient, George Bynum (Josef Sommer, seen in frequent flashbacks). Just as he feels like a failure regarding his marriage, he feels that he has failed with his murdered patient, whom he suggests would have been better off with a priest or a rabbi.

Early in the film, Rice is visited by the murdered patient's mistress, Brooke Reynolds (Meryl Streep). She has come with her ex-lover's watch, hoping that the psychiatrist will see that it is returned to his widow. From that moment on, Rice becomes obsessed with Reynolds, who is the prime suspect in the murder, and he sets out to discover if she is indeed guilty. He continues his pursuit of the killer despite repeated warnings from the police that she is likely to kill him next. In a scene with his mother (Jessica Tandy), who is also a psychiatrist, he acknowledges that what he is doing may be irrational but that he must do it. He explains that he spent two years working with the murdered patient and that he wants to find out who killed him. As he begins to fall in love with Reynolds (Streep), he becomes progressively more involved in her case, and at one point, he even bids $15,000 to buy a painting at an auction as a way of assisting the heroine in her flight from arrest.

Flashbacks of therapy sessions with his deceased patient, Bynum (Sommer), shed a little more light on Rice's obsession with Reynolds. Bynum first refers to her in the session as "your type—stiff." He then continues to refer to her in all subsequent therapy session as "your girlfriend." Bynum repeatedly taunts the psychiatrist provocatively with comments such as "I have been to bed with your girlfriend." As this taunting continues, the patient begins to believe that Rice is having a problem with Reynolds. He points out that while Rice asks him questions about every other significant individual in his life, he never asks him about Reynolds. Hence, the audience sees that the patient has created an imaginary special relationship between Reynolds and the psychiatrist, apparently out of a transferential need to provoke jealousy in his therapist. The movie shows Rice actually colluding with this ploy both in the sessions, through his absence of comments about Reynolds, and following the patient's death, by his obsessive pursuit of her vindication.

The film does not provide a simple answer for why Rice responds in this countertransferential manner. Only by attempting a systematic understanding of the nature of Rice's countertransference is his behavior understandable. One of several unconscious factors that may be at work in the mind of Sam Rice is an identification with his dead patient, especially since he pursues the same woman with whom his patient was sleeping. The psychiatrist's pursuit of Brooke Reynolds (Streep) makes for a suspenseful film, but it also seems odd that he should involve himself so closely with a woman who may have killed Bynum and who, according to the police, may make him her next victim. Freud (1923) said that identification may be the only condition under which a lost object may be given up. Rice, racked with guilt over his perceived negligence in treating Bynum, may have identified with his ex-patient as a way of dealing with his grief. Moreover, oedipal themes abound under the surface of *Still of the Night*'s plot. Bynum has created an oedipal triangle with Rice and Reynolds in his attempts to induce jealousy in the psychiatrist. Since Rice colludes in this triangle, one can speculate that he has a countertransference wish to eliminate his rival for Reynolds. Hence, when Bynum is murdered, Rice's guilt is activated because of his unconscious death wish toward his patient. The film then shows the parallel situation between Rice's relationship with Reynolds, where the "other man" has been murdered, and Rice's relationship with his mother, where the father is apparently absent. (We have not been able to locate the appearance of a female psychiatrist's husband in any American movies unless the husband is a former patient.) In fact, when the hero first kisses Reynolds in his apartment, the doorbell rings, and he says, "That's my mother." The doorbell interrupts the kiss, and his mother proceeds to warn him that he is getting too involved in investigating the murder. Oedipal destruction is further handed out in Reynolds's revelation late in the movie that she inadvertently killed her own father. Rice's wish to track down the murderer may be partly motivated by his wish to prove his own innocence. Finally, the oedipal theme is elaborated further in a crucial dream sequence. Bynum relates a dream in a therapy session where Reynolds is portrayed as a little girl pursuing Bynum as a father figure. A teddy bear, a prominent symbol in the dream, has its eye pulled out, allowing blood to flow freely from the remaining hole. Although the film does not offer any interpretation of this episode in the dream, the bleeding eye immediately calls to mind the Oedipus myth since Oedipus blinds himself with a brooch (an upward displacement of castration) as punishment for having killed his father and slept with his mother.

In summary, the actions of Dr. Sam Rice in the film are puzzling and not well explained by the movie itself. They are somewhat clearer if we understand Rice, in the throes of a divorce and hence vulnerable to countertransference feelings, as recapitulating the oedipal situation with his older male patient and that patient's younger mistress. His quest to exonerate Reynolds and locate the murderer, then, is a compromise formation of sorts; that is, he achieves an oedipal victory of winning over Reynolds for himself while expiating his own unconscious guilt by tracking down the real murderer. While the general public may see him as a slightly unconventional private-eye hero, a psychiatrically sophisticated audience member sees him as out of control and dangerously self-destructive. As with many of Hitchcock's films, the happy ending does not entirely resolve many of the darker psychological aspects of the film.

The genre to which *Lovesick* belongs demands a cute, funny hero and a young, uncorrupted heroine. *Frances*'s genre demands a sympathetic but unconventional protagonist surrounded by forces wishing to confine her because of cruelty, intolerance, or, perhaps, countertransference. *Still of the Night* demands a handsome, pensive hero and Hitchcock's worldly, cool blonde heroine. Hence the needs of the genre in Benton's film produce our paradoxical hero, who is, confusingly, devoted to his patients at the same time that he is out of control with his acting out of countertransference feelings. For the audience of a thriller, however, the complex problems encountered in psychoanalysis are finessed by drawing attention to a crime that when solved provides the feeling that *all* problems—even psychological ones—have been disposed of. This is exactly what happens in *Spellbound,* although that film takes itself somewhat less seriously, even offering the audience a comic ending in the final shot. *Still of the Night,* on the other hand, has a lifelessness at its center, which may have resulted from Benton's efforts to work in Hitchcock's genre without fully understanding the master's vision. Much of the same thing can be said of the several Hitchcockian films directed by Brian De Palma. Nevertheless, the confusion in Sam Rice's character can be understood as a result of Benton's desire to make a psychiatrist into a conventional Hitchcockian hero. Mel Brooks, by the way, attempted the same transformation in his tongue-in-cheek homage to Hitchcock, *High Anxiety* (1977), and for many of the same reasons, that film stands as one of the least successful of Brooks's genre parodies.

The naive audience member leaving *Still of the Night* who wishes to pursue the film's implications might make the following assumptions: (1) if analysts like their patients and enjoy working with them, they will forgo insisting that the patient pay his fee; (2) when a patient is murdered, the therapist is likely to feel like a failure and feel that his patient would do as well with a clergyman; (3) a patient can "set up" his therapist to have a special interest in the patient's lover; (4) the therapist may in turn develop an erotic obsession with the patient's lover and may "move in" on this lover if the patient dies; (5) a therapist is much like a private eye in his pursuit of truth and will risk life and limb to get to the bottom of a murder when it involves his patient; (6) to protect a former patient's lover, a psychotherapist will conceal evidence from the police and spend thousands of dollars of his own money. This kind of behavior might be dismissed as outrageous in a different context, but in *Still of the Night*, Sam Rice is portrayed so sympathetically and so heroically that the audience believes he is a good man who is simply loyal to his patients.

These three films, *Lovesick, Frances,* and *Still of the Night,* bring little that is new to the portrayal of psychiatrists in American cinema. Except for some brief nudity and strong language, there is virtually nothing in *Frances* that would have been out of place in a 1960s film about a doomed but vital hero. *Lovesick* can also be seen as a 1960s film, specifically an antiestablishment escapist comedy like *The Graduate.* Saul Benjamin, who even shares a name with the character played by Dustin Hoffman in that film, could be The Graduate grown up, although, as we have pointed out, this attempt at translating sixties myths into the 1980s does not appear to be a feasible project, at least not for *Lovesick.* *Still of the Night* looks back even farther. Without its high-tech visual style and graphic violence, Robert Benton's film could be *Spellbound* with the sex roles reversed. These films—like so many that have come before—continue to undermine the claim of psychiatrists that they can operate without succumbing to countertransference feelings. This trend has been in full force for over twenty years now, and in the next chapter, we will assess its impact on the actual treatment of psychiatric patients.

Clinical Implications

6

Our inquiry into cinematic visions of countertransference leaves a number of questions unanswered. What is the relevance of these images for the clinical practice of psychiatry? Are patients or potential patients significantly influenced by these depictions? Can we assume that audiences are sufficiently discriminating to know the difference between the celluloid image and what they actually encounter in therapy? Do screen portrayals adversely affect patients by causing them either to overidealize or to distrust their psychiatrists? Do the depictions of movie psychiatrists affect psychiatrists themselves and the way they practice their art? Finally, could the treatment of psychiatry in the movies be, at least in part, a cause for the decline in the public image of psychiatry, or conversely, is it the *result* of that decline?

Unfortunately, we do not have all the answers to these questions. However, we do feel that these issues deserve consideration and that psychiatric movies are not irrelevant either to the interactions of doctors and patients or to the public's understanding of psychiatry. The cinema is the great storehouse for the intrapsychic images of our time, and movies touch on fundamental human psychological processes with which patients and therapists alike identify. Film serves many of the same functions for modern audiences that tragedy served for fifth-century Greeks: in addition to providing catharsis and *anagnorisis,* the mythological (i.e., political, ideological, and spiritual) dimensions of film unite audiences with their culture as profoundly as the Aeschylean and Sophoclean visions of man in the universe were a major part of the civic and religious life of every Athenian citizen.

Perhaps the consideration of these questions should begin with another question: are the screen portrayals of psychiatrists really accurate? In our historical overview, we attempted to avoid judgments on whether or not a particular portrayal was "realistic." Clearly, such judgments are made according to some notion of what normally goes on in the consulting room of the competent, well-trained psychiatrist. Through our experience with numerous workshops for mental health professionals and symposia at national psychiatric meetings, however, we have come to realize that the characterization of typical psychiatric practice is a highly subjective process. We have been repeatedly impressed at how frequently psychiatrists disagree about whether or not a particular movie realistically depicts how a psychiatrist functions. For example, while some mental health professionals feel that *Ordinary People* provided a realistic glimpse of what a human, compassionate, and effective psychiatrist is like, others laughed heartily at the idea that Dr. Berger would come out to his office in the middle of the night to see Conrad under the circumstances depicted in the movie.

It is just these kinds of disagreements that have contributed to the public skepticism about the scientific status of psychiatry (Fink 1983). When millions of Americans read news reports of the Hinckley trial and the Patty Hearst trial, they are privy to "expert" psychiatric testimony that presents diametrically opposed arguments for the sanity or the insanity of the defendant. The expert psychiatric witness on each side claims that because of his training, experience, and knowledge, his diagnosis and formulation is accurate, while the psychiatric expert on the opposite side of the case is thoroughly confused and inaccurate in his appraisal of the data.

The problem of establishing realistic screen portrayals is even more difficult for movies such as the films portraying psychiatric abuses that were discussed in our previous chapter. *Frances,* after all, is based on a true story, one might argue, and reports of psychotherapists having affairs with patients as in *Lovesick* are not at all uncommon (Davidson 1977). Horror stories about the abuses of psychotropic medications, electroconvulsive therapy, and psychosurgery in state hospitals around the country surface with regular periodicity. Are these depictions distortions? Yes and no. On the one hand, they are not distortions, because there really are psychiatrists here and there who are sadistic and punitive toward their patients; there really are psychoanalysts who act on their erotic feelings toward their patients; and there are probably even instances of homicidal psychiatrists who have murdered their own patients. On the other hand, these portrayals are distortions in the sense that they misrepresent the typical, average, well-intentioned psychiatrist, who attempts to understand and harness his countertransference feelings in the service of what is ethical and best for his patients. To the uninformed audience member, who may or may not have contact with a psychiatrist outside a movie theater, the movies may not be portraying just one particular psychiatrist but rather *the* psychiatrist, just as many moviegoers regard James Bond as *the* secret agent or Vito Corleone as *the* Mafioso. Without knowing what the customary and modal behavior of a psychiatrist is, the audience has no standard by which to judge the appropriateness and the frequency of what it witnesses on the screen. Returning to the comparison of the American public's reaction to movies and that of the ancient Greeks to Sophocles and Aeschylus, audiences may perceive characters and situations as archetypes: just as Oedipus is Man, and Thebes is the Polis, Americans may regard a particular character as representative of an entire profession, conveying its core characteristics. Hence the psychiatrist in the cinema is a psychiatric Everyman, who is likely to make the audience member think to himself, "So that is what psychiatrists are like."

For both filmmakers and audiences, the movie psychiatrist is a transference object. Brenner (1982) notes that transference is pervasive—the only difference between transference in the analytic situation and transference in life outside the consulting room is that it is analyzed in the clinical setting. In other words, we are all transforming those around us into various objects from our past at an unconscious level throughout the course of our personal and professional lives every day. Conceptualizing the film psychiatrist as a transference object may be more valuable than quibbling about which movie psychiatrist comes closest to an accurate portrayal of the real-life psychiatrist. If it is true that transference is pervasive in all human relationships, it is also true that every relationship is a mixture of real aspects and transference distortions. The psychiatrist, whether in movies or in real life, is perhaps particularly subject to transference distortions. As Paul Fink has pointed out: "While all physicians have their roots in the priesthood and in the rites of the society, they do not retain the mantle of magic incantation as do psychiatrists. Aesculapian authority has evolved in a nonverbal direction. Psychiatry is often called upon to deal with mental pain such as guilt (which is more akin to priestly authority than Aesculapian authority)" (1983, 673). After all, translated directly from its etymological origins, psychiatrist means "doctor of the soul." Perhaps psychiatrists are more prone to significant transferential distortions because they can so easily be regarded as supramedical mind readers who understand the dark workings of the human psyche in a way inaccessible to others. It is just this quality that is so often depicted in movies about psychiatrists. Similarly, as Fink points out, such powers are frightening and people may devalue or ridicule them in order to deal with their anxiety over these perceived superhuman powers.

While the attribution of magical powers to psychiatrists is certainly a distortion, mental health professionals must acknowledge their own contribution to fostering such distortions. The similarities between the mystique of psychoanalytic institutes and that surrounding secret societies are the object of many humorous comments. The reluctance among psychoanalysts and other psychotherapists to make themselves accountable for what they do may encourage the belief that the therapeutic process is intuitive and magical rather than rational and empirical. Historically, psychiatry may have contributed to its own idealization and mystification by affecting omniscience and by promising remedies for highly complex social problems that were well beyond its purview (Fink 1983). The growth of psychiatry following World War II was partly related to its ability to explain behavior, such as malingering among soldiers, in a psychodynamic manner. Hence what was previously condemned as immoral or evil behavior was now understood as psychopathological. This phenomenon provided psychiatrists, as Fink puts it, with "the external superego power of absolution usually reserved for priests." (1983, 677). Psychiatrists have thus been blamed, and not entirely without just cause, for being the harbingers of an era of situational ethics and the self-proclaimed experts on social issues beyond the scope of the consulting room. In 1960, Stephen Sondheim's lyrics in *West Side Story* took note of this trend in the unforgettable song "Officer Krupke," in which juvenile delinquents urge a policeman to go easy on them since they are "misunderstood" and "psychologically disturbed" rather than criminal or antisocial.

Another area in which satirical portrayals of psychiatrists are disconcertingly close to reality is their use of obfuscating jargon. As early as 1931, the alienist in Lewis Milestone's *The Front Page* utters the phrase "dementia praecox," even as he is collapsing to the floor with a bullet wound in his leg. Unfortunately, psychiatrists must plead nolo contendere to the charge that they have enhanced the trend toward mystification by talking and writing in a tongue that is as unfamiliar as a foreign language to most outsiders. Another frequent fantasy, that psychiatrists are always analyzing those around them, even at social situations, is neatly captured in the scene from Claudia Weill's *It's My Turn* (1980) in which a psychiatrist condescendingly refers to another man's beard as "a classic case of compensatory displacement." While psychiatrists would like to view this behavior as only a movie stereotype, anyone who travels in psychiatric circles is familiar with individuals who offer free and wild analyses of persons who are not their patients in an effort to impress their friends over cocktails. Hence, the psychiatrist in *It's My Turn* is certainly a stereotype and a figure laden with transference distortions, but he is nevertheless based on a kernel of truth.

In the final analysis, of course, art owes no debt to reality. Filmmakers and screenwriters are in no way obligated to present portraits of psychiatrists that are acceptable to the psychiatric profession. And as we have attempted to demonstrate throughout this study, the question of "realism" may even be a red herring in the study of cinema, a medium that seems to communicate almost entirely through myths and conventions. Furthermore, while there is surely some relationship between cinematic art and its sociohistorical moment, too many other factors complicate the specific issue addressed in this study, the image of psychiatry. While filmmakers are certainly free to portray psychiatrists in any way they wish, the graver question is to what extent they influence patients' or potential patients' inclinations to seek or accept psychiatric help.

THE REACTION OF PATIENTS

We have known mental health professionals who are highly skeptical when we suggest that cinematic images of psychiatrists may seriously influence a person's attitude toward his current or future therapist. Any intelligent person, the argument goes, can discriminate between the celluloid image and the real thing. We strongly disagree with this argument, which paints the moviegoer as a sophisticated and rational thinker who is beyond the influence of unconscious forces. We would submit that media images work on us unconsciously throughout our lives, even if we consciously reject the film stereotypes that we see. The cumulative effect of viewing film after film is the creation of a mental warehouse full of internal stereotypes stored in preconscious and unconscious memory banks. The laconic cowboy, the mad scientist, the whore with a heart of gold, and the socially inept intellectual are all examples of such internal stereotypes. Madison Avenue has long been aware of the power of these subliminally perceived and stored images, and its denizens have used them to sell everything from toothpaste to political candidates.

While we would argue that the *average* person may not be adept at distinguishing the objective reality of a particular occupation from its distorted image in the media, it is intuitively obvious that the ability of emotionally disturbed individuals, who may already experience compromised reality testing, is even more impaired. We have seen numerous clinical examples of this phenomenon. After viewing *One Flew over the Cuckoo's Nest,* a patient in a psychiatric hospital revoked his previously given consent for electroconvulsive treatments. He explained that after seeing ECT administered in the film, he wanted no part of such treatment, thus depriving himself of a badly needed and clearly indicated intervention. Another hospitalized patient walked out of *Frances* after a scene in which patients are raped by a series of sailors who have been smuggled into the hospital by a psychiatric aide. The patient, who reported that the film made her feel "like the whole world was out to get me," said she had previously felt her own hospital unit to be a safe place, but that the movie made her question both the motives of mental health professionals and their worthiness of her trust. We are also familiar with a case in which the family of a hospitalized patient refused to consent to ECT because of its depiction in *Cuckoo's Nest*.

Psychiatric patients come to the consulting room with expectations of how a psychiatrist should behave based on what they see in movies. After witnessing Elizabeth McGovern's forbidden wish acted out with Dudley Moore in *Lovesick*, one female analytic patient told her analyst that she was haunted by the thought that the boundaries of the psychoanalytic situation might not be as clear as she had thought. She commented that if she developed erotic feelings in the transference, she might not be so willing to talk about them. These thoughts came from a patient who was relatively sophisticated in terms of her knowledge of psychoanalytic and psychiatric ethics. One can only speculate on the impact of such a movie on prospective patients who have never seen a psychiatrist or who do not know one. A male patient in psychotherapy with a female therapist had spent over two years working through a highly sexualized transference. Near the end of his psychotherapy, he also saw *Lovesick* and reported that it was deeply disturbing to him. He said that if he had seen it when he first came to treatment, he would have been much less likely to discuss his feelings so openly with this therapist. He told his therapist that the movie left him with the impression that different therapists apply different ethical standards to their relations with their patients.

Just as portrayals of negatively tinged stereotypes may lead patients to expect that their psychiatrists will somehow violate them, more positive portrayals may similarly result in a patient developing unrealistic expectations of an idealized sort. A young female college student who had seen *Ordinary People*, for example, came to psychotherapy for a variety of interpersonal difficulties. After several weeks of therapy, the patient, who carried a diagnosis of borderline personality disorder, was growing increasingly frustrated with her therapist. She insisted that he should behave more like Judd Hirsch in *Ordinary People*. She wanted him to be less formal, and more specifically, she wanted him to hug her, just as Judd Hirsch had embraced Timothy Hutton. The therapist made an educational comment about his reasons for thinking that hugging her would not be in her best interests. The patient was not satisfied with his explanation and demanded, "If Judd Hirsch can do it, why can't you?" Her therapist maintained his position, and a split transference developed early in the psychotherapy, with Judd Hirsch's Dr. Berger representing the idealized, all good object and the actual therapist representing the devalued, all bad object. The behavior of the former was continually referred to as a standard that the therapist was failing to live up to.

This vignette demonstrates how even positive portrayals of psychiatrists in films may have adverse clinical implications because they may lead to false and overidealized expectations of what a psychiatrist can and will do for them. Patients who have seen dramatic results from the cinematic version of the cathartic cure are often prone to expect similar results in their own psychotherapy. Numerous patients come to psychotherapy fully expecting to immerse themselves in detective work, collaborating with their therapists to uncover the single repressed traumatic memory that has created all their symptoms. These patients may beg their therapists to hypnotize them so that they can delve into the dark recesses of their minds to locate the missing link between etiology and cure. The belief that the derepression of a buried traumatic memory will lead to cure can serve as a powerful resistance to therapeutic or analytic progress if patients repeatedly take flight from the here-and-now transference situation in search of dark secrets in their past. Patients near the end of lengthy psychoanalytic treatments often express some disappointment that they have almost completed their treatments without a blinding flash of insight, accompanied by the uncontrolled affective storm depicted in the movies.

In the vignette describing the college student's infatuation with the Judd Hirsch character in *Ordinary People,* her psychiatrist eventually felt that he must see the movie so that he could understand more of what she was talking about. After viewing the film himself, he felt much better equipped to deal with the patient's demands and to understand her expectations of him. One of the clinical implications of movie depictions of psychiatrists is that therapists ought to have some familiarity with their screen images so that they are in tune with the meanings of these images to patients. A knowledge of relevant films can be a significant benefit in one's work with patients. One striking example of this benefit occurred when a young professional woman, in her third year of analysis, brought the following dream to her analyst: "I was standing naked in a bedroom drying myself off after a shower. A menacing sort of man was in the room with me. At first I was embarrassed; then I was not. I sat on his lap, and he had some sort of mask on his face so that I could not see who he was. I became increasingly frightened as he sat down on the bed with me. He leaned his head back on my breasts; and his mask fell off, revealing the face of Michael Caine. I woke up in a state of panic." The analyst asked for the patient's associations to the dream as he would any other dream. The patient's associations were not particularly productive in deepening the material or in shedding light on the meaning of the dream. The analyst, remembering that she had made a reference to having seen *Dressed to Kill* not long ago, interpreted to her that the appearance of Michael Caine in the dream could be understood as a way of symbolizing her analyst in disguised form, since she had recently seen Michael Caine play the role of a psychiatrist in a movie. This interpretation resulted in a breakthrough in the patient's associations. She expressed intense anxiety that, just as in *Dressed to Kill,* there would be destructive consequences were she to reveal her sexual feelings toward her analyst. She worried that her father had physically abused her because she had been seductive toward him and was terrified that the same situation would be repeated in the transference even though she rationally and consciously knew that her analyst would not actually be violent toward her. Hence the movie image of Michael Caine as a psychotic and violent psychiatrist had been appropriated by her unconscious to represent a not yet conscious tranference fantasy about her analyst. Her analyst's knowledge of that film enabled him to be in better touch with her unconscious and to make an appropriate intervention that led to a deepening of her associations. While it is certainly not realistic to think that all psychiatrists should keep up with the current cinematic releases, this dream beautifully demonstrates how screen images come to inhabit the unconscious minds of the moviegoers and surface in the consulting room.

These clinical vignettes illustrate how psychiatric patients leave movies with conscious and unconscious expectations of certain behavior from their psychiatrists. But is only the patient half of the therapist-patient dyad affected by these depictions? To some extent characters in movies teach us all how to function in our respective roles in society. John Wayne showed generations of men how to be manly. Marilyn Monroe taught women how to be sexy. Even though we may abhor these stereotypes, we cannot question their influence on how people function with one another and how they view themselves. Psychiatrists have no professional immunity from this influence. A resident psychiatrist told his psychotherapy supervisor somewhat sheepishly that he had been so taken by Judd Hirsch's engaging portrayal that he had tried to affect some of those qualities in his own behavior toward patients. He even confessed that he had borrowed some lines from the character of Dr. Berger verbatim! An elderly analyst admitted that he had originally chosen psychiatry because of Claude Rains's portrayal of Dr. Jaquith in *Now Voyager.* Most likely he was responding to the character's aura since Dr. Jaquith engages in virtually no psychotherapeutic work in the film. Another middle-aged psychiatrist acknowledged that his viewing of *The Three Faces of Eve* as a teenager had convinced him to become a psychiatrist. This same psychiatrist recalled his early disenchantment with the painstakingly slow pace of psychotherapy as compared to his expectations that it would be as dramatic as that depicted in the movies of his adolescence. One can only speculate on how many therapists may secretly have nagging doubts that they are not living up to the standards of their favorite movie psychiatrist. The influence of cinematic portrayals of psychiatry cannot, then, be dismissed as trivial. Its impact on patient, therapist, and the treatment itself may be protean and elusive at times, but it is a significant and far-reaching one.

THE IMAGE OF PSYCHIATRY

Psychiatry's image problem in the twenty years since the Golden Age has certainly not been confined to the movies. Statistics reflecting the trends in recruitment of medical students into the specialty of psychiatry are particularly revealing in terms of the decline in respect for the discipline. A consistent figure of 7 percent of medical school graduates entered psychiatry from the post–World War II period through the 1950s and into the early 1960s (Nielsen 1980). Beginning in 1965 there is a noticeable drop in the number of medical school graduates specializing in psychiatry. This decline continues gradually right on through into the 1970s, when a 50 percent decrease in the percentage of graduates entering psychiatry is recorded by the end of the decade. Although psychiatry, particularly psychoanalysis, is one of the least remunerative medical specialties in terms of rewards for time spent in training, there are other reasons for the decline in medical student interest. Yager and Scheiber (1981) found that the negative public image of psychiatry was one of the primary reasons that students were shunning psychiatry as a specialty. They specifically cite media images of evil or foolish psychiatrists as contributing to these negative feelings.

A corresponding decrease in federal funding of psychiatric research and education can be documented in the same historical pattern. Adjusting for inflation, grant support from the National Institute of Mental Health leveled off around the mid-1960s after almost two decades of dramatic increases (Pardes and Pincus 1983). This plateau was followed by a steady decline from the mid-1960s to 1980. A parallel but even more dramatic pattern can be traced for the amount of money NIMH set aside for its clinical training budget designated for psychiatric education (Pardes and Pincus 1983).

This decline in the public image of psychiatry, in the career interest of medical students, and in the funding of psychiatric research and education parallels the historical trend we have outlined in the cinematic attitude toward psychiatrists with uncanny synchrony. Whether the fall from grace in the movies is the partial cause or the partial result of the parallel pattern in society at large is a "chicken-egg" question that is probably unanswerable. Presumably, both processes mutually influence each other. Students clearly come to medical school with the same biases against psychiatry that characterize most graduating medical students. In another study, Yager et al. (1982) found no significant differences between the attitudes of first- and fourth-year medical students toward the specialty of psychiatry. The students surveyed viewed psychiatry as unscientific and imprecise as well as less prestigious than other medical specialties. These preconceived biases are apparently further reinforced through the negative opinions expressed by other specialists during their training years. If these negative views are preexisting, one can assume that they must, at least in part, stem from negative portrayals in the media, including movies. As Linter (1979) has pointed out, while the electronic media cannot be entirely responsible for the prejudicial attitudes toward psychiatrists, they play a prominent role in perpetuating and broadening the stigma.

Despite the historical trends we have outlined in the cinematic portrayal of psychiatrists, the public at large has always maintained a split view of psychotherapists and psychoanalysts. On the one hand, there is awe at their perceived knowledge of the mysterious workings of the unconscious mind. Existing side by side with this idealization and reverence is contempt for their limitations, disappointment related to their failure to solve all of the social ills of the world, and devaluation associated with their inability even to solve the personal ills of the individual. Depending on the social and psychological forces of the time, the idealized or the devalued aspect may predominate, but underlying all historical epochs there is this pervasive contradiction in our attitudes toward psychiatrists. Their perceived omniscience is envied and feared, so mental health professionals must be continually ridiculed and put in their place to neutralize these negative feelings. Movies reflect this process by continually seeking to demonstrate that psychiatrists, and analysts in particular, are vulnerable to the same human frailties as everyone else. Those of us in the mental health professions may simply respond with, "So what? We already knew that." However, the fantasy that psychoanalysts and psychotherapists are somehow perfect or superior to everyone else dies hard; and there seems to be a need to confirm repeatedly that they are not perfect. One is reminded of the humorous definition: "A psychoanalyst is someone who pretends he doesn't know everything."

When psychiatrists react with hurt and defensiveness to the celluloid images on the screen, they probably do little to help their cause. The choice of psychotherapy as a profession entails the acceptance that one must serve as a target for a variety of primitive feelings in one's patients. If the therapist can accept that his role as transference object transcends the consulting room and spreads onto the movie screen, one can view the distortions with detached curiosity, with empathy, and with understanding, just as one approaches transference reactions in patients. As Fink (1983) points out, several recent surveys of public attitudes convey a predominant message that there is still basically a positive image of the profession despite all the negative publicity. In the meantime, psychiatrists and other psychotherapists can content themselves with the fact that the rash of films made about them reflects an intense interest in psychiatry on the part of filmmakers and on the part of film audiences. To paraphrase Oscar Wilde, the only thing worse than being portrayed in movies negatively is not being portrayed in movies at all.

PART·TWO

The Psychiatrist at the Movies

Methodology and Psychoanalytic Film Criticism

7

■ As Robert B. Ray (1985) has written, American movies are "massively overdetermined." Numerous, often overlapping forces—ideological, sociological, financial, historical, technological, political—have governed what Americans see at the movies. In part 1 we attempted to identify how the changing images of psychiatrists in American movies can be understood in terms of many of these forces. In doing so, we occasionally made use of psychoanalytic interpretations, suggesting, for example, that Freud's understanding of "displacement" in the dream work can explain how movies often displace forbidden subjects, such as sex or politics, into sanctioned conventions of melodrama (Eckert 1974). But as we hope the previous chapters have demonstrated, many other forces lie behind the repertory of conventions with which the American cinema has portrayed the psychiatrist.

In the four chapters that follow, we rely almost exclusively on psychoanalytic thinking to interpret several recent films. These films address unconscious forces so compellingly that we have found psychoanalytically informed methodologies to be the most effective means toward understanding them. The best complement to a study of the cinema's mythology of psychiatry is a psychoanalytic inquiry into how movies actually play on the mind.

The application of Freudian and post-Freudian thought to movies, however, has recently become a controversial subject, especially in the wake of the semiotic revolution in film studies. Originally the study of the sign systems which generate language and communication, semiotics now embraces how meaning is generated in any system, including human gestures, road signs, literature, painting, and music as well as film. The particular kind of emphasis that semiotic film critics place on theoretical constructs is a relatively new phenomenon, especially in the United States. In the early 1970s, when film study first became a recognized discipline in American universities, there were few American documents purporting to establish a poetics for the movies. The principal film theorists were Europeans such as Eisenstein, Pudovkin, Bazin, and Kracauer, but in America there was little except the films themselves. The theoretical writings of D. W. Griffith, for example, seem somewhat absurd today: the most important principle of filmmaking, according to Griffith, was matching the action to the "human pulse beat" (Monaco 1981, 311). (The most seminal statements by American film critics are collected in Mast and Cohen 1985.) Systematic examinations of American movies first began to appear in French periodicals, most notably *Cahiers du cinéma* (Hillier 1985). In the 1950s, the contributors to this journal included François Truffaut, Jean-Luc Godard, Jacques Rivette, Claude Chabrol, and Eric Rohmer, all of whom would go on to make movies, almost always engaging in some kind of dialogue with the classical Hollywood cinema. These filmmakers took American movies much more seriously than did Americans themselves, largely because they saw film in terms of the "politique des auteurs" rather than as entertainment or as sociological document. The *auteur* theory of cinema—which sees the director as the true author of a film—can be understood as another way of "centering" the reading of a film around a single artistic vision, giving movies the same aesthetic legitimacy as, for example, a symphony of Beethoven or a painting of Van Gogh. But these filmmakers and subsequent *Cahiers* theorists also incorporated ideas from thinkers who worked at "decentering" critical study away from a unifying subject. They appropriated Italian semiotics as well as the work of French-speaking theorists such as Ferdinand de Saussure, the founder of modern linguistics, and the structural anthropologist Claude Lévi-Strauss. After France was struck by the cultural upheavals of 1968, the *Cahiers* critics incorporated the more politically charged ideas of Louis Althusser, Roland Barthes, Julia Kristeva, and the most eminent philosophical critic of centers, Jacques Derrida. They also began reading the post-Freudian psychology of Jacques Lacan, whose most important student in the field of film theory has been Christian Metz (1982). All of these thinkers concerned themselves in some way with the "deep structures" that film theorists saw at work in the movies. The *Cahiers* critics have been extremely successful if only in terms of their influence: by the mid-1970s, a new generation of film critics with roots in French theory and semiotics was writing prolifically about film in England and the United States as well as in France. Other journals, such as *Screen* in England, *Communications* in France, and *Camera Obscura* in the United States, began printing articles that drew almost exclusively upon methodologies established by the *Cahiers* critics.

One of the most fascinating effects of the semiotic revolution in film criticism has been the rediscovery of Freud in the academy. Many professors of psychology were telling their students in the 1960s and 1970s that Freud's writings were obsolete at the same time that, as we have demonstrated in the previous chapters, the prestige of psychoanalysis was declining in the Hollywood cinema. Curiously, attacks on psychiatrists in the movies were most pronounced during the same years that Freud was becoming increasingly important to film theorists. The writings of Lacan have been extremely fashionable in American universities for several years now, and Metz has made Freudian thought a crucial ingredient in semiotically based film theory. As of this writing, Metz's work verges on orthodoxy in many university cinema study programs.

Nevertheless, psychoanalytic film criticism is controversial because of the often pugnacious stands of both the semioticians and their detractors. Some of the psychoanalytically inclined writers who embrace French theory insist that all previous film criticism, especially in America, is hopelessly impressionistic and unsystematic. Furthermore, the theorists charge that earlier film criticism seldom has a valid methodological basis and that it borrows its operating principles haphazardly from disciplines such as literature, theater, or sociology. Film semioticians claim to find a rigorous, scientific methodology in the actual language of film rather than in, say, the stale formalism of 1950s literary criticism. Obviously, writers who find themselves the objects of these attacks do not enjoy being told that everything they have written is outdated and useless. Critics outside the semioticians' circles argue that the new methodologies are so top-heavy with theoretical formulations (concentrating on what Metz calls "cinema" rather than "film") that the actual movies themselves become secondary: the analysis of specific films becomes the handmaiden of theory. Moreover, as William Rothman (Nichols 1976, 438–51) has argued in his critique of a semiotic analysis of cinematic codes by Daniel Dayan (Nichols 1976, 451–59), the methodological principles of the French theorists can lead to the same kinds of imprecise generalizations with which "impressionistic" critics have been charged.

Perhaps the most important contribution of the French theorists and their disciples has been the creation of an intellectual climate that compels critics to lay their methodological cards on the table, robbing them of the assumption that their readers share the innumerable unspoken judgments that are made long before the actual writing takes place. Later on in this chapter we will attempt to spell out the methodological principles which govern part 2 of this study, but first we will survey the important psychoanalytic elements of contemporary cinema semiotics in order to establish how our approach is different. It is difficult, however, to locate the precise boundaries of current trends in psychoanalytic film theory because so many writers have so thoroughly incorporated Freud's legacy into the larger semiotic project. In fact, Kaja Silverman has argued that Freudian psychoanalysis should be considered "a branch of semiotics" (1983, 194). Like many other writers in this tradition, Silverman's film criticism overlaps psychoanalysis with linguistics, Marxism, feminism, and the theories of kinship structures developed by Lévi-Strauss.

Jacques Lacan, the most important writer in this psychoanalytic component, presents problems for even the most advanced student of contemporary film criticism. As devout a reader as Silverman has written: "Lacan's prose is notoriously remote, and his presentation deliberately a-systematic. Many of the terms to which he most frequently returns constantly shift meaning. These qualities make it almost impossible to offer definitive statements about the Lacanian argument; indeed, Lacan himself almost never agreed with his commentators" (1983, 150). It is therefore impossible to define clearly the terms from Lacanian theory that have proven the most useful for semiotic film criticism. Without attempting even a superficial survey of Lacan's work, we will nevertheless touch upon his concepts of the "mirror-stage," the "Imaginary," the "Symbolic," and the subsequent use of his ideas in the concept of "suture" in the cinema.

In his revision of Freudian theory, Lacan locates the Imaginary in the newborn child's pleasure in the sense of complete union with its mother. The child makes no differentiation between itself and its surroundings—blankets, pillows, milk, or nurse as well as mother. "At this point the infant has the status of what Freud describes as an 'oceanic self,' or what Lacan punningly refers to as 'l'hommelette' (a human omelette which spreads in all directions)" (Silverman 1983, 155). Somewhere between the ages of six and eighteen months, the child sees its image in a mirror and experiences this reflection as the first illustration of a unified self-concept (Laplanche and Pontalis 1973, 250–52). The child, however, *misrecognizes* its image in the mirror as more coordinated and focused than it actually is, projecting this reflected body outside itself as an ego-ideal. Later, when this ego-ideal has been introjected, the child acquires the desire to identify with others, a crucial aspect in the experience yet to come of finding pleasure in identifying with characters in movies.

For our purposes, the most important element in this formulation is the child's exclusive understanding of itself through projection and hence its inability to see itself except in terms of the Other. Lacan also suggests that the infant develops a dramatically ambivalent relationship with this reflected self, both loving it (for possessing the child's ideal image) and hating it (for being outside the child's body). Consequently, the child gains a facility that it will later use at the movies, the ability to identify alternately with the exhibitionist and the voyeur, the master and the slave, the victim and the victimizer. Lacan has called this ambivalent order, with its extremes of love and hate, "the Imaginary." Metz takes one of his most important titles from this concept: *The Imaginary Signifier* (1982) suggests that identifying ourselves with the visual images we encounter in the cinema replicates our childhood experiences. The irresistible appeal of movies resides in their close relationship with the mirror stage, a moment in our development when we first begin confusing self with Other.

Only when we acquire language and the structures that go with it do we enter into what Lacan calls "the Symbolic" even though the images produced during the Imaginary stage are still present. The Symbolic serves merely to control these images and to derive meaning from them. Lacan posits a close association between the Symbolic order and the oedipal crisis; in fact, he even goes so far as to suggest that the primordial law of the oedipus complex is identical with the order of language (Lacan 1977, 66). Since language is the means by which we structure the world, and since the oedipal crisis is only resolved by assimilating the patriarchal values by which this structuring takes place, the child acquires a controlling awareness of sexual difference along with the Symbolic order. In particular, Lacanian discourse involves the concept of "lack," both as the phallocentric key to sexual difference and in the more symbolic sense of seeing the world in terms of absence and presence.

Over the last few decades, semiotics has influenced numerous disciplines by deflecting study away from the "meaning" of a text and toward the processes through which any assumed meaning is generated. Similarly, the appropriation of Lacanian psychoanalysis by cinema semioticians centers on how audiences experience movies, particularly the narrative films of classic Hollywood. Rather than psychoanalyzing the characters or the filmmakers, students of Lacan address the complex means by which the cinematic apparatus invokes the Imaginary and Symbolic orders of the typical viewer. The key word in this process is "suture," a controversial term whose validity is difficult to verify since it grows out of theory rather than empirical observation. The cinematic application of this Lacanian concept was first developed in a pair of articles published in 1969 in *Cahiers du cinéma* by Jean-Pierre Oudart (1978). Oudart's ideas have been appropriated variously and perhaps incompletely: David Bordwell, for example, argues that Oudart's commentators have overlooked the most interesting aspects of his theory (1985, 111). At any rate, suture is usually understood in terms of a medical metaphor implying that cinematic gaps created by cutting or editing are "sewed" shut to include the viewer, who identifies himself with some aspect of the "gaze" created by the camera (Dayan in Nichols 1976, 451–59). Instead of asking "Who is watching this?" and "Who is ordering these images?" the viewer accepts what he is seeing as natural, even when the camera's gaze shifts most abruptly from one character or scene to another. Suture works because of the cinematic code that makes each shot appear as the object of the gaze of whoever appears in the shot that follows, the most commonly cited example being the "shot/reverse shot" formulation in which each of two characters is viewed alternately over the other's shoulder. We do not ask "Who is watching?" because each shot answers the question for the previous shot. The Israeli theoretician Daniel Dayan calls this "the tutor-code of classical cinema": "Unable to see the workings of the code, the spectator is at its mercy. His Imaginary is sealed into the film" (Nichols 1976, 449).

The operation of suture within a particular film determines the unique way that we experience that film, especially how we are affected by its subtext. From our limited understanding of this constantly redefined concept, we offer examples of how a semiotician might describe the operation of suture in two Golden Age films, *Suddenly, Last Summer* (1959) and *Psycho* (1960). A crucial scene in *Suddenly, Last Summer* takes place when Dr. Cukrowicz (Montgomery Clift) first meets Catherine (Elizabeth Taylor) while she is under the supervision of a nun in a mental hospital. Clift is in the foreground of the shot when Taylor enters without seeing him. He drifts out of the frame to the left, stationing himself behind a bookcase while he observes an exchange between the victimized Taylor and the victimizing nun. Although the audience cannot see Clift, and although the camera shifts back and forth between Taylor and the nun, the entire scene is played out under his gaze. When the tormented Taylor unintentionally burns the nun's hand with a cigarette, Clift emerges from the left side of the frame and saves her from imminent punishment. Later on when the corrupt hospital director, Hockstader (Albert Dekker), demands that Taylor be lobotomized, he cites the hand-burning incident as evidence of her violent behavior. Clift insists that "she was provoked," a judgment that the audience can verify, having seen the entire episode from his point of view. We identify with Clift because we have become him, watching the same scene with his compassionate perspective and projecting him as our surrogate into the action to rescue the helpless and pulchritudinous heroine.

To our knowledge, no feminist film critics have written on *Suddenly, Last Summer,* but the work of Mulvey (Mast and Cohen 1985, 803–16), Doane (1982), Kuhn (1982), and de Lauretis (1984) establishes the basis for a feminist/Lacanian reading of the scene we have just described: the cinematic apparatus of the commercial cinema has historically served the interests of patriarchy, privileging the gaze of the male hero and subordinating the heroine as the object of the gaze. When Montgomery Clift emerges from behind the camera to save Elizabeth Taylor, he is part of a system that dominates and determines the behavior of the female while simultaneously using her for voyeuristic pleasure. One of the most essential—and one of the most controversial—elements of Lacanalysis is the suggestion that the female body creates anxiety for men because it represents the possibility of castration. In her extremely influential essay "Visual Pleasure and the Narrative Cinema," Laura Mulvey (Mast and Cohen 1985, 803–16) has suggested that the patriarchal camera style of classical Hollywood can assuage this anxiety only by submitting women to the male order or by fetishizing their bodies. Although Mulvey devotes her attention primarily to films by Sternberg and Hitchcock, her thesis would explain the voyeuristic abstraction of women's bodies that takes place throughout the history of the American cinema, most notably in the final reels of numerous Busby Berkeley musicals.

Psycho provides a more complex example of suture. As in Busby Berkeley's fanciful dance sequences, Hitchcock's camera seems to take on a life of its own even though we are expected to understand Hitchcock's films as a much closer replication of the "real" than we are Berkeley's production numbers. Specifically, Hitchcock's camera seems to perform feats that destroy any possibility that it might possess the gaze of a character in the film. In fact, *Psycho* begins with several establishing shots of Phoenix, Arizona, in which the camera seems to float across the city, searching for one specific window. It ultimately closes in on this window, finding a small opening beneath the venetian blinds, which have been pulled down almost all the way. The camera then appears to glide through this tiny space and into a hotel room occupied by two partially clad lovers (Janet Leigh and John Gavin). Not only has the camera (and the spectator) violated the laws of gravity; the impossible entrance into the room also constitutes a violation of the lovers' privacy, one which recalls the primal scene and its subsequent anxieties. We identify with the gaze of the camera at our own peril.

Another example of a purposeful camera operating in *Psycho* without the gaze of a predetermined character takes place just after the famous shower murder: a close-up of the dead Marion (Leigh) alone in her motel room is the point of departure for a tracking shot that leaves the bathroom, traverses the bed, pauses to glance at the newspaper containing the stolen money, and then looks out the window to the house where Norman Bates (Anthony Perkins) can be heard shouting, "Mother! Oh God, Mother! Blood, blood!" Silverman has described this shot as essential to the complex system of suture, keeping the narrative going after we have lost our heroine. We identified with her in the shower even though the camera frequently threw us back into the Imaginary by letting us experience the murder from several points of view, from that of the victim, the victimizer, and even the shower head. The extent of our complicity in the murder becomes clear when the camera becomes the only "living" thing in the bathroom. Silverman describes the tracking shot that closes momentarily on the stolen money as the promise that the narrative will continue: "What sutures us at this juncture is the fear of being cut off from the narrative" (Silverman 1983, 212). To satisfy us, the shot continues out the window to the house from which Norman Bates appears, the next object with whom we can identify. Spectators at a screening of *Psycho* are so hungry for suture that they do not rebel against a film that not only implicates them in murder and voyeurism but even exposes its own workings. What they eventually get for their trouble is narrative closure, the comforting statements of a psychiatrist who exorcises their terror with the authority of science. Critics who scoff at the pronouncements of Dr. Richmond call attention to the transgressions into which we have voluntarily let ourselves be sutured as well as to the final shot of Anthony Perkins, which once again makes us identify with a missing Other. This Absent One (Oudart 1978) is the same unattached camera that has brought us into the terror of the Imaginary and that is completely outside the discourse of the psychiatrist.

Not every critic has agreed with this account of how the viewer is constructed in classical cinema. Robin Wood, for example, alluding to studies by feminist/ Lacanian critics such as Mulvey, rejects the notion that the camera of Hitchcock and others instructs women both to collude in the punishment of transgressing women and to accept the dominant male order (Wood 1986, 247). He argues that something quite different often takes place, citing Hitchcock's *Vertigo* as an extreme case: "From the moment when Hitchcock allows us access to the consciousness of Judy/Kim Novak, the male identification position is undermined beyond all possibility of recuperation; no spectator of either sex, surely, acquiesces in Judy's death or perceives the male protagonist's treatment of her as other than monstrous and pathological" (Wood 1986, 247). Raymond Durgnat goes even farther, questioning Lacan's comparison of the spectator's mental operations to pathological conditions: "Lacan's theoretical scoptophilia is fatal to the study of film, since its logical correlative is self-castration by superego forces" (1982, 61).

As we suggested earlier, psychoanalytic film criticism seldom exists in a vacuum. The most interesting theoreticians of suture, such as Dayan and the

Screen critics Stephen Heath (1981) and Colin MacCabe (1985), have expanded the concept to include a Marxist perspective, particularly Althusser's reading of Lacan. In "Ideology and Ideological State Apparatuses (Notes towards an Investigation)" (1971), Althusser argues that ideology represents the Imaginary relationship of individuals to their material conditions. The system of suture, relying on a highly complex technology manipulated by a major commercial industry, is responsible for "naturalizing" the ideology articulated artificially but persuasively by this industry. These critics frequently succeed in demystifying Hollywood movies, revealing the psychological means by which they bind audiences to their cultures. The *Screen* critics have probably made the most important contributions to film theory in recent years even if their prose often renders their writings inaccessible to many film students. Nevertheless, their theoretical positions are becoming increasingly influential, providing critics with the basis for many of the most thorough readings of American films.

We should point out that many critics who rely upon psychoanalysis do not depend exclusively upon the semiotic methodologies of Lacan, Metz, and Althusser. Stanley Cavell (1981b) and Robin Wood (1986) read Freud for quite different purposes, but both have worked psychoanalytic thought into original and convincing readings of specific films. Some of the most interesting work of the last few years has been in the relationship between film and the "dream screen," an area researched by Bruce Kawin (1978), Marsha Kinder (1980), and Robert Eberwein (1984). Jane Feuer (1982) has even appropriated dream analysis into a study of the Hollywood musical. Robert B. Ray (1985), whose book we cited at the beginning of this chapter, has transcended the rigidly theoretical orientations of the *Screen* and *Cahiers* critics, taking from them what he needs while developing a method for discovering the basic paradigms of the American cinema. What distinguishes a critic such as Ray is the clarity of his prose and his thorough readings of important films. He adopts a pluralistic approach based primarily in the deep structures discovered by Freud, Althusser, and Lévi-Strauss, but without the "mixture of over-precision and vagueness" that characterizes much of semiotic film theory (Durgnat 1982, 62). Too often cinema semioticians are so locked into one system that they tend to find the same set of signs over and over again in each film. Unlike a more versatile writer such as Ray, Lacanian film critics return repeatedly to motifs of castration and absence even when a film's content may suggest other approaches.

In the chapters that follow, we hope to illustrate the potential for pluralism in psychoanalytic film criticism. We have based our work in this section on concepts derived from a wide array of clinical psychoanalytic literature. Like the clinician who adopts different theoretical positions according to the needs of different patients, we have used a variety of perspectives to illuminate several quite different films. While the Lacanian approach has produced intriguing accounts of film as process, we are more interested in the films themselves, in their texts, subtexts, themes, and characters. Each of these films invites different degrees of explanatory power from a variety of theoretical formulations. In addition, we have attempted to flesh out our interpretations by drawing upon relevant information that may not always be grounded in psychoanalysis. For example, we frequently quote statements that the filmmakers have made to interviewers, realizing that the artists themselves may have much to tell us even if we do not subject their statements to psychoanalytic interpretation.

The methodological problems encountered in the psychoanalytic understanding of film are essentially no different than those intrinsic to the field of applied psychoanalysis as a whole. This bastard child of clinical psychoanalysis has always been viewed ambivalently by critics within psychoanalysis itself, by those skeptical of Freud's work, and certainly by the semioticians. Clinical psychoanalysis is anchored to the here-and-now phenomena of transference and resistance and to the associations of a patient who attempts to put aside his psychological censor and say whatever comes to his mind. Applied psychoanalysis runs the risk of losing its way once the consulting room has been left behind. From Freud's earliest forays into the application of psychoanalytic ideas to art, literature, and biography, these difficulties have regularly been acknowledged. Artistic creations, books, letters, and diaries have been used as substitutes for free associations and transference material. As Freud himself realized, these substitutes could in no way compare with bona fide clinical data from the consulting room. He noted in *Moses and Monotheism:* "I am very well aware that in dealing so autocratically and arbitrarily with Biblical tradition—bringing it up to confirm my views when it suits me and unhesitatingly rejecting it when it contradicts me—I am exposing myself to serious methodological criticism and weakening the convincing force of my arguments. But this is the only way in which one can treat material of which one knows definitely that its trustworthiness has been severely impaired by the distorting influence of tendentious purposes. It is to be hoped that I shall find some degree of justification later on, when I come upon the track of these secret motives. Certainty is in any case unattainable, and moreover it may be said that every other writer on the subject has adopted the same procedure" (1939, 27).

Coltrera (1981), in an elegantly argued essay on the methodological problems inherent in the application of psychoanalytic principles to biography, emphasizes that Freud never claimed that his proposed reconstructions regarding such historical figures as Leonardo (Freud 1910) were meant to be taken as historical facts. Critics tend to overlook, Coltrera argues, that Freud's only claim was psychoanalytic validity, rather than historical truth, a critical methodological distinction. From Freud's point of view, the Leonardo construction was best viewed as a *Romandichtung,* a fiction intended to be understood as analogical rather than as a literal reconstruction of the artist's actual childhood. "The point is really that Freud's construction is a psychological explanation meant to facilitate understanding and is not an empirical statement about causality. As such, it is valid in that it is consistent within the conditions of its premises; but one may fairly ask whether it is useful as a biographical construction" (Coltrera 1981, 19). Like the semioticians, we make no claims that we have arrived at the definitive reading for each of the films we discuss in the chapters that follow. We are more interested in providing a variety of means for making sense of particular characters or particular movies. More specifically, our emphasis is on how clinical psychoanalytic theory can illuminate the text, the characters, and the subtext of a film as well as the way in which an audience experiences it. Following Coltrera, our aims are to be psychoanalytically valid and internally consistent.

In chapter 8 we apply the knowledge gained from clinical work with narcissistically disturbed patients to shed light on the psychology of the protagonists in two recent cinematic autobiographies, Bob Fosse's *All That Jazz* and Woody Allen's *Stardust Memories.* While some authors, notably Berman (1985), have effectively transformed the creative product of the artist into a window to the psyche of the author, we have avoided analyzing either Fosse or Allen in our approach to these films. Rather, we attempt to analyze the fictional protagonists in these films as though they were real people by applying our understanding of narcissistic character pathology. Even though these films are obviously autobiographical, we do not assume that there is a direct one-to-one psychological correlation between the screenwriter/director and his fictional alter ego on the screen. Furthermore, we have tried to understand the characters in Fosse's and Allen's films in terms of larger cultural patterns that psychoanalytically inclined writers such as Lasch (1979) have identified.

Celebrity worship is such a pervasive phenomenon in our media-dominated culture that we may take it for granted without reflecting on its psychological origins. In chapter 9 we examine three films that explore the theme of the celebrity: Martin Scorsese's *King of Comedy* and two films of Woody Allen, *Zelig* and *The Purple Rose of Cairo.* Through a careful examination of the themes and characters in these three quite different movies, we seek to demonstrate how narcissistic needs and existential anxieties dovetail in the public's creation of idols to love and worship. We believe that our approach provides at least as complete a reading of a film such as *Zelig* as does the recent Lacanian analysis of the film by Feldstein (1985).

In chapters 10 and 11 we approach two films as though they are overdetermined products of the unconscious similar to a dream. Ridley Scott's *Alien* is a powerfully effective horror/science fiction film because it brilliantly evokes primal anxieties of a paranoid nature that lurk in all of us. Just as a dream disguises the unconscious concerns from the dreamer, so does Scott's film present these anxieties in somewhat disguised form that a psychoanalytic reading lays bare. While our approach relies heavily on the formulations of Melanie Klein, it is noteworthy that Dervin (1985) has successfully applied a more classical interpretation, one focused on primal scene imagery, to this film and others. Both levels of interpretation are psychoanalytically valid and internally consistent, and together they reflect the extent to which the themes in movies are multiply determined by issues from various levels of psychosexual development.

Chapter 11 approaches Robert Altman's somewhat obscure chamber movie *3 Women* as though it literally is a dream. Again we do not claim that the interpretation we provide is a literally accurate formulation of Robert Altman's unconscious motives in writing and directing the film. Instead, we claim that looking at the film as though it were the dream of a pubescent girl provides a coherent framework for making sense out of what is otherwise an abstruse and elusive movie.

These four chapters illustrate the multiplicity of theoretical paradigms available to the student of psychoanalysis. The conceptual framework applied to a particular film or films is chosen according to its usefulness in explaining characters, themes, or the text. Self psychology and object relations theory illuminate the films in chapters 8 and 9 because narcissistic issues are of paramount importance. The Kleinian model of pre-oedipal development, specifically the paranoid-schizoid position, provides a basis for understanding the pervasive anxiety generated by *Alien*. Finally, a classically Freudian approach involving oedipal themes elucidates the dreamlike ambiguities of *3 Women* described in chapter 11.

Narcissism in the Cinema I: The Cinematic Autobiography

8

■ Early in Bob Fosse's film *All That Jazz* an aspiring actress (Deborah Geffner) tells director Joe Gideon (Roy Scheider): "I want so to be a movie star. Ever since I was a little kid, I wanted to see my face on the screen, forty feet wide." This comment is whispered into the ear of Gideon as she is in the process of seducing him in exchange for his casting her in his Broadway show. The exchange between them is a microcosmic glimpse of the narcissistic culture in which we live. Christopher Lasch (1979) has compellingly described this culture as one in which there is a worship of celebrity, a fascination and obsession with electronic images produced by the media, a ruthless pursuit of being "visible" and "recognized" despite the fact that there may be no substantive content beneath the image. Moreover, within the corrupt value system of the narcissistic society, the supremacy and security of intimate personal relationships brings disillusionment as well as the exploitation of others for one's own ends.

One of the unique characteristics of our self-absorbed contemporary culture is a pervasive kind of "stage fright," an acute sense of self-consciousness related to a fantasy of a ubiquitous audience (Gabbard 1979 and 1983). As Lasch puts it, "All of us, actors and spectators alike, live surrounded by mirrors. In them, we seek reassurance of our capacity to captivate or impress others, anxiously searching out blemishes that might detract from the appearance that we intend to project" (1979, 2). This sense of always being "on," always performing, always trying to impress has led to an intense self-scrutiny that has resulted in a rapidly increasing flow of confessional writing. Autobiographical and confessional statements now come not just from the great writers and famous actors but from mere show business personalities who are far from being household names.

An even more recent phenomenon is the cinematic autobiography. The medium of film lends itself to narcissistic self-display even better than the novel or the play. What could be more exhibitionistic than to expose one's intimate

189

and private self on the great silver screen and charge admission for people all over the world to bear witness to it? Fosse's *All That Jazz* (1979) and Woody Allen's *Stardust Memories* (1980) have successfully utilized the form of the cinematic autobiography to depict the lives of two troubled artists. Bob Fosse directed and wrote *All That Jazz*, the portrayal of a self-destructive director-choreographer played by Roy Scheider. (Veteran screenwriter Robert Alan Arthur, who shares the film's writing credit with Fosse, died while *All That Jazz* was in production.) Even the sketchiest acquaintance with Fosse's own life reveals that the life of the film's protagonist, Joe Gideon, has striking parallels to Fosse's marriage with dancer Gwen Verdon, his work on the film *Lenny*, his near-fatal heart attack, and his own peculiar contributions to musical comedy choreography, most notably the forward thrust of the female pelvis.

Woody Allen directed, wrote, and starred in *Stardust Memories*, a look at a few days in the life of Sandy Bates, a director struggling with life, love, success, and death while fighting those who condemn his new preference for making serious films instead of funny ones. Allen has denied that the film is directly autobiographical, but Pauline Kael (1980) has made the following observation: "Woody Allen calls himself Sandy Bates this time, but there is only the nearest wisp of a pretext that he is playing a character; this is the most undisguised of his dodgy mock-autobiographical fantasies." Andrew Sarris (1980), on the other hand, while hyperbolically calling *Stardust Memories* "the most mean-spirited and misanthropic film . . . in years and years from anyone anywhere," argues that the film is, in effect, not autobiographical enough because it omits any reference to the more sympathetic people who have cooperated with Allen on his films and because Allen, unlike Sandy Bates, does not appear at retrospectives of his films.

Both films owe an immense debt to Federico Fellini's 1963 masterpiece *8 $\frac{1}{2}$* as does another recent autobiographical film, Paul Mazursky's *Alex in Wonderland* (1971), which actually features Fellini himself in several scenes. Unabashedly autobiographical, Fellini's *8 $\frac{1}{2}$* moves in and out of flashback and fantasy to explore the often funny, often tragic tensions between an artist's life and his work. Allen and Fosse have accepted a number of conventions from *8 $\frac{1}{2}$* almost as if Fellini's film has provided the obligatory framework upon which an autobiographical movie must be constructed. All three films share the cataloging of lovers and wives, the caricaturing of critics and producers, the ceaseless searching for answers to grave problems, the idealizing of the protagonist's innocent youth, and the blurring of distinctions between illusion and reality. In one way or another, both *Stardust Memories* and *All That Jazz* appropriate the double ending of 8 ½, in which Guido (Marcello Mastroianni), the surrogate Fellini, appears to die while at the same time participating in a fantasied procession of the people from his life, which culminates in a reconciliation with loved ones. We should also point out that all three films have made critics uncomfortable—they have all received bitterly negative reviews from many quarters—and that they have provoked speculation about the psychology of their directors.

While writing and directing a movie about one's self may not in and of itself be narcissistic, the point we wish to stress is that *All That Jazz* and *Stardust Memories* both portray protagonists with severe narcissistic problems. The narcissistic difficulties are presented somewhat differently in the two movies, and the vicissitudes of the protagonist's narcissism provide an absorbing experience for the viewer. We will systematically examine the narcissistic themes in each of the movies, comparing them and contrasting them with one another, and we will illustrate how they reflect certain intrapsychic, interpersonal, and cultural phenomena.

Narcissistic Object Relations

Unlike the neurotics of nineteenth-century Viennese culture, the narcissist is less likely to complain of symptoms and more likely to report difficulties in his interpersonal relationships. "The symptomatology of patients with narcissistic personality disturbances . . . tends to be ill defined, and the patient is in general not able to focus on its essential aspects, but he can recognize and describe the secondary complaints (such as work inhibitions or trends toward perverse sexual activities)," reports Kohut, who also describes "subtly experienced, yet pervasive feelings of emptiness and depression" as typical of the narcissistic personality (1971, 16). Kernberg (1974) has identified the type as one who may be superficially smooth and effective in social situations but has serious disturbances in more intimate relationships with others. He may be extremely ambitious to the point of being grandiose, while at the same time feeling inferior and being extremely dependent on the applause and admiration of those around him to maintain his self-esteem. Furthermore, Kernberg states: "Along with feelings of boredom and emptiness, and continuous search for gratification of strivings for brilliance, wealth, power and beauty, there are serious deficiencies in their capacity to love and be concerned about others. This lack of capacity for empathic understanding of others comes as a surprise considering their superficially appropriate social adjustment. Chronic uncertainty and dissatisfaction about themselves, conscious or unconscious exploit-iveness and ruthlessness towards others are also characteristic of these patients" (1974, 215).

Kernberg's words precisely describe Joe Gideon, the central character in *All That Jazz*. Gideon is a womanizing, chain-smoking, heavy-drinking, amphetamine-popping workaholic whose relationships with women are as love-less as they are exploitative. In one of the many fantasied conversations with Angelique, the Angel of Death (Jessica Lange), Gideon is asked if he believes in love. Gideon responds, "I believe in saying I love you. It helps you con-centrate." And furthermore, "It works," meaning he can manipulate the woman in question to obtain the desired results. In a later scene he is arguing with his girlfriend Kate (Ann Reinking) about his infidelity. While Kate angrily expresses her jealousy and her love for Joe, Gideon approaches the interchange as though it were a scene in a play. Kate even coaches him on the reading of his lines to her while he utters stage directions for his statements as though sincerity were a quality that can be taught and affected. Similarly, when he engages in an otherwise serious confrontation with his ex-wife, the entire scene is choreographed, with Gideon making suggestions while his ex-wife works her frustrations into stylized gestures in the dance. When asked by his daughter why he does not get married, Gideon explains that he does not dislike anyone enough to inflict that form of torture on her.

Near the end of the film, when he lies close to death in the hospital, Gideon says to Kate that he really does love her. When Angelique questions his sincerity, he frankly acknowledges that he does not know if he meant it or not. He does not know "where the bullshit ends and the truth begins." In the elaborate fantasy production number prior to his death (plates 29 and 30), Gideon is introduced as a man who "allowed himself to be adored, but not loved." His success in show business, it is said, was matched by a dismal failure in his personal relationships. Even in his wake-up ritual each morning, he looks at himself in the mirror and says with a stylized gesture, "It's show time, folks." Life itself is theater, where feelings are manufactured to "con" the "audience."

Fosse takes a split view of women in *All That Jazz*. On the one hand, the women around Gideon are degraded, exploited sexual playthings, inspiring neither loyalty nor empathy. In contrast, the fantasied Angelique is portrayed as the ideal woman. Dressed in a virginal white wedding gown, she serves as his Horatio in his frequent internal dialogues. This splitting of object repre-sentations is quite typical of the narcissistic personality, as Kernberg (1974) has pointed out. The wise, pure, understanding but seductive Angelique is the idealized representation of woman split off from the devalued sexual objects in

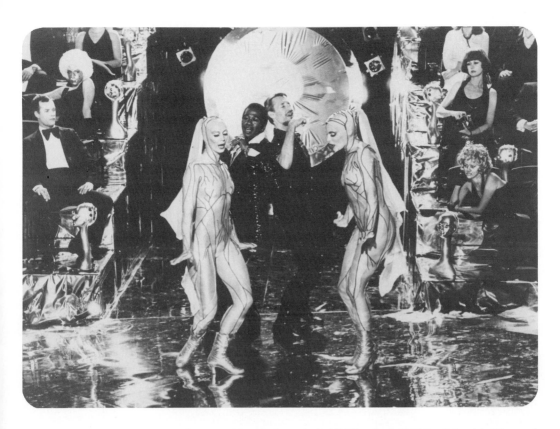

PLATE 29. Bob Fosse's modernist, allegorical musical *All That Jazz* (1979). Columbia Pictures/ Twentieth Century–Fox. The Museum of Modern Art/Film Stills Archive.

external reality. By putting the scenes of Angelique in the setting of a dusty old attic, Fosse suggests that Angelique is an archaic internal object, that is, the good idealized mother who continues to haunt Gideon and who is quite separate from the devalued bad maternal object representation. Appropriately, Angelique is also, like the Belle Dame Sans Merci, both lover and destroyer.

Gideon's devaluation of those about him does not know sexual distinction, however, as almost everyone in Gideon's world is viewed with contempt. This haughty disdain for others, so characteristic of the narcissistic personality, is strikingly revealed in his scene with the producers, composers, and writers of his Broadway show. Fosse makes these other characters into repulsive caricatures with no redeeming qualities. Similarly, in the initial read-through of the show, Gideon is definitively set off from the actors and other staff of the production. Apparently in the first throes of heart disease, Gideon's slightest gesture is greatly magnified by the sound track while an entire roomful of people makes no sound whatever. When he is actually diagnosed as having heart disease and told that he must stay in the hospital, he contemptuously shouts, "What do doctors know?" He denies his condition and repeatedly disobeys the doctor's orders. Kernberg (1974) has noted that chronic and intense envy is often at the core of the narcissist. To avoid envying those around him, Gideon has to devalue the people with whom he comes in contact and to view them as having nothing to offer him. The paradox is, of course, that he is then unable to have his needs met by other people.

Stardust Memories would seem to be based not only on 8 ½ but also on *Sullivan's Travels,* a 1941 American film written and directed by Preston Sturges. Surprisingly, Woody Allen has told Diane Jacobs (1982) that he saw *Sullivan's Travels* only after he had made *Stardust Memories* and Sturges's son sent him a copy. He was, of course, impressed at the "amazingly similar points" that the two films address (Jacobs 1982, 150). In *Sullivan's Travels,* Joel McCrea plays Sullivan, a Hollywood director whose earliest films have been comedies with titles like *Hey Hey in the Hay Loft* and *Ants in Your Pants of 1939.* However, at the outset of the film, he is in a struggle with the studio bosses, who seek to prevent him from making a serious film about human suffering called *Oh Brother Where Art Thou?* In particular, the opening scene of *Sullivan's Travels,* which

PLATE 30. Joe Gideon (Roy Scheider) choreographs his own death in Bob Fosse's *All That Jazz* (1979). Columbia Pictures/Twentieth Century–Fox. The Museum of Modern Art/Film Stills Archive.

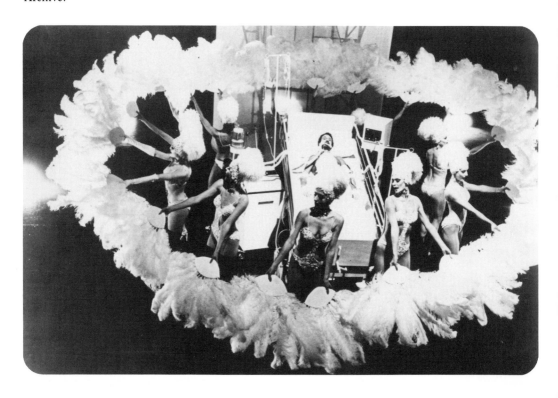

begins with the final moments of Sullivan's film, strongly anticipates the beginning of *Stardust Memories*. However, in *Sullivan's Travels,* after some intense suffering of his own, Sullivan happily decides to return to making funny films. He also enjoys a traditionally romantic and wholesome relationship with a starlet played by Veronica Lake. Although some of the people he encounters wish to exploit him, in general Sullivan fits quite well into his world. By comparison, we can see the extent to which the life and loves of Sandy Bates are involved with narcissistic problems.

The first scene in *Stardust Memories* shows significant differences between Allen's and Fosse's portrayals of narcissism. The opening scene of Allen's film, which plays with images both Bergmanesque and Felliniesque, shows Bates sitting in a chillingly sterile railway coach with an assortment of misfits (plate 31). Another coach on a nearby track is filled with partying beautiful people, and Bates finds himself on the outside looking in. Hence we immediately see that Allen is much less defended against his envy and much more open to acknowledging that other people have good things that he lacks. Allen is more aware of shallowness in interpersonal relationships and much more inclined to poke fun at himself than is Fosse. In *Stardust Memories* a reporter even says that he is doing a piece on the shallow indifference of celebrities and would like to include Bates in the story. Later, Allen's protagonist participates in a brief and degrading sexual relationship with a female groupie, but he has an observer's distance about these affairs. He berates the groupie who wishes to go to bed with him by asking her if she really wants to engage in "mechanical sex with a stranger." When she responds that "empty sex is better than no sex," the film implies that he goes along with her to bed anyway. The difference here is that Allen discourages the entire process and pokes fun at it whereas Fosse seems more serious in his depiction of a strikingly similar scene. When the ambitious female dancer whom we quoted at the opening of this chapter seduces Joe Gideon, Fosse uses nudity and romantic music to invite the audience to participate in the sensual pleasure of the encounter. Unlike Allen, Fosse asks the audience, at least its male members, to identify with the narcissistic pursuits of his protagonist.

Similarly, Allen is more inclined to make a joke out of his character's pathological grandiosity. At several points in the movie he shows himself as a child, on one occasion putting on a cape (possibly a reference to the caped child who represented the young Guido in 8 ½) and flying off like Superman. Later we see the child performing magic tricks in a send-up of the posturing show business magician. The archaic grandiose self described by Kohut (1971) as central to the understanding of narcissism is here parodied in the embodiment

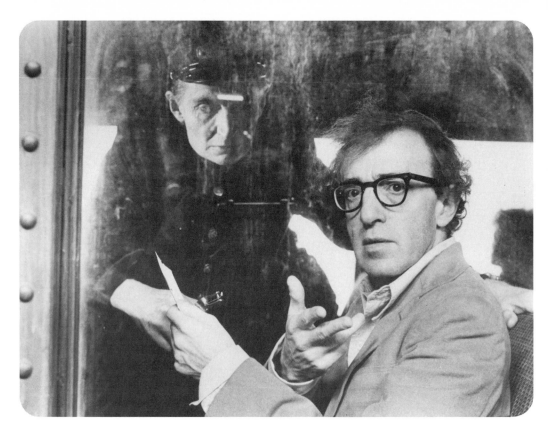

PLATE 31. Woody Allen is on the wrong train (although they both lead to the same place). *Stardust Memories* (1980). United Artists. The Museum of Modern Art/Film Stills Archive.

of this self in a young boy with magical and superhuman powers. One of the clearest examples of Allen's ability to take comic distance from his own narcissism, and also one of the funniest lines in the movie, comes in response to a fan who asks Bates what he thinks of the criticism that his movies are narcissistic. Bates replies that if he were to associate himself with any figure from Greek mythology, it would be Zeus rather than Narcissus.

Although Fosse seems much more angry in his satirical attacks, Allen's protagonist shares some of Fosse's contempt for those around him. The multitudes of fans surrounding Sandy Bates at the Hotel Stardust are characterized by distorted facial features and inane chatter. Bates is portrayed as superior to all of his revolting and flawed admirers. Moreover, he feels himself a victim of the masses of people who want to use him or take something from him. On the one hand, Allen's Bates is committed to humanitarian concerns: he contributes to cancer research, committees to help Russian dissidents, etc. But it is his awareness of human suffering that makes so much of his success unsatisfying, and of course this awareness exists on a highly abstract level.

Sandy Bates shares Joe Gideon's problems with women although, once again, Allen appears to have more compassion for his female characters than Fosse has for the women who pass through the life of Gideon. Allen shows us a world where Bates's needs can never be met. He is in relentless pursuit of the perfect woman although he is, by his own admission, "fatally attracted" to women for whom a sustained, stable relationship is impossible. As a result, his relationships with women begin with idealization only to be followed by disillusionment. This dilemma too he approaches with humor. When asked if he really thinks there is such a thing as a perfect mate and are not good relationships based on compromise anyway, he replies that all good relationships are based on luck. Significantly, the film ends with Bates making what appears to be a sincere commitment to Isobel (Marie-Christine Barrault), the one woman in the film who shows the potential for a mature relationship. However, this scene turns out to be a film within a film, and as in 8 $\frac{1}{2}$, we are unsure of the extent to which it represents a satisfying end to the romantic problems that the film presents. Throughout most of the film, Sandy is regularly reminded of how much he loved the hopelessly manic-depressive actress Dorrie (Charlotte Rampling).

The notion of celebrity is central to the culture of narcissism, according to Lasch (1979), and we will examine three different films in this context in the next chapter. In *All That Jazz* Gideon wallows in the fringe benefits of his celebrity and enjoys it, but in *Stardust Memories* Sandy Bates feels beleaguered by the multitudes of his fans as well as ill-served by the many people whom financial success has placed in his service. When a policeman questions him about a gun for which he has no permit, Bates informs the policeman that he can make an exception in his case because he is a celebrity. The next scene shows him sitting in a jail cell, showing Allen's ability to take an ironic distance from his sense of entitlement related to being a celebrity. Nevertheless, the many scenes in which Allen caricatures Sandy Bates's admirers seem to have upset many of his fans, perhaps because they construed these uncharitable portraits as attacks by Woody Allen upon them personally. Allen's treatment of his fans also prompted some of the most bitter attacks from critics and reviewers. In his conversation with Jacobs, Allen touched on the fan/celebrity question: "So many people were outraged that I dared to suggest an ambivalent, love/hate relationship between an audience and a celebrity; and then shortly after *Stardust Memories* opened, John Lennon was shot by the very guy who had asked him for his autograph earlier in the day. I feel that obtains. The guy who asks Sandy for his autograph on the boardwalk and says, 'you're my favorite comedian' in the middle of the picture, later, in Sandy's fantasy, comes up and shoots him. This is what happens with celebrities—one day people love you, the next day they want to kill you. And the celebrity also feels that way toward the audience; because in the movie Sandy hallucinates that the guy shoots him; but in fact Sandy is the one who has the gun. So the celebrity imagines that the fan will do to him what in fact he wants to do to the fan. But people don't want to hear this—this is an unpleasant truth to dramatize" (1982, 147–48). In spite of Allen's recognition of the troubling relationship between fan and celebrity, the celebrity phenomenon is handled primarily with irony throughout *Stardust Memories.* The movie focuses on the public's fascination with celebrity and how empty that obsession is, grounded as it is in fantasy. Real life and life in the movies seem to be indistinguishable; both are impressionistic flashes and images. At the very end of the movie an old Jewish man says, "I don't understand. He makes a living doing this? I like melodramas and musicals."

The final scene in the film finds Bates in an empty theater with an empty screen, again reflecting his own internal emptiness. The image is probably meant to emphasize the artist's ultimate isolation from the public, but it may also recall the sad clowns of the silent cinema like Charlie Chaplin, who were often left alone at the ends of their films. As we have pointed out, Allen has not, in the final analysis, made a "serious" movie in the way that Fosse has. Allen pokes fun at himself throughout, and this humor distances him from self-indulgence and self-aggrandizement.

MIDLIFE CRISIS

Seen from the perspective of adult developmental phases, the protagonists in both films find themselves facing midlife issues. As Kernberg (1980) has persuasively argued, the midlife crisis is largely a crisis of narcissism. One needs to come to terms with one's mortality, one's limitations, and one's inability to attain all that one wished to achieve in one's lifetime. One must mourn one's own death, mourn the death of loved ones, and overcome one's envy of the youth who have supplanted oneself. Individuals with narcissistic personalities typically experience a worsening of their narcissistic sufferings in midlife, becoming increasingly aware of their inability to satiate themselves. As Kernberg describes it, "The patient's relentless greed, his avid and yet destructive incorporation of what he envies, the consequent deterioration of his object representations, his wanting things because they are not his rather than because of their intrinsic value, all increase endless greed while impoverishing and destroying what he receives. This affects the narcissistic patient's relationship to his past and to the future. He longs for a new narcissistic refueling, but discovers that lasting satisfaction is never to be found; consequently he restlessly hopes for and yet fears the future" (1980, 136). Furthermore, as the narcissistic individual reaches middle age he becomes envious of what he himself was in the past and has a profound sense of having lost what he once had.

Jaques (1965), in his classic paper on the midlife crisis from a Kleinian perspective, points out that a shift characteristically occurs in artists and writers around the age of thirty-five to forty. While pre-midlife work tends to reflect an optimistic youthful idealism about the inherent goodness in man, the later, post-midlife work reflects acknowledgment of and resignation to the fact that hate and destructive forces exist as well. For Jaques the successful resolution of the midlife crisis involves overcoming an early adult idealism built upon unconscious manic defenses against two inescapable aspects of human life: (1) personal death and (2) the existence of hate and destructive impulses within all of us. The depressive position must be worked through once again; that is, love and hate must be integrated into an ambivalent view of one's self and one's relationships.

In examining the narcissistic struggles of our two protagonists from the standpoint of the midlife crisis, there are considerable differences. Allen's protagonist has dropped the youthful manic defenses and has become acutely aware of suffering and death. Allen himself has said that the movie is about "a filmmaker/comedian who's reached a point in his life where he just doesn't find anything amusing anymore and so he is overcome with depression" (Moss 1980, 43). He sees the suffering everywhere around him epitomized by the death of his high school friend Nat Bernstein from amyotrophic lateral sclerosis. Moreover, as Allen himself acknowledged in the conversation with Jacobs cited above, Bates has a sense of his own destructive potential. *Stardust Memories* includes a satirical sketch from one of the director's films in which Bates joins police and hunting dogs in pursuit of a monster representing his narcissistic rage and his potential destructiveness. All around him and the monster are dead bodies. His pessimism about being helped is dramatized by an ineffectual analyst's attempts to deal with the monster.

Allen's protagonist is also represented as an artist who has gone through the kind of transition that Jaques describes. He is a comedian who has recently turned to more serious themes in his movies, much like Allen in real life. After a series of unpretentious comedies such as *Take the Money and Run* (1969) and

Bananas (1971), Allen's films turned slowly toward the bittersweet romance of *Annie Hall* (1977) and *Manhattan* (1979). His most serious film was *Interiors* (1978), a Chekhovian drama about the tensions between and within the members of an affluent New York family. Though not without humor, *Interiors* was much grimmer than his audience had dared to expect. In *Stardust Memories*, Bates comments, "I don't want to make funny pictures anymore. I look around and all I see is human suffering. Didn't anyone else read that piece on the front page of the *Times* about how matter is decaying?" Even when extraterrestrial beings appear to Bates in one of his fantasies, the film again expresses an ambivalent attitude toward the changes in Bates's career when the spacemen inform him that they liked the early, funny movies best. Moments later, Bates faints after another fantasy in which his adoring fan shoots him.

Fosse's Joe Gideon faces midlife with much less openness. He continues the use of his youthful manic defenses to ward off depression, acknowledgment of death, and an acceptance of his own destructive potential. Jaques notes that some individuals attempt to avoid midlife crisis by strengthening manic defenses: "The compulsive attempts, in many men and women reaching middle age, to remain young, the hypochondriacal concern over health and appearance, the emergence of sexual promiscuity in order to prove youth and potency, the hollowness and lack of genuine enjoyment of life, and the frequency of religious concern are familiar patterns. They are attempts at a race against time. And in addition to the impoverishment of emotional life contained in the foregoing activities, real character deterioration is always possible" (1965, 511). So while Allen has seen beyond his manic defenses to the despair beneath, Fosse's protagonist is desperately involved in a flight of overactivity in an effort to maintain his manic defenses. In *All That Jazz* we see Gideon dealing with the important midlife issue of his own mortality in a scene from a film he is making called *The Standup*. (Fosse made a similar film about the life of Lenny Bruce called *Lenny*. The film received mostly unfavorable reviews, and like Gideon, Fosse underwent coronary bypass surgery shortly after its opening.) In the scene from *The Standup*, a comedian played by Cliff Gorman does a blackly humorous parody of Kübler-Ross's five stages of dying. The most memorable stage in Gorman's rendition is "denial." In fact, one of his doctors says of Gideon, "Everything he does is a denial of his condition." Hence Gideon does not see himself as middle-aged, dying, and in need of treatment.

Klein (Segal 1964) maintains that the manic relation to objects is characterized by a triad of feelings: control, triumph, and contempt. These feelings serve the defensive function of warding off guilt, mourning, a sense of loss, and feelings of having depended upon a valued object. This manic triad manifests itself in Gideon's response when his doctor informs him that his condition is serious. In his fantasy he stages an elaborate production number involving the doctors as characters. He is in control now that he is the director, no longer a passive victim of the medical treatment but rather the active master of his own destiny. Moreover, he is able to deny his dependence on the doctors by imagining that he controls the entire proceedings. Contempt is present in his portrayal of them as know-nothing performers in a production number. Triumph is seen in his denial of his depressive feelings about what is happening to him and about the impending losses of those he values. His narcissistic injury is graphically portrayed as Gideon, watching a television critic assail *The Standup*, becomes pale and short of breath, finally collapsing with an apparent myocardial infarction.

DEATH

The extinction of consciousness through death is the ultimate narcissistic injury, and the terror of death is one reason the narcissist does not age well. In the two movies, both protagonists are deeply concerned with death. After staving off his anxieties about death with drugs, alcohol, hypersexuality, workaholism, and the manic defenses mentioned above, Gideon finally shows a touch of despair after open-heart surgery when he says to himself about his life, "I'd like to run the whole thing over again." In another of these many blurrings of the line between show business and life, Gideon ventilates his anger at God by plaintively asking, "What's the matter, don't you like musical comedy?" However, this brief glimpse of the despair underneath is rapidly sealed over by a massive denial of death. His death becomes a manic triumph where as director he stages one production number after another (plates 29 and 30). His ex-wife, his girlfriend, and his daughter perform for him as he lies in bed, while his double sits in the director's chair in charge of the proceedings. This doppelganger effect allows us to see that, while part of him experiences the passive helplessness of dying, another split-off part omnipotently imagines itself to be in control of everything happening to him. In a cynical eulogy that is a parody of show business sincerity, O'Connor Flood (Ben Vereen) says that Gideon spent his life bullshitting until he did not know what was real and what was bullshit. The only reality for Gideon was death. When the production numbers have ended, and he breathes his last, he finds himself floating up a tunnel toward the outstretched arms of Angelique, who waits to greet him with death's embrace. Here Fosse has appropriated elements of the often-reported "near-death experience" (Gabbard, Twemlow, and Jones 1981) to say something about

Gideon's (and perhaps Fosse's) view of death. Even death itself is viewed with manic defenses as a joyous reunion with the idealized, all-good, internal mother. Fosse further defends against death through sexualization as the seductive Angelique begins to disrobe as Gideon approaches death.

As in the running joke about Alvy Singer's obsession with death that was central in *Annie Hall,* Allen views death in a much more sober fashion, as the ultimate narcissistic injury. He sees it as the inevitable outgrowth of the inherent destructiveness in human beings. When he is told that the public adores him, he responds by saying, "Today they adore you; tomorrow it's one of these," and he makes a gesture of shooting himself in the head. Paradoxically, though, while Allen's Bates has more insight into the reality of his own personal death than Fosse's Gideon does, Allen treats it with more humor. Gideon's self-destructive life is humorlessly portrayed as a form of slow suicide. In contrast Allen presents the self-destructive workaholic in the person of a comic character riding an exercycle who says that he had two heart attacks before he started exercycling and two after (plate 32). When he finishes his exercycling, he lights up a cigarette. Allen seems to be saying that death is relentlessly stalking us

PLATE 32. Absurdist therapy: Woody Allen with Anne de Salvo and Jaqui Safra in *Stardust Memories* (1980). United Artists. The Museum of Modern Art/Film Stills Archive.

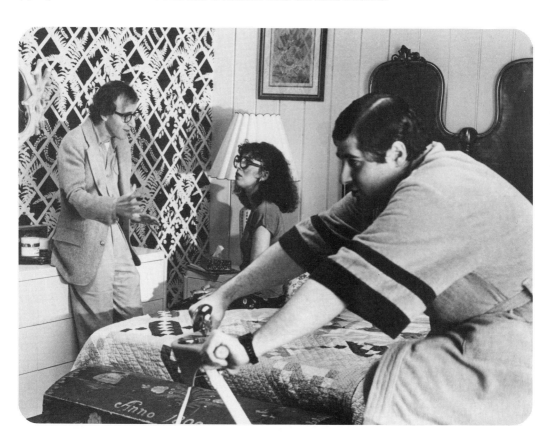

no matter what steps we take to prevent it. While Gideon's death is real despite his manic attempts at denying it, Sandy Bates's death is simply a fantasy in *Stardust Memories*.

In Woody Allen's film a psychoanalyst indicates that Bates's problem is that he has dropped his defensive denial and sees too much reality. Gideon's problem may be the converse in that he does not see reality but continually uses manic defenses to avoid it. Both situations are tragic in a sense. Gideon's is tragic because the manic defenses prevent him from seeing his own destructiveness, whereas Bates's is tragic because he is aware of his depression but feels impotent to affect it in any way. Because of his severe narcissistic impairment, he cannot allow his love to overcome his sense of destructiveness and his consequent suffering.

We have discussed two contemporary cinematic autobiographies that present the narcissistic struggles of the protagonists. Whether Bob Fosse and Woody Allen are themselves suffering from narcissistic character pathology is unknown to us although Fosse's treatment of his narcissistic protagonist seems much more an apologia than does Allen's self-consciously ironic treatment of his main character. Our main goal, however, has been to enlarge our understanding of current cultural and intrapsychic narcissistic phenomena through an examination of how Joe Gideon in *All That Jazz* and Sandy Bates in *Stardust Memories* approach relationships with significant figures in their lives, how they deal with the midlife crisis, and how they struggle with the knowledge of the inevitability of personal death. Both films provide unique insight into the vicissitudes of narcissism at a particular point in the male adult life cycle.

Narcissism in the Cinema II: The Celebrity

9

As we noted in the previous chapter, the fascination with celebrity is one of the dominant themes of our narcissistic culture. The cinematic medium, perhaps more than any other facet of modern society, has been instrumental in the creation of this infatuation with the rich and famous. Spinoffs from the phenomenon of the movie star—including the television personality, the rock star, the sports hero, the evening news anchorperson, and even the media-created political personality—are so thoroughly entrenched in contemporary popular culture that we may easily forget their origins: all of these versions of the celebrity owe a large debt to screen images, which have created or greatly enhanced their fascination for the public. An examination of narcissism in the cinema would be incomplete without an analysis of the notion of celebrity.

While the idea of celebrity is to a large extent the child of the twentieth century, it is simply the latest transformation of an archetypal figure as old as human culture itself—the hero. A quick glance at the earliest extant literary works, for example, the Gilgamesh epic and the works of Homer, reveals that an obsession with heroes was a fixture in the human psyche at the dawn of man's intellectual awareness. As William James (1958) commented at the beginning of this century, when television was only the dream of a visionary inventor, "Mankind's common instinct for reality . . . has always held the world to be essentially a theatre for heroism" (1958, 281). Ernest Becker (1973) has persuasively argued that the problem of heroics is the central existential issue of human life. Unlike his fellow creatures in the animal kingdom, man lives with the terrible knowledge that amidst all the ambiguities of life, one thing is certain: he will cease to exist at some point in the future. This unbearable certainty of extinction leads man to invent various immortality strategies. Religion is one. The heroic quest is another. Man longs for cosmic significance. He hungers to be "somebody," a hero who will be remembered and talked about long after he has gone to his grave.

Becker points out that narcissism is fundamental to the understanding of this human urge to heroism. From early childhood, the whole human organism demands to be the center of the universe, to be noted, admired, loved, praised, and even worshiped. In Becker's own words, this developmental phenomenon is "too all-absorbing and relentless to be an aberration, it expresses the heart of the creature: the desire to stand out, to be the one in creation. When you combine natural narcissism with the basic need for self-esteem, you create a creature who has to feel himself an object of primary value: first in the universe, representing in himself all of life" (1973, 3). As we grow and become socialized, the quest for heroism undergoes transformations that disguise it in one form or another; but as Becker has observed, society creates hero systems that provide external validation for each individual who lays claim to his or her own heroic act: "Human heroics is a blind drivenness that burns people up; in passionate people, a screaming for glory as uncritical and reflective as the howling of a dog. In the more passive masses of mediocre men, it is disguised as they humbly and complainingly follow out the roles that society provides for their heroics and try to earn their promotions within the system: wearing the standard uniforms" (1973, 6).

Today our heroes are no longer warriors, conquerors, or generals. Nor are their achievements equivalent to the vanquishing of armies. The criteria for success have been redefined with the advent of the pervasive influence of the media. Lasch has characterized it thus: "The good opinion of friends and neighbors, which formerly informed a man that he had lived a useful life, rested on appreciation of his accomplishments. Today men seek the kind of approval that applauds not their actions but their personal attributes. They wish to be not so much esteemed as admired. They crave not fame but the glamor and excitement of celebrity. They want to be envied rather than re-spected. Pride and acquisitiveness, the sins of an ascendant capitalism, have given way to vanity" (1979, 59). Today's hero is someone who has successfully manufactured a winning image that so appeals to the masses as to catapult him into a position of celebrity. The substance behind the image is of little concern either to the celebrities themselves or to those who worship them. Political campaigns, for example, are no longer issue-oriented but rather geared to the politicians' use of television to package an image worthy of the voters' confi-dence. During the 1984 presidential election, commentators observed repeat-edly that voters often disagreed with Ronald Reagan on the issues he supported but nevertheless voted for him because of his appeal as a media personality. One wag even suggested that the only candidate who could have beaten Reagan in 1984 was Clint Eastwood, a comment which proved slightly prophetic in

1986 when Eastwood was overwhelmingly elected mayor of Carmel, California. When media correspondents interviewed voters at polling places, people seldom commented on Eastwood's politics, addressing themselves instead to his charisma. Lasch makes the following observations:

> What a man does matters less than the fact that he has "made it." Whereas fame depends on the performance of notable deeds acclaimed in biography and works of history, celebrity—the reward of those who project a vivid or pleasing exterior or have otherwise attracted attention to themselves— is acclaimed in the news media, in gossip columns, on talk shows, and magazines devoted to "personalities." . . . Success in our society has to be ratified by publicity. The tycoon who lives in personal obscurity, the empire builder who controls the destinies of nations from behind the scenes, are vanishing types. Even non-elected officials, ostensibly preoccupied with questions of high policy, have to keep themselves constantly on view; all politics becomes a form of spectacle. It is well known that Madison Avenue packages politicians and markets them as if they were cereals or deodorants. (1979, 59–60)

Cinematic art has now developed the capacity to comment intelligently and critically on what the medium itself has created, as if Dr. Frankenstein had begun writing scholarly treatises on the adverse consequences of monster-building. Three recent films, *Zelig* (1983) and *The Purple Rose of Cairo* (1985), both written and directed by Woody Allen, and Martin Scorsese's *King of Comedy* (1983), provide penetrating insights into the phenomenon of celebrity as well as the contribution of the electronic media themselves to the contemporary obsession with celebrity. However, the psychologically astute makers of these films have avoided implying that the problems developed de novo with the advent of movies and television. Rather, they treat the quest for heroism as a pervasive, preexisting human frailty that easily accomodated itself to the American media explosion.

King of Comedy

Written by Paul D. Zimmerman and directed by Martin Scorsese, *King of Comedy* points the camera at a most single-minded individual in contemporary Manhattan who bears the improbable name of Rupert Pupkin (Robert De Niro). Rupert is a 34-year-old messenger boy who lives in his own special fantasy world. He writes and rehearses stand-up comedy routines in front of an imaginary audience in the privacy of his basement, where reality only occasionally intervenes whenever his mother loudly demands that he quiet down. The principal idealized object that peoples his fantasy world is Jerry Langford (Jerry Lewis), a character based closely on Johnny Carson although the original script for the film, dating from the early 1970s, had been written for Dick Cavett (Frank and Krohn 1983). Pupkin has a life-sized photograph of Langford (Lewis) at his talk show desk tacked to the wall next to an equally large photo of Liza Minnelli. He lives out his grandiose fantasies of glory and fame by sitting next to his Langford and Minnelli pictures while carrying on an imaginary dialogue with the famous host and affecting all the mannerisms of a regular guest on late-night talk shows.

Rupert Pupkin is an embodiment of the primary importance of maintaining one's self-esteem through the mirroring validation of others. He exemplifies what is perhaps Kohut's (1971, 1977) greatest contribution to our understanding of narcissism—that the regulation of self-esteem ranks with sexuality and aggression as one of the major forces in the human psyche. His fantasy life does not depend on aggressive or sexual conquests but rather on throngs of cheering fans worshiping him and on the idealized Langford begging him to take his place for six weeks while Langford vacations. He looks to acclaim and admiration as the panaceas for his anxiety and his internal emptiness.

King of Comedy opens to the sound of Ray Charles singing the old torch song, "I'm gonna love you like nobody's loved you, come rain or come shine." We then see Rupert threading his way through a crowd of hungry autograph seekers outside the studio door through which Langford will soon pass. As Pupkin shoves his way to the front of the crowd, he strives to distinguish himself from his acquaintances in the odd subculture of autograph hounds, telling one repeatedly that acquiring the signatures of stars is "not my whole life." Rupert's flamboyant wardrobe is also much more elaborate than that of the rest of the crowd, and he affects an air of superiority to the others. When he manages to work his way into Langford's car, he asks the renowned talk show host for a chance on his show. Barely able to tolerate Pupkin's unrelenting pleading, Langford tells him to call his office. Brimming with self-confidence, Pupkin goes home and prepares a tape for Langford's assistant, now convinced that his wildest fantasies are about to be fulfilled. He seeks out Rita (Diahnne Abbott), an idealized woman from his past, who now works as a bartender. He takes her to dinner and courts her with his "talent register," a book of autographs of the famous, many of whom he blithely insists are his personal friends. Even though Rita fails to find his book fascinating, Pupkin shows her page after page of signatures culminating with a page that bears his own scrawl. Kernberg (1975) has noted how the narcissist, experiencing himself as fundamentally worthless, must attach himself to idealized objects in order to bask in the reflected glory of these objects. Rupert hopes to impress Rita by persuading her that the luster of the stars has rubbed off on him and that he lives in their shadows. He makes no effort to court her by selling her on his own qualities—only his association with those whose attributes are beyond question. Rita is singularly unimpressed by his name-dropping and is, ironically, more interested in Rupert himself. But Rupert seems unaware of his own charms and proceeds relentlessly to win her over in the only way that has meaning for him.

Rupert indulges in an elaborate fantasy about his meeting with Langford to discuss his tape. He imagines that Langford raves about his talent, proclaiming his envy for Rupert. In the fantasy, Jerry even invites him to his country house for the weekend. But when Rupert's tape is rejected by Langford's assistant (Shelley Hack), Rupert confuses fantasy with reality, eventually taking Rita on the train with him to Langford's house in the Hamptons, assuring her that he has been invited and that he and Langford are the best of friends.

The couple's ill-fated trip shows us the dark side of the celebrity's life. Early in the film the camera reveals Langford in his sumptuous Manhattan apartment, eating alone at a long table while three television sets play silently in the background. The emptiness of Langford's life recalls the widely publicized divorces of Johnny Carson, the personality Langford most clearly suggests. In fact, after abandoning the original script for *King of Comedy* written for Dick Cavett, Scorsese asked Carson to play the role. Carson refused, saying in effect that he was too accustomed to taping a show each night in one take and that he had no desire to enter into a process that required repeated shootings of the same scene: "If I wanted to make a film and repeat the same scene nineteen times, I would make it myself" (Frank and Krohn 1983). Some commentators subsequently praised Carson for his caution, arguing that *King of Comedy* might inspire some fan to kidnap Carson, and some criticized Scorsese, whose earlier film *Taxi Driver* provided the fantasy that inspired John Hinckley to attempt the assassination of Ronald Reagan. However, it may also be that Carson understood Scorsese's intentions all too well and demurred at associating himself with a project that so thoroughly examined the nature of his celebrity status.

When Rupert and Rita arrive at Langford's country house, the audience witnesses again the emptiness and sterility of Langford's inner life, symbolized by the white-walled starkness of his home. Langford is called in from the golf course when they arrive, and he is uncompromising in his annoyance at this invasion of his privacy. He angrily explains to Rupert that he too has a life and that he resents this violation by the intruders. Rupert is blind to Langford's rage until Jerry is forced to tell him point-blank that when Rupert gained entrance to his limousine, Langford seemed to encourage him only in order to be rid of him. As Rupert leaves, he tells Langford how disappointed he is to find out what Jerry is really like. He tells him that he is going to work fifty times harder than Langford and become fifty times more famous. Langford's final comment to the intruder is "then you're going to have idiots like you plaguing your life."

Rupert responds to this devastating injury to his self-esteem with narcissistic rage, although Scorsese's oblique style of storytelling omits any scenes in which Pupkin's confident exterior is actually ruffled. Instead, we see Rupert plotting with another devoted autograph hunter, Masha (Sandra Bernhard), whose sense of reality is even more profoundly askew than his. They plan to kidnap Langford so that Rupert can blackmail the producers into allowing him to deliver the opening monologue on Jerry's show. After successfully carrying out his scheme, Rupert tells the FBI men who have been called in on the case that he will release Langford and surrender to their custody only after he has been allowed to watch the tape of his monologue in the presence of Rita at the bar where she works. Rupert's performance impresses Rita and the denizens of the saloon only slightly more than it does the FBI agents, one of whom says that he would also like to arrest the man who writes Rupert's material. Nevertheless, Rupert Pupkin has accomplished his goal, and he goes off to meet his fate cheerfully.

In Rupert's monologue, he admits that he has kidnapped Jerry Langford in order to appear on his show. The audience laughs, not understanding that the man they are watching is not just another of the comedians who regularly attempt to amuse the television audience on Langford's program. They also laugh when he tells them that his rash act is worth it since it is better to be "king for a night than schmuck for a lifetime" (plate 33). The film ends with a newscaster intoning that the incident has made the name Rupert Pupkin a household word. His picture appears on the cover of *Time, Newsweek, Life, Rolling Stone,* and *People* magazines, and he writes his best-selling autobiography while serving two years and nine months of a six-year prison sentence. In the open-ended conclusion to the film, Rupert is introduced as "the legendary, the inspirational, the one and only king of comedy, Rupert Pupkin." The camera slowly zooms in on Rupert as he receives the audience's enthusiastic applause, his impassive face suggesting that he may already be aware of the ambiguous rewards of celebrity.

The publicity for *King of Comedy* noted that Robert De Niro had prepared for the role of Rupert Pupkin by studying stand-up comedians in order to learn the secrets of their timing and delivery, just as he had learned to play the saxophone for Scorsese's *New York, New York* (1977). For the same director's

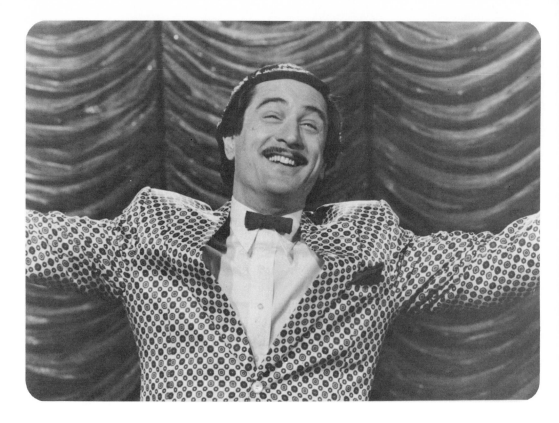

PLATE 33. Rupert Pupkin (Robert De Niro) accepts the adulation of Jerry Langford's audience in *King of Comedy* (1983). Twentieth Century–Fox. The Museum of Modern Art/Film Stills Archive.

Raging Bull (1980), De Niro had studied boxing and then gained forty pounds so that he could play the fighter Jake La Motta later in life. But the comedy routine that De Niro actually delivers in *King of Comedy* does not rise much above the level of mediocrity established through the years by run-of-the-mill performers who daily fill up the schedule of "The Tonight Show." Scorsese has told interviewers that one of the elements of the film's first script that attracted him most was the monologue: because it is neither good nor bad, audiences have no way of evaluating the potential talent of Pupkin, who has, after all, scrupulously avoided performing in public until he reaches the big time on the Langford show (Henry 1983). Scorsese has intentionally left open the question, is Pupkin a truly funny comedian who merely took an unconventional road to stardom, or is he just another desperate, vapid individual seeking the prize of celebrity? It would seem that he is just as empty as Jerry Langford, who is in fact not portrayed as much of a comedian either. Scorsese had taped Lewis performing a monologue for the beginning of the film, but the director says that he excised it from the final print because it raised distracting questions about the relative merits of Pupkin and Langford as comedians (Frank and Krohn 1983).

Scorsese and his screenwriter Zimmerman have made a film about how our fascination with celebrity has led us to confuse genuine talent with a kind of chutzpah or daring, which may be neurotic or even criminal. The increasingly sensationalistic world of American entertainment invites the blurring of distinctions between what is legitimate and what is not, and the case of Rupert Pupkin provocatively exposes this confusion. The crucial moment in *King of Comedy* may be the scene at Langford's country house in which Rupert shows himself to be incapable of understanding Langford's question about how he would feel if someone barged in on him the way Pupkin has intruded on Langford. The narcissistically disturbed individual's inability to empathize with the feelings of others is beautifully illustrated here as is Pupkin's extreme idealization of Langford's life: Rupert cannot imagine how anything in Langford's domain could be unpleasant even when he himself has caused the unpleasantness. Scorsese suggests that only someone as confused as Pupkin could envy someone like Langford.

However, Scorsese is working in a marketplace where subtle questions about American attitudes are seldom associated with big box office. He has apparently sought to make two films: one for a naive or "right" audience, who may find De Niro's Pupkin to be as adept as any other stand-up comedian presented by Johnny Carson, and who may assume that the film is another in a long series of American entertainments about a little guy who beats the system. The other film that Scorsese has made with *King of Comedy* is addressed to the ironic or "left" audience, who are more acquainted with cinematic codes. Scorsese has asked this audience to think more critically about America's television heroes, particularly in terms of the issues that have been raised in this chapter. Even though *King of Comedy* was not a box-office smash, Martin Scorsese understands that he can be both an artist and a commercially successful director if he makes his films in this way. Scorsese achieved his greatest financial success with *Taxi Driver*, the twelfth largest grossing film of 1976 (Steinberg 1980). Although most audiences and even some critics lumped it with "street westerns" such as Michael Winner's *Death Wish*, Robert B. Ray has shown that *Taxi Driver* reveals the psychosis that can lie beneath the unruffled exteriors of America's vigilante heroes. The film's large naive audience may have perceived it as another glorification of violent revenge, but *Taxi Driver* represents a powerful attack upon "the belief in the continued applicability of western-style, individual solutions to contemporary complex problems" (Ray 1985, 351).

If we are right about Scorsese's dual intentions, we must not then be surprised that *King of Comedy* has many moments of ambiguity. For one thing, episodes of fantasy are interwoven with episodes of reality. Since Scorsese does not use musical or cinematographical clichés to announce that the film is about to fade into a fantasy sequence, we are not even sure if the renown that Pupkin enjoys at the end of the film is in his head or in reality. Some critics have made the same observation about Scorsese's *Taxi Driver* (1976), in which the rise of Travis Bickel (De Niro again) to hero status at the film's end could be the fantasy of a man dying from gunshot wounds. Scorsese himself says that he likes "open endings" (Henry 1983).

If Scorsese and screenwriter Zimmerman did intend for the ending of *King of Comedy* to be taken literally, they may be telling us that Rupert's narcissistic quest for heroism is no more or less absurd than society's need to make such personages into the objects of fascination and admiration. As Lasch puts it:

> The media have conferred a curious sort of legitimacy on antisocial acts merely by reporting them. . . . The criminal who murders or who kidnaps a celebrity takes on the glamor of his victim. The Manson gang with their murder of Sharon Tate and her friends, the Symbionese Liberation Army with its abduction of Patty Hearst, share with the presidential assassins and would-be assassins of recent years a similar psychology. Such people display, in exaggerated form, the prevailing obsession with celebrity and the determination to achieve it even at the cost of rational self-interest and personal safety. (1979, 84)

Rupert Pupkin can be viewed as a narcissistic Everyman. As Kernberg (1975) has written, the narcissist sees society divided into two groups consisting of famous celebrities on one side and mediocrities like himself on the other. The narcissist is "nobody" if he is not in the company of the great. The average or mediocre person is viewed contemptuously, as though he has no redeeming features and cannot lead a meaningful life. Rupert's efforts to link up with Langford are an attempt to confer greatness upon himself. Bob Fosse developed this same theme in his 1983 film *Star 80,* in which Paul Snider (Eric Roberts), filled with self-contempt and self-loathing, aspires to become "somebody" by exploiting his relationship with Playboy's sweetheart Dorothy Stratten in order to gain proximity to Hugh Hefner and the Playboy crowd. In hopes of gaining passage into the inner sanctum of the Playboy mansion, Snider cultivates an image through hours of rehearsal in front of a mirror and through excessive attention to his wardrobe. When both Hefner and his circle reject him, he reacts with murderous and suicidal narcissistic rage. If one is not a celebrity, one is an abject failure without a reason to live.

From analytic observations in a clinical context, Kohut (1971) has described the narcissist's problem as an arrest of normal development of the bipolar self. Narcissistic patients typically form two kinds of transferences in the consulting room: (1) the mirror transference linked to an archaic grandiose self that performs for mother hoping to recapture the lost perfection of infancy by winning her approval and thus an empathic validation of the self and (2) the idealizing transference linked to an effort on the part of the undeveloped self to recapture the lost perfection by merging with an idealized parent image. While Rupert Pupkin certainly embodies the grandiose self's efforts to obtain mirroring validation from an audience of approving parental figures, we also see how Jerry Langford functions as an idealized parent imago for Rupert's friend Masha. While Rupert is off at the studio conducting the negotiations for his appearance on Langford's show, Masha is reveling in her private audience with Langford, whom she has tied up in her dining room chair. As she undresses in front of him, she tells Jerry that she loves him, something that she has never even told her parents, who, she poignantly tells him, never loved her. She sings to him, "You're gonna love me like nobody's loved me, come rain or come shine." In this scene she pathetically reveals an important dynamic in the worship of celebrities, i.e., the fantasy that the love between the celebrity and the follower would be of a pure and reparative nature, making up for the absence of love experienced as a child. Masha knows virtually nothing of the real Jerry Langford, but she does know that she loves him as she loves no one else. Langford is the object of an idealizing transference on Masha's part, and in her fantasy she can shore up her fragile self-esteem by merging with this all-loving and all-giving parent of her dreams through the act of making love.

Sandra Bernhard made her first film appearance as Masha in *King of Comedy*, and it is a memorable one. When Langford, bound with several yards of masking tape, sits helplessly before a meal that Masha has prepared for him, she suddenly rakes her arm across the table and shoves the dishes to the floor so that she can recline on the table before him. The violence in her gesture momentarily suggests that the film may turn as violent as many of Scorsese's earlier films. However, even the gun that Masha had earlier trained upon Langford turns out to be a toy, and he has no difficulty escaping from her. Masha plays out her ambivalent relationship with Jerry in an earlier scene when she contemplates which color looks best on the talk show host while she dresses her prisoner in a sweater knitted especially for him. Masha has lost track of the difference between contemplating her idol on a television set and contemplating him as a hostage in her house.

In the throes of this idealizing and erotic transference confusion, Masha believes that she is successfully seducing Langford. While her idealization of Jerry is dependent on his ongoing love for her, Rupert's idealization is much more transparently a narcissistic exploitation of Jerry for his own self-aggrandizement. Rupert is only interested in Langford as a means of establishing himself as the "King of Comedy." The transferential natures of both Rupert's and Masha's attachments to Langford make them unable to see that his *real* characteristics starkly contrast with the fantasied qualities they attribute to him. In fact, Jerry Lewis plays Langford throughout the film as a character singularly lacking in personal charm.

Becker (1973) believes that the phenomenon of transference is a fascination with the fatality of the human condition. The essence of transference, as Becker sees it, is a taming of terror. Just as the infant deals with his helplessness by believing in his parents and ascribing to them an omnipotent control over fate, so does the adult connect himself with transference figures to deal with his anxiety over the seeming randomness of the universe. Becker notes: "The use of the transference object explains the urge to deification of the other, the constant placing of certain select persons on pedestals, the reading into them of extra powers: the more they have, the more rubs off on us. We participate in their immortality, and so we create immortals. . . . Man is always hungry . . . for material for his own immortalization" (1973, 148). Celebrities represent immortality to their followers. How else can we understand the extraordinary mass grief reactions to the passing of idols such as John Lennon or Elvis Presley? The throngs of mourners are not so much crying for their heroes as for themselves. A bulwark against death has been ripped away, or as Becker comments, "The people apprehend at some dumb level of their personality: 'our locus of power to control life and death can *himself* die; therefore, our own immortality is in doubt' "(1973, 149). The movie star is preserved forever on celluloid, never to be erased from memory, captured in the zenith of his splendor and beauty, safe from the decaying effects of disease and age. Regardless of his own qualities, Jerry Langford provides meaning for Masha and for Rupert, just as the Reverend Jim Jones provided meaning for his followers in Guyana and Hitler provided meaning for his countrymen in Nazi Germany. To find meaning man must look outward for an externalized projection of what he lacks in himself. In one of Rupert's fantasies, he appears on the Langford show as a guest and is surprised when Jerry arranges for him to be married to Rita on his show. The justice of the peace who performs the ceremony thanks Rupert for giving meaning to everyone's lives as the "King of Comedy" marries his "Queen." The justice of the peace wishes them a successful reign as Rupert imagines himself bringing meaning to the lives of millions as Langford has brought meaning to his own life. His fans will live forever through their attachment to their immortal "King."

ZELIG

The brilliance of Woody Allen brings a different perspective to the celebrity phenomenon in his 1983 film *Zelig*. Here we have another unprepossessing nebbish, Leonard Zelig, the film's protagonist. But whereas Rupert Pupkin sought fame and glory, Zelig desires nothing more than to be accepted by those around him. His chameleon-like ability to change his physical appearance and personality in order to blend in with his companions catapults him into celebrity in spite of himself. Allen works minor miracles with cinematographer Gordon Willis and editor Susan Morse in creating the ambience of newsreels and photographs from the 1920s, the setting for the film (plate 34). With the

PLATE 34. Zelig (Woody Allen) becomes a Republican. *Zelig* (1983). Orion Pictures Company/ Warner Brothers. The Museum of Modern Art/Film Stills Archive.

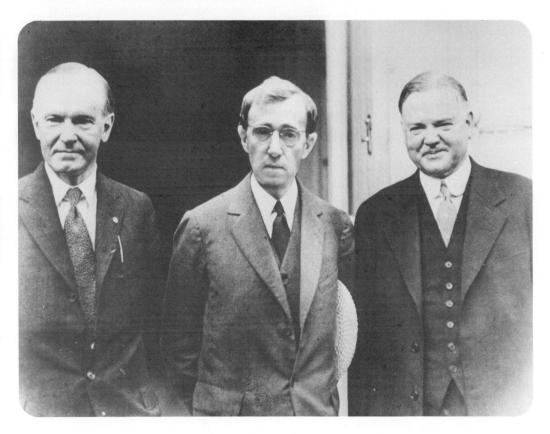

booming voice of a narrator accompanying the grainy footage, the rise and fall of Leonard Zelig is charted almost entirely as a major news story of the Jazz Age, an ingenious conceit that underscores the media's role in creating this unlikely celebrity. Throughout the film Allen interjects comments on the Zelig phenomenon from real-life intellectuals Bruno Bettelheim, Saul Bellow, Susan Sontag, Irving Howe, and John Morton Blum. They speak with great authority as though they actually knew Zelig, a parody not only of the witnesses in Warren Beatty's 1981 film *Reds* but also of Allen's own mock-documentary style in his first directorial effort, *Take the Money and Run* (1969).

When Zelig comes to the attention of a psychiatrist, Dr. Eudora Fletcher (Mia Farrow) (plate 6), she embarks on a heroic effort to cure him of his tendency to take on the characteristics of whomever he is with. His case receives extensive media attention, and various experts from the medical field expound their theories about his illness. Meanwhile, he is the object of the American public's intense fascination. A man interviewed in a barbershop paradoxically proclaims, "I wish I could be Leonard Zelig, the changing man, and be different people, and maybe someday my wishes would come true." Another man interviewed describes Zelig as "one of the finest gentlemen in the United States of America." The adulation and the envy hardly seem warranted given Zelig's real characteristics—he is a simple man who explains that he assumes the characteristics of others because "I want to be liked." Nevertheless, a dance called "The Chameleon" is created to celebrate him, and a movie of his life is made in Hollywood. Allen shows us a few scenes from the imagined movie, called "The Changing Man," an accurate parody of the B-movies of the 1930s. "The Changing Man" is also a glamorous distortion of Zelig's real situation, a further comment by Allen on how movies encourage the public in their transference distortions.

Zelig's rise to celebrity reflects the public's need to believe in someone. Society is fascinated by a man who has no self, no personality of his own. He is literally the projected image of themselves, a mirror that reflects back the person's own reflection. In one scene the film shows Zelig sitting alone, staring into space, as the narrator comments: "Though the shows and parties keep Zelig's sister and her lover rich and amused, Zelig's own existence is a nonexistence. Devoid of personality, his human qualities long since lost in the shuffle of life, he sits alone quietly staring into space, a cipher, a nonperson, a performing freak. He, who wanted only to fit in, to belong, to go unseen by his enemies, and be loved, neither fits in nor belongs, is supervised by enemies and remains uncared for."

As the plot develops, Zelig disappears following the murder of his sister, and everyone easily forgets him. The one exception is Dr. Fletcher, who launches an exhaustive search for him. When she finally discovers him, she has her cousin make a film of her work with Zelig because, "I'm planning to make history." The film even questions the motives of Dr. Fletcher, who wants to exploit Zelig's freakish qualities to make herself famous. Moreover, Allen once again points out how the medium of film itself turns Dr. Fletcher and her bizarre patient into famous celebrities. In search of an understanding of the psychopathology of Leonard Zelig, Bruno Bettelheim is interviewed in one of the witness shots. Bettelheim makes the following comment: "The question of whether Zelig was a psychotic or merely neurotic was a question that was endlessly discussed among his doctors. Now I myself felt his feelings were really not all that different from the normal, what one would call the well-adjusted, normal person, only carried to an extreme degree, to an extreme extent. I myself felt that one could really think of him as the ultimate conformist." For Bettelheim, Zelig's celebrity is the outgrowth of his effort to conform himself to everyone around him. This situation is, of course, only slightly removed from the situation of the present-day politician, who tries to conform to every imaginable constituency to gain sufficient popularity to be elected. The real personality and the real beliefs may be as difficult to discern as the real identity of Leonard Zelig. (The fact that Allen was able to persuade people like Bettelheim, Bellow, and Sontag to participate in his project makes a strong statement in and of itself. The lure of being preserved on celluloid is tempting even for the most prestigious and well established.)

A breakthrough in Dr. Fletcher's treatment of Zelig comes when she begins to emulate the qualities of the chameleon man herself. Zelig is acting like a psychiatrist, of course, since he is in the company of a psychiatrist. Recalling an earlier confession of Zelig's, she tells him that she has lied about having read *Moby Dick* because she was with an erudite group of people and wished to impress them. She says to him, "I want so badly to be liked, to be like other people so I don't stand out." Zelig breaks down and says, "I'm nobody. I'm nothing." Indeed, Zelig is in reality nothing, serving the same function as an inkblot on a Rorschach card, that is, the role of a container into which people project aspects of themselves. In that regard he functions as an ideal celebrity since he has little personality of his own to interfere with the transference feelings of his adoring public. As Dr. Fletcher's cure begins to take effect, however, he allows himself to disagree with others. He carries the cure too far and begins to disagree violently with another doctor about the weather, even to the point of striking the doctor with a rake. The narrator tells us matter-of-factly that Zelig has become "overopinionated."

When the cure is complete, Zelig is once again a hero because he has *stopped* being a chameleon. He now preaches to schoolchildren, "Be yourself." The masses who once loved him for being a chameleon with no personality of his own now love him for having stopped his "as if" transformations. It matters little what Zelig is or says; he is merely a repository for innumerable projections. He is not loved or adored for what he is but only for what he represents to those who adore him. One of the witnesses, historian John Morton Blum, identified here as "author of *Interpreting Zelig*," says that Zelig is a man of symbolism—he was one thing to Marxists and another to the Catholics. The American people, in the throes of the depression, "found in him a symbol of possibility, of self-improvement and self-fulfillment. And of course, the Freudians had a ball—they could interpret him in any way they pleased. It was all symbolism. But there were no two intellectuals who agreed about what it meant." Elsewhere, the announcer tells us that to French intellectuals, Zelig was a symbol for everything.

As the saga continues, Zelig disappears after a series of exposés about his sordid past, which includes polygamy and the abandonment of women he had impregnated. The public turns on him, and he is universally condemned. Idealization rapidly crumbles into devaluation because he has not lived up to their images of him. When he eventually turns up in Nazi Germany, Saul Bellow comments that his presence in that country made eminently good sense because "although he wanted to be loved, craved to be loved, there was also something in him that desired immersion in the masses, anonymity; and fascism offered Zelig that opportunity so that he could make something anonymous of himself." While Rupert Pupkin in *King of Comedy* embodies the narcissistic quest for recognition and fame, the character of Zelig demonstrates another aspect of the narcissist's wish for approval, that is, the wish to blend in with those around him so that he feels a sense of acceptance. The approval of one's peers may be the ultimate desire of the narcissist, and he may do whatever is necessary, including distorting his own personal beliefs, to gain approval. Lasch (1979) notes how conscious emulation of role models is superseded in the narcissistic character by an unconscious and automatic imitation of those around him, reflecting not a true search for a role model but rather the emptiness of the narcissist's reservoir of self-images. As his own identity is obliterated, the narcissist cannot identify with someone else without seeing the other person as an extension of himself and thereby obliterating the other person's identity as well. *Zelig* demonstrates the two-way process of narcissistic mirroring. While

Leonard Zelig attempts to please others by becoming like them and gaining their approval, others see themselves in the character of Zelig and idealize what they see. By attaching themselves to this idealized parental imago projected onto Zelig, they feel their own self-esteem enhanced, just as Zelig feels enhanced by the approval of those with whom he blends. The process might be likened to a hall of mirrors in which each distortion is reflected back in a reverberating chain of constantly changing images.

As Dr. Fletcher rescues Zelig from Nazi Germany, he makes a dramatic escape from a squadron of Nazi fighters by flying upside down across the Atlantic. Zelig is once again an instant hero—his past philanderings seemingly forgotten and forgiven—and he is awarded the Medal of Valor. In another scathing satire on the inanity of the public's creation of celebrities, Allen has Zelig make the following comment in his acceptance speech: "It shows exactly what you can do if you're a total psychotic." In other words, the patient's psychiatric disorder makes him a hero and the object of worship and envy for the masses. Leonard Zelig, like Rupert Pupkin in the closing scene of *King of Comedy,* is adored and idolized despite obvious and pathetic character flaws. Both Pupkin and Zelig are men who have "made it," an accomplishment that trivializes all of their many shortcomings.

THE PURPLE ROSE OF CAIRO

Two years after the appearance of *Zelig,* Woody Allen again explored the theme of celebrity in *The Purple Rose of Cairo.* It may be useful to conceptualize *Stardust Memories, Zelig,* and *The Purple Rose of Cairo* as Allen's "celebrity trilogy" since the filmmaker's attitude toward the phenomenon of celebrity undergoes an evolution in these three films. The contemptuous attitude toward celebrity worshipers that Allen conveys in *Stardust Memories* is transformed into empathic understanding by the time of *The Purple Rose of Cairo.* In this latter film Allen recognizes that the fascination with celebrities serves an almost religious function in our secular society. It fulfills one of mankind's strongest psychological and spiritual needs and may be an essential antidote to the toxins associated with the vicissitudes of life. Moreover, *The Purple Rose of Cairo,* more than the other two members of the trilogy, acknowledges the centrality of movies and movie stars in our construction of life-sustaining illusions. Although Allen himself has indicated that he prefers *Stardust Memories* (Ansen 1986), most critics find *The Purple Rose of Cairo* to be a richer and more complex work. It simultaneously operates on many different levels: comedy, tragedy, a feminist commentary on sexual relationships, a quasi-religious existential statement, a psychological examination of the meaning of movies to the human psyche, an ironic and self-parodic commentary about the shallowness of movies and movie people, a simple love story, and a Pirandellian exploration of the nature of reality and illusion. As he did in *Zelig,* Allen returns to the Great Depression as the setting for his film, perhaps drawing some parallels between the financial bankruptcy of that era and the spiritual and psychological bankruptcy of our own.

Cecilia (Mia Farrow), the protagonist of *The Purple Rose of Cairo,* lives in a reality that is unbearable. She is married to an out-of-work slob named Monk (Danny Aiello) who beats her whenever the spirit moves him. She is stuck in a dead-end job in an era when people are lining up to jump out of windows rather than face the financial hardships that are upon them. For Cecilia, the movies represent an alternative to this harsh reality. Relationships are easy in the movies. Boy meets girl; boy falls in love with girl; and boy and girl live happily ever after. Sexual anxieties do not exist in the movies because there is a fade-out after the first kiss. At one point in the film, a woman in a movie house comments that her middle-aged husband comes to the movies because he is a student of the human personality. She goes on to emphasize that he has trouble with real-life human beings, but he is much more successful in relating to celluloid characters.

After losing her job and walking out on her adulterous husband, Cecilia sits in the darkened movie theater for one showing after another of *The Purple Rose of Cairo,* a film-within-a-film that transports her from her desperate situation in New Jersey to a romantic adventure on another continent. She becomes particularly fascinated with the handsome and naive hero of the film, Tom Baxter (Jeff Daniels). After multiple viewings of the film, the heroine's fantasy becomes reality: Tom Baxter comes off the screen and into the movie house to sweep Cecilia off her feet. Without a moment's hesitation she flees with him through a back alley as he attempts to escape from the cinematic world of fantasy into the stark reality of Cecilia's world.

The stranger-in-a-strange-land theme of *The Purple Rose of Cairo* is as irresistible to audiences as it is to filmmakers. There are numerous other films about a visitor from another world or another dimension, who arrives on earth as an incorruptible innocent, unfamiliar with the ways of the world. This visitor may be a mermaid, an extraterrestrial, a foreigner, or, in the case of *The Purple Rose of Cairo,* a celluloid character who exists only on the screen. The following films appeared just in the two years preceding the release of *The Purple Rose of Cairo:* John Carpenter's *Starman,* Stephen Spielberg's *E.T.,* Ron Howard's *Splash,* Paul Mazursky's *Moscow on the Hudson,* and John Sayles's *The Brother from Another*

Planet. The prototype of this story of innocence among the corrupt is, of course, the Christ story. Woody Allen is obviously aware of this parallel as he pans to a shot of a crucifix when Tom Baxter visits a church on his tour of Cecilia's world. Indeed, it is in the church that Cecilia's husband confronts Tom Baxter and challenges him to fisticuffs (plate 35). Tom gets the better of his opponent as long as the fighting is fair. But when he offers to shake Monk's hand and apologizes for the pain he has inflicted, Cecilia's husband knees him in the groin. Tom crumples to the ground, complaining in disbelief that his rival is not engaging in fair fighting.

Tom Baxter only knows the principles of fair play: deceit and dishonesty are alien to him. When he wanders innocently into a bordello, he is on unfamiliar ground. As the prostitutes surround him and listen intently, he speaks to them about the wonders of childbirth and the mysteries of existence. So taken with this inspirational young man, the ladies offer to service him for free. He thanks them for their offer but turns them down in deference to his love and loyalty for Cecilia. The denizens of the brothel are duly impressed, and one expresses a wish that there might be other men like Tom in the "real" world.

The parallels with Christ and the plethora of Christ figures in literature and film are obvious. Perhaps our strongest psychological need is for the illusion

PLATE 35. Different styles of combat: Jeff Daniels and Danny Aiello in *The Purple Rose of Cairo* (1985). Orion Pictures Corporation. The Museum of Modern Art/Film Stills Archive.

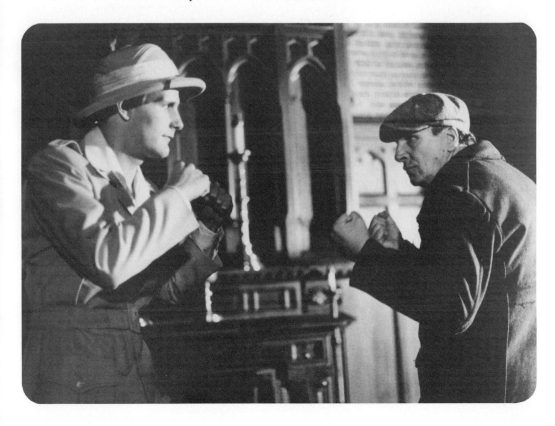

that somewhere, whether it be in a stable in Bethlehem or on the great silver screen, there exists an individual with transcendent, near-perfect qualities. The most salient feature of the movie hero is that he is not like us. He is unfettered by human selfishness and greed, by the baser instincts characteristic of the dark side of man. Hence, in the midst of perhaps the blackest era of United States history, Allen illustrates how the film idols provided hope that a transcendent realm existed where a young man and young woman would meet, fall in love, and dance around the room in stunning fashion to the accompaniment of "Cheek to Cheek."

George Bernard Shaw once observed, "There are two tragedies in life. One is not to get your heart's desire. The other is to get it." Cecilia would undoubtedly agree. When her movie idol descends from the heavens to profess his love for her, more problems are created than solved. Tom is unable to function in a world where stage money is not accepted as currency, where cars do not start just because one sits behind the wheel, and where people do not behave as though they are the inventions of screenwriters. Moreover, Gil Shepherd (also played by Jeff Daniels), the actor who portrays Tom Baxter in the film within the film, appears on the scene. The producers of the movie are livid at Tom's departure from the screen and have enlisted Shepherd's assistance in persuading Tom to return to the film. Gil pursues Cecilia in an intensive effort to court her away from Tom (plate 36). If he can win Cecilia's heart, he can save his career from ruin by forcing Tom back to the screen. As we get to know Gil, we are stunned to find that the transcendently flawless Tom Baxter is a creation of an actor who is not fit to wear Tom's pith helmet, let alone his halo. Gil Shepherd is a man of extraordinary vanity. Like Monk, he is a man of the real world, who exploits Cecilia according to his own needs, with little regard for the impact of the exploitation on Cecilia.

The climax of the film occurs when the heroine must choose between Tom and Gil in the empty movie theater while the characters on the screen look on. Reality and fantasy have reversed themselves. The action is now taking place in the darkened house while the audience consists of a group of actors peering out from the movie screen. Gil Shepherd seems aware of the strange state of affairs and comments, "I know this only happens in the movies, but I love you." Faced with an agonizing decision, Cecilia chooses Gil and says to Tom, "I have to choose the real world." A hard-bitten actress warns her from the screen, "You're throwing away perfection." Cecilia would have been wise to listen to this prophetess of doom. After Tom returns to the screen, Gil slips off to Hollywood without even a word of explanation. To Cecilia's horror, she

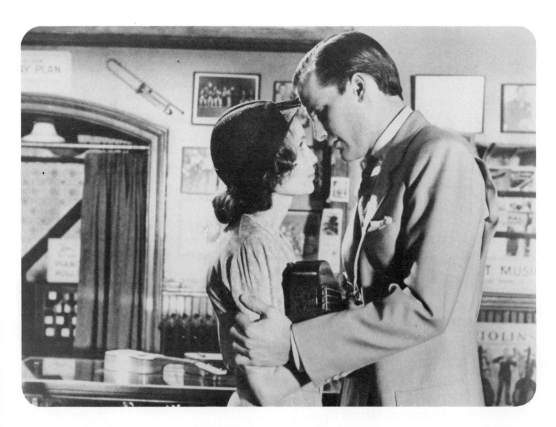

PLATE 36. Mia Farrow with the real thing (Jeff Daniels) in *The Purple Rose of Cairo* (1985). Orion Pictures Corporation. The Museum of Modern Art/Film Stills Archive.

discovers that she has made the wrong choice and is once again taken advantage of by a callous and self-serving man of the real world. She is left with a reality that is too grim to face, so she returns to the movie theater and immerses herself in yet another escapist fantasy of dancing with Fred Astaire. The film ends as it began, with the camera glued to Cecilia's face, her eyes transfixed with an almost beatific glow as she worships in her cinematic sanctuary.

As he does in *Stardust Memories* and *Zelig*, Allen again illustrates the folly of celebrity worship. We all know that Tom Baxter does not exist independently of the actor playing him. While Tom may be a virtuous and loyal boy scout, he turns out to be the creation of a narcissistic and insensitive boor, who exploits and victimizes our heroine. However, whereas our sympathies lie primarily with the celebrity protagonists of *Stardust Memories* and *Zelig*, in *The Purple Rose of*

Cairo our hearts are with the celebrity worshiper. We empathize with her predicament and with her psychological need to believe in Tom Baxter and Gil Shepherd. One way Allen plays on our sympathies is to demonstrate our own vulnerability to believing in the illusions that movies offer. Like Cecilia, we find ourselves believing and hoping that Gil and Cecilia will go off into the sunset to live happily ever after at the end of the film. Even though we know rationally that such an outcome would never realistically come to pass, we are willing to suspend our disbelief to collude with the filmmaker's illusion. After we are jolted by the harsh reality of Gil's departure, we must accept that we are vulnerable to the same escapist fantasies as Cecilia.

Allen also helps us understand Cecilia's need to believe in Tom Baxter. As with Masha and Rupert's transference to Jerry Langford, Cecilia's transference to Tom represents the only available means of alleviating her despair. Just as the analysand may perceive his analyst as having idealized characteristics that bear litle resemblance to the normal human flaws of the analyst's true personality, so does Cecilia perceive Gil Shepherd. By the ingenious device of splitting the fictional character and the actor into two different people, Allen provides us with a graphic example of the difference between transference and reality. Tom is the idealized transference creation while his counterpart Gil represents the nonfictional man behind the transference. When Cecilia looks at Gil, all she can see is Tom. Never mind the fact that Gil's real attributes in no way resemble those of his doppelganger, Tom. Cecilia is blind to the vanity of Gil because she needs the transcendent Christ-like qualities of Tom to tame the terror of her existence.

Tom Baxter is for Cecilia what Jerry Langford is for Masha in *King of Comedy*. Both manifest idealizing transferences to their respective male celebrities. Each woman is made whole simply by standing close to their illustrious heroes and basking in the reflected glory. Kohut (1971) originally described this form of transference as typical of patients suffering from narcissistic personality disorder. However, in his posthumously published third book (Kohut 1984), he revised his thinking because of his increasing awareness of the ubiquity of such trans-ference phenomena. He came to realize that even the healthiest person has a normal narcissistic need for idealized self objects in his environment. They are as necessary for psychological survival as oxygen is for physical survival. Cecilia's idealization of Tom Baxter is then a matter of survival. After reeling from the devastating blows to her self-esteem inflicted by her husband and her boss, Cecilia could enter the movie theater and revel in a buoyant sense of well-being because of her connection with this transference figure. When her self-esteem plummets after she realizes that Gil Shepherd has deceived her, she rapidly restores a cohesive sense of self by returning to the movies and sitting in the shadow of Fred Astaire and Ginger Rogers.

In film after film, Woody Allen sends this recurring message: there is no special luster to celebrities. They are far more similar to us than they are different. Rock Hudson may have been a handsome, virile leading man, but he succumbed to AIDS. Dick Van Dyke is an alcoholic. Johnny Carson has the same marital problems the rest of us have. Marilyn Monroe committed suicide. Dustin Hoffman is short and difficult to get along with. Elvis was a drug-crazed paranoid. The list goes on and on. Despite his sobering vision of the folly of celebrity worship, Allen's world view has evolved to the point in *The Purple Rose of Cairo* where he realizes that Cecilia would probably have been better off living in her fantasy than opting for the reality of the vain, self-serving Gil Shepherd. Perhaps the movies represent an opportunity for us to fulfill in a harmless way the need for fantasy and illusion that is intimately linked to our primal terror associated with the meaninglessness of existence.

Although *The Purple Rose of Cairo,* like *Zelig,* appears to be a film about a particular period in American history, the themes of the films reverberate with images of our contemporary culture. Near the end of *Zelig,* Irving Howe appears as a witness and makes the following observation: "It was absurd in a way. He had this curious quirk, this strange characteristic, and for a time everyone loved him. Then people stopped loving him; then he did this stunt with the airplane; and then everyone loved him again. And that was what the twenties were all about. And if you think about it, has America changed that much? I don't think so."

In his keen summary of the Zelig phenomenon, Howe brings us back to the present. Indeed we have *not* changed that much since the 1920s. We live in an age where thousands of screaming teenagers worship rock stars who spit blood and blow up Oldsmobiles on stage, where daredevils scale skyscrapers in defiance of the law but in full view of the television cameras, and where ordinary citizens perform death-defying stunts in order to appear on television shows with names such as "Real People" and "That's Incredible." Many of these people are admired because they have not settled for the mediocrity of the masses, for being "nobody." They have made something of themselves through their own idiosyncratic version of the American dream. *King of Comedy* and *Zelig* depict two such protagonists who emerge from anonymity into celebrity. The irresistible folly of their rise to stardom, like the irresistible folly of Cecilia's attraction to her movie idol, touches something profound and human in all of us as we sit in the darkened movie theater, knowing that our own existence is shortened with each unrelenting tick of the clock.

Alien and Melanie Klein's Night Music

10

■ *Alien,* Ridley Scott's hugely successful science fiction film of 1979, is at some moments so horrific that it might more appropriately be classified a horror film. Indeed, *Alien* may share with John Carpenter's *Halloween* (1978) the dubious distinction of having brought the graphic violence of marginal or "cult" movies such as *The Texas Chain Saw Massacre* and *Night of the Living Dead* to mainstream audiences. Regardless of its genre, however, the success of Scott's film—it was the fourth largest grossing film of 1979 (Steinberg 1980)—may not depend entirely on its fascination with grisly death. Large audiences do not go to theaters simply to gaze at bleeding intestines, even if this does appear to be the lesson that many in the business of filmmaking have learned from *Alien.* Clearly the film is more professional than the rash of monster and mad-slasher movies of recent years, but *Alien* also draws much of its power from its perhaps unintentional evocation of infantile anxieties best described in psychoanalytic terms by Melanie Klein. As Noël Carroll (1981) has pointed out, psychoanalysis "is more or less the *lingua franca* of the horror film and thus the privileged critical tool for discussing the genre." Particularly useful are Klein's theories on part-objects, introjection, and projection. If Klein is right, none of us ever completely overcome the angst of our earliest childhood imaginings. More so than most films of its kind, *Alien* skillfully evokes these early but imperfectly repressed anxieties about nurturing figures that can turn against us, about our own aggressive tendencies that can punish us from within or without, and about our tenuous relationship to bodies with no discernible beginning or end.

Many horror and science fiction films besides *Alien* can be understood in terms of Klein's work, most obviously her account of how the infant utilizes introjective-projective mechanisms in order to deal with primitive annihilation anxieties, including derivatives of the death instinct and of early oral aggressive drives. In *The Exorcist* (1973), as well as in its sequels and imitations, the Devil or some other possessing spirit moves back and forth among child and adult victims in ways quite consistent with this fantasy. This evil spirit is analogous to the bad, persecutory object, which is alternately projected and re-introjected.

Other films have played upon a child's ambivalence toward his love objects in somewhat different ways. For example, in a B-movie from 1953 called *Invaders from Mars,* a boy witnesses the gradual takeover of his community by alien forces. His own parents are the first to be transformed: one day they return home visibly unchanged but exhibiting the conventional affectless behavior of alien-inhabited humans in science fiction films. The child is portrayed as well behaved and affectionate, but he is abused by his possessed parents even when he attempts to demonstrate his love for them. The boy learns that the infected members of his community can be identified by means of a small wound at the back of the neck, clearly the site of penetration by the Martian invaders. Eventually the boy seeks help from a pair of parent surrogates—his female teacher and an archetype from the 1950s, an oracular space scientist. He explains to them that his real parents are "wonderful" and would never behave so unpleasantly without foul play from aliens. When he encounters the aliens themselves, their leader appears as a large head inside a transparent sphere. Attached to the head are phallus-like tentacles, which undulate slowly within the globe. This nightmare combination of parental betrayal and disembodied part-objects in fact turns out to be the child's dream at the film's conclusion. By comparison, Tobe Hooper's 1986 remake of *Invaders from Mars* contains several in-jokes for sci-fi film buffs but shows little understanding of the original. Unlike Philip Kaufman's 1978 remake of *Invasion of the Body Snatchers,* Hooper's film makes no attempt to update the odd combination of infantile anxieties and anti-Communist hysteria that created an especially fertile soil for science fiction films in the 1950s. Kaufman, by moving the action of his film to San Francisco, changed the McCarthyist politics of the original *Invasion of the Body Snatchers* into an amusing satire of 1970s hedonism and human potential plat-itudes. The film did not, however, dilute any of the power that the original derived from depicting the paranoid states in which the characters constantly find themselves. Hooper's remake of *Invaders from Mars,* on the other hand, keeps its tongue in its cheek throughout, poking appropriate fun at the original's plot but also frittering away the film's potential power by joking with the child's terror. Even in a summer of weak competition from undistinguished action films, *Invaders from Mars* quickly vanished from theaters.

Film scholars have identified the original *Invaders from Mars* and a handful of other American films from the 1950s with the politics of the McCarthy era. The first *Invasion of the Body Snatchers,* the most commonly cited example of this trend, can also be considered from both a political and a Kleinian perspective. The belief that Communists could and would project themselves into a loved one and overnight transform him or her into a soulless and hostile creature finds its metaphors in the same science fiction conventions that touch on the childhood anxieties identified by Klein. One of the films that played on the generalized xenophobia of the McCarthy period was *The Thing,* directed by Christian Nyby in 1951. The creature from outer space—part plant, part animal—manifests itself in unusual ways and threatens to break into the protected domain of the intrepid heroes. Central to Klein's understanding of infantile development is the tendency to split off the "bad" or aggressive aspects of the self and project them into objects in the environment, thus producing paranoid anxiety about external attack within the infant. This concept operates in audiences' responses to *The Thing* as well as to virtually any film about destructive creatures trying to break into the fragile safety of our immediate surroundings. (A Kleinian analyst would have much to say about the "monsters from the id," which Walter Pidgeon unconsciously projects in *The Forbidden Planet.*) John Carpenter's 1982 remake of *The Thing* takes us even deeper into a uniquely Kleinian world where evil forces are introjected by people and even transformed into grotesque combinations of human body parts. The suspense in this film derives from the paranoid tension concerning whether the invader from space is inside or outside the members of the team of Arctic scientists.

The protagonists in all of these films contend with a similar dilemma: they cannot be sure if their family members, colleagues, and loved ones are who they say they are. In both versions of *Invasion of the Body Snatchers,* no one can be trusted, because familiar bodies have been transformed into pod people. The police and even the psychiatrist in the film cannot be counted on since they have become part of "them." In *The Exorcist* Regan (Linda Blair) has the same body but is no longer the same person. Similarly, in George Romero's *Night of the Living Dead,* when an injured and helpless little girl is left alone in the basement with her father's corpse, she is later discovered to be making a meal out of her father, having been transformed into a flesh-eating zombie. In Carpenter's *The Thing* the protagonist (Kurt Russell) must resort to a blood test to determine which members of the Arctic crew are "really themselves" and which have been invaded by the alien force and taken over from inside.

Part of the horror in these films lies in their obsession with the notion of the double—the idea that a good person can be transformed into an alter ego or doppelganger of an unrelentingly evil nature. The protagonists then must assume a hypervigilant stance toward all their familiar friends and acquaintances to discern which of them can be trusted and which of them must be destroyed.

In clinical psychiatry a rare nosologic entity, known as Capgras' Syndrome (Lehmann 1980), describes just this state of affairs. The person afflicted with this syndrome is consumed with a variant of paranoia in which he believes that friends or family in his environment are actually impostors. The Capgras victim may point out that there are minute differences between the impostor and the actual person. While Capgras' Syndrome represents an extreme at one end of the continuum, the cinematic theme of the double in horror films is chilling to the audience because it touches on a normal developmental experience that is universal. As infants mature, they experience the mother as alternately good and bad, depending on the extent to which she is satisfying their needs. The transformation of the good, loving mother into the bad, persecuting mother is clearly a source of intense anxiety for the infant. This developmental moment, in which mother is split into a good mother and a bad mother, may well be perceived in the infant's mind as a transformation similar to the one portrayed in the horror films we have described. Hence many of the most effective horror films replay the Kleinian theme involving the transformation of a good object into an identically appearing evil object, which Klein would understand as a projection of the split-off bad self. This motif achieved a tasteless if inevitable fulfillment in the 1984 Christmas release *Silent Night, Deadly Night,* in which Santa Claus is transformed into an ax-murderer. When the television commercials advertising this film created a grass roots protest movement, the film was withdrawn from many theaters. Parents made it clear that this was one good object that would not be taken over from within by evil forces.

No science fiction or horror film, however, has evoked the full range of Kleinian anxieties so thoroughly as *Alien.* It may be more than an interesting coincidence that approximately midway through the film, Tom Skerritt as Captain Dallas of the star ship *Nostromo* is relaxing in "the shuttle," listening to the second movement of Mozart's "Eine kleine Nachtmusik." This lovely serenade is especially disarming because it is the only music in the film that is not part of the background score, and because its courtly associations are jarringly inappropriate to the grim, automated world of the space vessel. There are a number of explanations for the presence of this music in *Alien.* First, it is in the shuttle—a small ship attached to the enormous hulk of the *Nostromo*— that Ripley (Sigourney Weaver) makes her escape back to the earth and away from the dangers of outer space: we should not be surprised that earlier in the story it is shown to be a place where a character might find solace from the troubling events of the rest of the ship. Also, since *Alien* is part of the grand tradition of technically sophisticated space adventures, which began with Kubrick's *2001: A Space Odyssey* (1968), it is possible that the film's makers are paying tribute to the earlier film. *2001* was remarkable for its association of classical music with spaceships, and in its final scenes it placed an astronaut in a drawing room from the eighteenth century, the era of Mozart.

The use of a few measures of "Eine kleine Nachtmusik" also reminds us that the action of the film takes place in the eternal night of space and that the film is full of nightmare imagery and, of course, nightmarish content. But the ironic fact that this nightmare movie begins with people waking up and ends with one going to sleep is paralleled by the inconsistency of Mozart's sublime night music with the tones of horror struck throughout the entire film. The title "Eine kleine Nachtmusik" implies an evening's entertainment, and because *Alien* is an entertainment that deals with the stuff of nightmare, and because the infantile anxieties described by Melanie Klein pervade the entertainment, we have called this chapter "*Alien* and Melanie Klein's Night Music."

Alien was one of the first films to make full use of the new technologies, which greatly expanded the film's impact on its audience: seventy-millimeter projection equipment and six-track Dolby sound have made *Alien* an over-whelming experience. The audiences who flocked to the film in the summer of 1979 did not object to a plot that awkwardly sent characters off by themselves to be done in by the monster. Nor were they scared away by the scenes of explicit violence, which unnerved the film's more squeamish critics. Most likely they were attracted by those scenes, which compellingly touched their most primal terrors. As Freud (1920) pointed out, there is a compulsion to repeat those traumatic events that were passively experienced in an effort to gain mastery over them. People line up to see movies like *Alien* in order to reencounter powerful unconscious anxieties while retaining a sense that they have some control of an active nature the second time around. Moreover, the movie provides an aesthetic distance so that the audience knows that the terror on the screen is not actually happening to them, and they can experience relief along with their fright. The successful reactivation of primitive universal fears also depends on the director's handling of his subject matter, and we should point out certain technical achievements of Ridley Scott and his coworkers that serve to present these infantile experiences in an effective and affecting manner.

Alien owes a debt to its two major predecessors, *2001* and *Star Wars* (1977): whether we see humans fighting machines, monsters, or other humans, all three films show a fascination with highly refined technology and how it creates a new kind of explorer/hero. Like *2001*, *Alien* alludes to a computer-oriented power structure in which human considerations can become secondary. But like *Star Wars*, *Alien* shows us a future in which technology lacks the antiseptic sheen covering the great inventions of *2001*. In the two more recent films, gadgets can show their age and even break, although as Miller and Sprich (1981) have written, *Star Wars* may have achieved its overwhelming success by speaking to a culture that has difficulty finding meaning in an increasingly technological society. *Star Wars,* set in a world that is even more technologically complex than our own, strongly affirms that meaning can be brought to our lives.

In *Alien* Ridley Scott has rejected the technological fairy world of *Star Wars* and created instead an entirely new vision of the future in which urban and rural blue-collar workers haggle about their shares of the company wages while rusty chains and leaky pipes clutter the untended corridors of the spaceship. This is in sharp contrast to the innumerable science fiction films in which citizens of spacious, spotless cities stroll about in Hellenic revival gowns. (Some science fiction films were still adopting this approach to design as late as 1976, for example, *Logan's Run,* but the look was already being parodied by Woody Allen in 1973 in *Sleeper.*) The motley crew of the *Nostromo* in *Alien* is the predecessor of the grimy working-class population of the lunar mining village in *Outland* (1981). Scott developed this vision even further with the fully realized chaos of twenty-first century Los Angeles in his next film, *Blade Runner* (1982).

The future that *Alien* creates is not just the dehumanizing computer culture of *2001* in which man must outwit his machines in order to climb to the next rung in the evolutionary ladder. As a revisionist science fiction film, *Alien* creates a genuine dystopia in which urban decay and frustration have expanded into outer space and in which a sinister "company" blithely declares its employees expendable at the whim of its "weapons division." The film transcends the idealism that generated the paranoid films of the post-Watergate years, such as Alan Pakula's *The Parallax View* (1974) and Sydney Pollack's *Three Days of the Condor* (1975). The conspiracies in these films create waves of indignation in their characters because of a belief that political conspiracies at the highest level do not take place in the West. But in *Alien,* the consummate cynicism of the characters and their world is voiced by Captain Dallas, who says, "I don't trust anybody." The crew of the *Nostromo* is primarily made up of malcontents who do their unpleasant work purely for money and who show absolutely no ideals about family, country, or company. The only real human feelings in the film are directed by Ripley toward her cat.

The social and political setting of *Alien,* which has been extensively elucidated by Harvey Greenberg (1983), is an especially effective background for the nightmare action of the film. Just as there is no place in the ship to hide from the monster, there is no familiar, consoling institution to give meaning to the persecution of the characters. Even in *Outland,* Sean Connery had a wife and child to keep in mind when he went out to preserve his self-respect *High Noon*–style against the forces of evil, and *Blade Runner* ends with the hero escaping into a vernal paradise with his android lover.

Furthermore, Scott has used a number of cinematic devices to create a powerful sense of foreboding and anxiety. For one thing, he has frequently made the actors' dialogue incoherent. Even the characters themselves deliberately obscure their words: when Ripley goes to the lower deck to check on repair work undertaken by Brett (Harry Dean Stanton) and Parker (Yaphet Kotto), she has to shout over the noise of steam escaping from a valve. As soon as she leaves, Parker laughingly turns off the steam. Parker is much like the director himself, who does not care if everyone's exact words are understood.

The sound of the film (which won a British Academy Award for Derrick Leather, Jim Shields, and Bill Rowe) is also confusing, especially in the multitrack Dolby version. At many moments it is difficult to distinguish between what sounds are part of Jerry Goldsmith's atonal score and what are actual sounds on the ship. Furthermore, sounds frequently come from isolated corners of the sound system, and of course, one never knows when that corner is the one from which the alien will make its terrifying appearance.

Scott has also intensified the film's effects by using close-ups where we would expect establishing shots. Filmmakers have always used this technique for the creation of suspense, but Scott's technological expertise and stylization set him apart from conventional directors. For example, in the scene in which Brett goes looking for Jones, Ripley's cat, the audience never really sees much of the remote part of the ship in which Brett finds himself. Instead, Scott gives us suffocatingly tight close-ups of Brett's face and vertiginous tracking shots of the leaky heights of the ship rather than of the floor-level environs, which could conceal a lurking alien. We never see the expected establishing shots, and consequently we never even have an idea of what objects could do the concealing. Much the same effect is achieved toward the end of the film when Scott's camera closes in on Ripley's face even though we are much more concerned about the proximity of the monster.

Most notably, Scott and his cinematographer Derek Vanlint never give us the opportunity to examine carefully the fully grown monster, which dominates the action of the last half of the film. Although the camera often lingers on the beast's fingers or teeth, the entire alien is glimpsed only briefly, sometimes in a shot with such bright backlighting that the monster in the foreground is obscured. Scott has learned from Joseph Conrad that what we do not know can be more horrifying than what we know all too well. (Conrad's short story "The Duellists" was the source of Scott's first film; the novel *Nostromo* gave its name to the ship in *Alien;* and Conrad's theme of the double dominates *Blade Runner.*) Just as the horrors Kurtz inflicts on the natives in *Heart of Darkness* are more disturbing for never being revealed, so the monster that we never quite see is all the more terrifying.

The movie opens within the womblike confines of the mother ship. The camera pans the inside of the craft in some detail and finally comes to rest on the sleeping bodies of the seven crew members. As we examine the inside of the spaceship, we hear unformed and atonal noises, reminiscent of intrauterine existence, which are not readily identifiable but eerily familiar. We then see the diaper-clad crew begin to wake up from their frozen sleep state (plate 37). From this symbolic birth at the beginning, the movie goes on to create a world much like Klein's view of the infant's early months of life. The cinematographic technique of omitting establishing shots contributes to a spatial disorientation, which may well be representative of the infant's early cognitive experience. Furthermore, we hear heartbeats and breathing throughout the film, echoes of the first few months of life, when the mother's heartbeat and breathing are essential to the infant's sensory world.

PLATE 37. The crew of the Nostromo wakes up at the behest of "Mother," the ship's computer in Ridley Scott's *Alien* (1979). Twentieth Century–Fox. The Museum of Modern Art/Film Stills Archive.

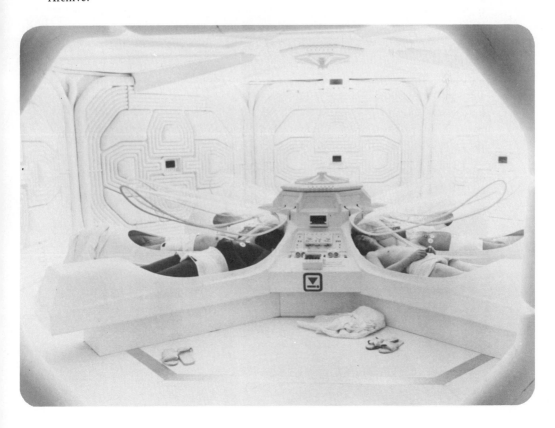

Klein indicates that the infant turns all of his libidinal desires and all his destructiveness onto his mother's body. Hanna Segal (1964), an articulate interpreter of Klein's writings, has observed that the infant's desires involve objects imagined to be inside the mother's body, including "fantasies of scooping out and possessing all of its contents, particularly . . . her babies" (1964, 7). This fantasy is portrayed early in *Alien* when the crew investigates the abandoned spacecraft on the remote planet. The inner lining of the ship is remarkably similar in appearance to the inside of a body (plate 38). The resemblance to the fantasied mother is all the more compelling because of the presence of egglike forms lying deep in the hold of the ship. When Kane (John Hurt) disturbs one of these eggs, he realizes the fulfillment of the scooping-out fantasy as well as its punishment when the alien leaps out of an egg and attaches itself to his face.

When Kane is returned to the *Nostromo,* diagnostic studies reveal that it is impossible to remove the creature from his face. One x-ray study reveals that the monster has extended an appendage down his throat and is keeping him alive. This situation can be understood in terms of the vicissitudes of early infantile development. The ego undergoes splitting and projects that part of itself containing the aggressive instinct, or the death instinct in Kleinian terms, into the original external object, the mother's breast. The infant then feels that the breast is bad, resulting in feelings of persecution. The terrifying but life-sustaining creature in *Alien* represents the bad persecuting breast: it is the recipient of the first projection of the child's internal aggressive drives, while at the same time it performs the traditional nourishing function.

Once the infant has projected his aggression into the mother's breast, he then lives in terror that the persecutory object will get inside him and destroy both him and his good internalized objects. Segal (1964) describes this fear as the leading anxiety in the paranoid-schizoid position, a normal phase in the first several months of infantile development. The terror of annihilation accompanying this phase of development leads to the evolution of defense mechanisms, principally the use of introjection and projection:

> The ego strives to introject the good and to project the bad. This, however, is not the only use of introjection and projection. There are situations in which the good is projected, in order to keep it safe from what is felt to be overwhelming badness inside, and situations in which persecutors are introjected and even identified with in an attempt to gain control of them. The permanent feature is that in situations of anxiety the split is widened and projection and introjection are used in order to keep persecutory and

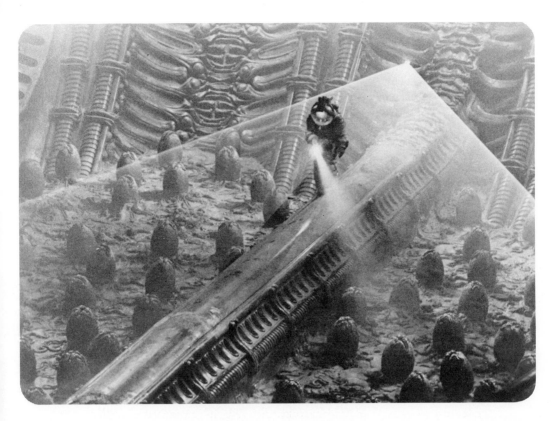

PLATE 38. Kane (John Hurt) explores the maternal body of a derelict ship in *Alien* (1979). Twentieth Century–Fox. The Museum of Modern Art/Film Stills Archive.

ideal objects as far as possible from one another, while keeping both of them under control. The situation may fluctuate rapidly, and persecutors may be felt now outside, giving the feeling of external threat, now inside, producing fears of a hypochondriacal nature. (Segal 1964, 26–27)

These defensive operations are graphically demonstrated in *Alien* when Kane is discovered to be free of the adhesive creature and is apparently back to his normal state of health. After sitting down to eat with his fellow crew members, he is destroyed from within when the alien ruptures his chest wall and escapes into the ship. To translate this sequence into the language of the paranoid-schizoid position, Kane introjected the bad persecutory object with the unconscious fantasy of gaining control over it. The dinner scene is characterized by much unnatural laughter, a kind of manic denial based on the fantasy that the persecutor has been annihilated. The dinner is disrupted by Kane's hypochondriacal concern about something within his body. The bad object is then re-projected—quite literally, when the alien rips through his chest wall—and is once again the source of persecutory anxiety as it disappears into the corridors of the spacecraft.

At this point, Scott's carefully crafted nightmare ambience can be seen as part of the persecutory anxiety that afflicts the remaining members of the crew, who are never sure where the alien, the projected bad object, is hiding and when it will strike. Captain Dallas's unwillingness to trust anyone is just one of the many manifestations of paranoia that strike all but two of the characters in the film. The first is Ash (Ian Holm), the science officer, who turns out to be an android. The second is the ship's computer, appropriately bearing the name "Mother." This maternal object also turns out to be bad when it reveals that it is in collusion with the company and is programmed to bring back the alien at all costs, even if the crew must be sacrificed for its capture. Just prior to the destruction of the ship, Ripley gives the computer an order, which it does not acknowledge. In a rage Ripley screams, "You bitch!" and smashes one of the computer's monitors.

Ripley's rage reflects the terror associated with the realization that she is living in a paranoid-schizoid world. It is a world devoid of good maternal objects. Nor are there any whole or ambivalently perceived mature objects in this chilling setting. The alien represents a thoroughly bad part-object, unrelenting in its evil and destructive nature. Ash, in commenting on this quality, expresses his admiration for the "purity" of the monster's devotion to the malevolent destruction of life. This ambience of part-objects, so typical of the paranoid-schizoid position, is heightened by the camera's tendency to show only part of the alien's anatomy at any one time. Here we see another version of the familiar Kleinian Capgras theme, as developed in films such as *Invasion of the Body Snatchers, The Exorcist,* and John Carpenter's *The Thing.* The crew naively trusted Ash, a science officer, to make judgments regarding the appropriate handling of the alien. They are shocked to learn that Ash is not who they thought he was. Rather, he is an android impostor with malevolent intentions. Moreover, "Mother," the ship's computer, is itself an evil force bent on their destruction rather than on their survival and safe return to earth.

To intensify the paranoid anxieties even further, the film shows all father figures being destroyed or, in the case of the robot Ash, working in tandem with the evil maternal computer. There is no rescuing father in this grim world of infantile terror. Contrary to the viewer's expectations, Captain Dallas, whom we assume to be the hero and the father figure of the ship, is killed relatively early in the movie, running counter to the convention of the science fiction or horror film. With the strong father figure now out of the picture, the crew has lost both its first and second command officers, leaving the strategy against the monster to be devised by two women, two childlike male figures, and the robot Ash.

The role of Ash in the movie leads us to another dimension of Klein's account of early infantile fantasies. Segal (1964) notes that the "infant's first dawning perception of the parental intercourse is of an oral nature, and the mother is conceived of as incorporating the father's penis in intercourse. Thus one of the riches of mother's body is this incorporated penis" (1964, 4). The mother, then, becomes a more terrifying object because of the infant's fantasy that she contains a penis in addition to the breast. These fantasies lead to anxiety about the "phallic mother," who is capable of destructive penetration, and to confusion about the equivalence between penis and breast. Indeed, the notion of the phallic mother is central both to children's stories and fairy tales and to a number of successful horror movies. The most obvious example of the former is the Halloween witch who rides with a broomstick between her legs. Movies such as Alfred Hitchcock's *Psycho* and Brian De Palma's *Dressed to Kill* portray female murderers who stab their subjects with sharp objects and who are later discovered to be men dressed as women. These terrifying figures resonate with the infantile concern that mother may possess a hidden phallus.

When Ash goes berserk in his confrontation with Ripley, he rolls up a girlie magazine and attempts to cram the phallic object down Ripley's throat, hence replicating the infantile terror that the mother's penis will be offered instead of the breast. Moreover, the monster itself is strikingly phallic, with its awesome tail, its long, tubular head, and its inner set of teeth, which extend and destructively penetrate its victims. The condensation of these oral and phallic elements is further illustrated by the fact that the monster also eats at least one of its victims.

The movie ends by fulfilling the audience's wish to master its infantile anxieties. Through an ingenious strategy, Ripley manages to overcome a considerable number of obstacles and extrude the monster from the shuttle, eventually blasting it out into space. Quite literally, Ripley has rid herself of badness via projection and then destroyed the projected badness. The film's last shot shows Ripley entering a blissful sleep with her cat, as though the extrusion of the all-bad part-object has allowed for an all-good world of symbiotic bliss to replace it. Hence the audience can vicariously experience not only the mastery of the paranoid anxieties associated with the persecutory object but also the achievement of the nonambivalent, all-good, blissful union with the all-good mother as the outcome of such mastery.

The special power of *Alien* is strikingly demonstrated by comparing it to the 1986 sequel, *Aliens,* which promises to be a greater commercial success than even Ridley Scott's original. With his producer and wife, Gale Ann Hurd, director James Cameron has infused *Aliens* with the same energy and imagination he brought to his first film, *The Terminator* (1984). In many ways a careful homage to the original, *Aliens* continually finds ingenious ways of inflating the plot, settings, politics, technology, and special effects of Scott's film. Cameron and Hurd are members of a new generation of commercially savvy and technically accomplished filmmakers who know exactly how to appeal to every segment of the audience. Their work is intelligent but not intellectual, involving but not challenging, startling but not unnerving, and is thoroughly enjoyable if not entirely admirable. In contrast to the comic book hyperbole of the sequel, Scott's *Alien* now seems like a pensive, scrupulously drawn chamber film.

In their most remarked upon departure from the original, Cameron and Hurd have more completely idealized women than perhaps any other filmmakers in recent memory. Not only is Ripley (Sigourney Weaver again) braver, tougher, smarter, and more resourceful than all the men in the film, so is at least one female marine. In addition, Ripley also excels in virtues traditionally associated with women: she is the only character able to communicate with a nine-year-old girl (Carrie Henn), the only survivor of an alien attack on a distant planet and the kind of innocent but streetwise child that exists only in Hollywood films. After promising to fulfill all the maternal needs of the little girl, Ripley saves her life by fighting to the death with another supermother, the alien queen bee. To further heighten the tension, the film has Ripley rescuing the child while the planet's nuclear destruction is seconds away.

Although *Aliens* quotes from the original in numerous ways, the film has excised almost all the Kleinianisms that made the first film so fiendishly effective. The change was probably intentional. Cameron and Hurd may have understood what made *Alien* successful, but they surely understand that most blockbuster hits do not stray as far from Hollywood's paradigms as does Scott's film. Whereas *Alien* did away with all reassuring father figures rather quickly, none are needed when the sequel's Ripley is the ideal mother and a better protector than the most attentive father. Furthermore, the romance that was so thoroughly missing from *Alien* has been provided not just in the sequel's gushy evocation of mother love, but also in the sexually charged conversations between Ripley and a soft-spoken marine (Michael Biehn) cut from an Alan Alda mold. Even the political paranoia of the original has been transformed: the horror of *Alien* was enhanced by the gradual realization that no institution could provide solace when the "company" was revealed to be as malevolent as anything lurking on the ship; a similar vision of an evil military-industrial complex is presented in the sequel, but its agent (Paul Reiser) is portrayed as just another movie bad guy, no match for the indomitable Ripley. *Aliens* ends on a deeply reassuring note as a man, a woman, and a child enter peaceful hypersleep, a postnuclear family returning to the bosom of Mother Earth. Audiences familiar with the original might have expected a baby monster to burst out of Carrie Henn's chest after she had been rescued from the aliens. This perverse touch might have been consistent with the introjection-projection motifs of the original, but it would have been completely inconsistent with the upbeat spirit of the sequel.

The plot of *Alien* is quite simple: a monster is at large and must be destroyed. But as we have shown, the film has developed a complex method of telling the story and has connected it—intentionally or otherwise—with the long-forgotten but still powerful anxieties of the audience. We have not argued that the film coherently works out a one-to-one correlation between its plot and these anxieties. Rather we have shown how images of these fantasies emerge variously in much the same way that images appear in primary process thought and how these images strongly suggest the infantile fantasies identified by Melanie Klein. Consequently, the film taps into the dark unconscious anxieties of the audience and produces a reaction that spectators might not quite understand, just as they are not quite able to understand much of the dialogue in the film. Clearly, the preverbal ambience of the paranoid-schizoid position is not dependent on a clear understanding of language. In more ways than one, the audience of *Alien* is kept profoundly in the dark.

3 *Women*: Robert Altman's Dream World

11

In the well-known fairy tale "Beauty and the Beast," a young girl must leave her father and journey to a remote kingdom where she is to live as the captive of a beast with a hideous aspect. Though she finds the monster terrifying, she also discovers him to be a most gracious host. He treats Beauty with kindness and consideration, catering to her every whim. The peace is disrupted only when the Beast makes his daily visit to Beauty to ask in vain if she has grown to love him. Finally, as the creature lies dying, Beauty acknowledges her love for him, and he is transformed into a handsome prince. If this enchanting fairy tale were a dream recounted by a young girl blossoming into womanhood, one might well speculate that the dream revealed the young girl's unconscious attempts to reconcile her anxieties about male genitality. The dream could be interpreted as a wish fulfillment in which the violent fantasies connected with the male genitals prove to be totally unwarranted, and sexual fears are conquered through the healing power of love.

3 Women (1977), written and directed by Robert Altman, can best be understood as another variation of the same dream, in which a girl verging on womanhood attempts to come to terms with the phallic aspect of male sexuality and to forge a new identity as an adult woman. Altman has in fact said that the movie came to him in a dream. His statement is useful because the film defies understanding when approached on the secondary process level of rational, left-hemispheric thinking. *3 Women* only becomes comprehensible when viewed at the primary process level of condensation, displacement, symbolization, dramatization, and the mobile cathexes of the dream work described by Freud (1900), Sharpe (1937), and others.

In interviews taken just after the release of *3 Women* (Jameson and Murphy 1977; Ciment 1977), Altman seemed genuinely uninterested in explaining the meaning of his film, a position consistent with his reputation as a thoroughly intuitive artist. In fact, Pauline Kael (1973) has said that Altman, more than

240

any other film director, is able to make contact with his unconscious. In a conversation with Roger Ebert, Altman explains how *3 Women* took shape. "I dreamed of the desert, and I dreamed of these three women, and I remember that every once in a while I'd dream that I was waking up and sending out people to scout locations and cast the thing. And when I woke up in the morning, it was like I'd *done* the picture. What's more, I *liked* it. So I decided to do it" (1978, 197). In an interview with the French critic Ciment (1977), Altman also explains that the three women of the film's title were originally (1) Millie, (2) Pinky, and (3) a synthesis of the two. However, the third woman, Willie (played by Janice Rule), originally an unnamed barmaid at the saloon visited by the other two women, developed into a central character as the production got under way. Nevertheless, the statements that Altman has made about the film suggest that a good deal of what appears on the screen in *3 Women* comes directly from his dream. The film is best understood as the dream of a young girl who is regressing from the pressures of fully sexual adulthood into a strange trio of roles that parody various stages of womanhood as well as familial relationship paradigms. Obviously, we are aware that what appears to be a young girl's dream originated in the mind of a middle-aged male. We could speculate here on how Altman and his coworkers may have reworked primary process material—at least as it was reported by Altman—in order to create a viable cinematic work of art. On the other hand, it is just as important to emphasize that we do not hope to analyze Robert Altman or his dream. As we stated in chapter 7, our goal is to apply the methodology of dream analysis to a film, all the while realizing that this application is analogical rather than literal.

Regardless of how thoroughly Altman transformed images that originated in his sleep, few other filmmakers have been quite so successful in translating their dreams directly into cinema, a medium that always reflects the personalities of producers, writers, editors, cinematographers, set designers, costumers, composers, and actors as well as directors. It is all the more remarkable that Robert Altman has made this extremely personal film since Altman is more likely than most directors to let his coworkers inscribe their own visions onto his films. Consequently, critics have difficulty generalizing about Altman's "style" or "vision." As Robert Self (1985) has written, Altman's films actually challenge notions of the self by which critics have conventionally established the identity of an *auteur*. Self singles out Altman's *Buffalo Bill and the Indians* as "the most postmodern of Altman's films" because it "asserts the difficulty of any unified, coherent identity of the self" (1985, 10). A similar claim can be made for *3 Women*, the film Altman made immediately after *Buffalo Bill*. Psychoanalytically informed dream interpretation provides a privileged view of the shifting selves in *3 Women,* and it may help us understand the ambivalences in Altman's work that make the conventional auteurist signature difficult to find.

According to Sharpe (1937), the dream work can transform the dreamer's self into different characters in the dream: for example, murderous wishes may be attributed to another character as the dreamer himself innocently observes the murderer in action. In *3 Women,* three aspects of the dreamer's psyche are represented by three different female characters; and with the freely shifting cathexes of the primary process, the dreamer seems to be identified with different portions of her psyche at different times during the dream. As befits an action so closely tied to the secret wishes of the unconscious, the film frequently appropriates the dream work to tell its story.

3 Women was shot in and around Palm Springs, California, and the action begins at the "Desert Springs Rehabilitation and Geriatrics Center," where Pinky Rose (Sissy Spacek) has just taken a job. The childlike Pinky is immediately fascinated by Millie Lammoreaux (Shelley Duvall), an employee at the spa who is assigned to show Pinky the ropes. Although the two never become friends in the usual sense, Millie quickly wins the complete adulation of Pinky, who calls her "the most perfect person I've ever met." Millie does little to court Pinky's devotion, but since she is looking for a roommate, she invites Pinky to move into her apartment. Millie, whose ambition is to become the next Breck girl, has decorated her apartment primarily in yellow to match her car and her wardrobe. But none of the residents of the singles complex where Millie lives share Pinky's intense feelings about Millie. In fact, the building is called Purple Sage Apartments, and the other singles keep Millie as far away as yellow is from purple on the color wheel.

The third of the three women, Willie (Rule), paints bizarre murals (created for the film by Bodhi Wind) and wears dark eye makeup, gray clothes, and a floppy sun hat. She is the taciturn wife of Edgar Hart (Robert Fortier), owner of the Purple Sage Apartments and "Dodge City," a hangout with a bar, a shooting range, and a motorcycle track. The three women represent three aspects of the evolving self of the young female dreamer: Pinky is the prepubertal latency child, idealizing and emulating the women around her, unconcerned about the perils of genital sexuality; Millie represents the genital and sexually alive adolescent/young adult who is not afraid of her own lust; and Willie, who is pregnant throughout most of the film, symbolizes the maternal, "postgenital" woman who has successfully negotiated male sexuality and is now preparing to take the consequences of the genital consummation. The highly permeable boundaries of these three figures is evident in the role reversals between Pinky and Millie halfway through the film and among all three at the end. The interchangeability of the three characters is reflected in the fact that both Millie and Pinky are Texans named Mildred and in the obvious clang association between the names Millie and Willie.

At the opening of the film the tension between the women and male genitality is clearly drawn. Behind the titles and atonal theme music we see Willie's gray-robed figure at the bottom of a dry swimming pool painting strange, colored creatures with tails and angry faces. Three of the figures have female breasts: two of them embrace while the third, like Willie, is pregnant (plate 39). The fourth figure is male with a large, dangling penis. The same four figures recur in at least two other murals that Willie has painted, including the one in the swimming pool at Purple Sage Apartments, each time with a male figure represented as a satanic and victimizing creature.

Basically the film has two parts. Although it often hints at the darker aspects of part 2, particularly by means of Gerald Busby's ominous music, part 1 primarily invites us to laugh at the two naive young women: Millie (Duvall) attempts to live out the two-dimensional life presented in slick magazines for

PLATE 39. Sissy Spacek and Shelley Duvall posing on the set of Robert Altman's *3 Women* (1977). Note Bodhi Wind's mural. Lion's Gate Films. The Museum of Modern Art/Film Stills Archive.

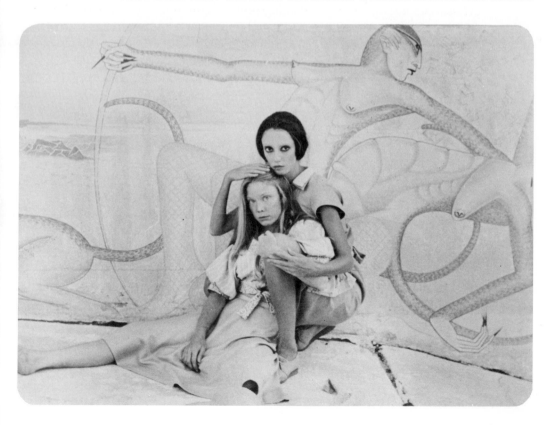

women, while the infantile Pinky (Spacek) merely marvels at the other's sophistication. As Altman laughingly suggested to Jameson and Murphy (1977), the middle half of the film could be the antics of a comedy team, Pinky and Millie, who would later appear in a sequel "Pinky and Millie Move to the City." There is even a kind of Laurel and Hardy pathos in the quaint, slightly sad manner in which they mimic a mother/daughter relationship.

Part 2 takes on a completely different tone as it opens with Pinky's attempted suicide and the overtly symbolic rescue by Willie. The compelling image of the pregnant Willie shivering alone in the pool after Pinky has been removed establishes her as a new mother-figure for Pinky. Altman himself has said that in this swimming pool scene, Pinky "floats in the water like a fetus in the maternal belly" (Ciment 1977, 14). Altman follows the image of Willie in the pool by cutting to Edgar walking down the stairs and then panning to the overbearing male creature that Wiliie has painted on the bottom of the swimming pool. This sequence is crucial because it unites Willie's painting with the characters of the drama at the same time that the film shifts away from satirical comedy and focuses on the conflict between Edgar and the three women. Henceforth the women begin turning away from traditional roles as natural mothers, daughters, and wives toward an artificial family unit without a threatening male presence. Before reaching this goal, the women act out an elaborate drama in which sex, death, and birth are intimately related.

After introducing Willie and her paintings at the beginning of the film, Altman cuts to still another swimming pool, this one full of water, the symbol of birth, death, and renewal that recurs throughout the film. In the pool aged bodies are guided about by much younger ones. It is a world dominated by pairs: the old people at the spa generally move in groups of two while the staff pairs off into sets of twins. Peggy and Polly, the blond identical twin sisters, are only slightly better matched than the inseparable Doris and Alcira—one Chinese, the other Chicano. Both are dark and members of minority groups. Equally compatible are Dr. Maas and Vivian Bunweill, whose intimacy seems more than professional and who jointly supervise the operations at the spa with the same degree of officiousness. (Later, we learn that Edgar was once Hugh O'Brian's "stunt double" on the set of television's "Wyatt Earp.")

Into this world come two women who would seem to be another matched set. Millie even tells Pinky, "You're a little like me," as the newcomer is fitted for a bathing suit. But the girls are not bound for the closed self-sufficiency of the other dyadic units. Although Pinky idolizes Millie, she is always on the outside looking in as when we first see her staring transfixed at Millie from behind a plate of glass. Millie too is an alienated individual with no family and no prospect of a satisfying relationship either with the medical students, who barely tolerate her presence at lunch, or with the denizens of Purple Sage, who ridicule her openly.

Millie and Pinky may not be a perfectly matched pair like those at the spa, but they consistently play at being big sister and little sister. Typically, when they first arrive at Dodge City, Millie expresses dismay when Pinky foreshadows her eventual symbolic death and rebirth by crawling in and out of a womblike tepee and then miming hanging at a prop gallows. (Pinky had earlier foreshadowed her suicide attempt by dunking herself in the geriatrics center pool, again to the embarrassment of Millie.) Throughout the first half of the film the sisterly relationship continues peacefully until the crisis of Edgar's late-night arrival with Millie. Pinky experiences something akin to the primal scene when she sees the two preparing to make love, but she receives the shock of a childhood nightmare when Millie rejects her for not being an adult: "You don't smoke, you don't drink, you don't do anything the way you're supposed to." In the context of the first half of the film the remark is mildly amusing because it once again reveals the irony in Pinky's adulation of a woman who so completely misunderstands adulthood. Within the dream logic of the film, however, Millie's forbidden tryst and her outburst concretize the worst fears of Pinky, who then attempts suicide.

Up to this point in the film, despite the clear establishment of Pinky and Millie as doubles of one another, their differences have been well drawn. Pinky is the wide-eyed little sister in awe of her classy older sibling. Millie is engrossed in efforts to involve herself with young doctors but occasionally deigns to offer Pinky some worldly advice. No competitiveness exists between them, because they are in entirely different leagues. So far, so good. But with the arrival of Edgar in the bedroom, a major shift occurs. Edgar clearly symbolizes the father since he is married to the maternal (and pregnant) Willie. The oedipal crime of incestuous sexuality is shared by both Millie and Pinky, and as a result, Pinky loses her innocence. Her introduction to male genitality and to sexuality is associated with the violation of an unspeakable taboo. While the manifest content of the film/dream indicates that Pinky attempts suicide because of her rejection by Millie, the latent content seems to be that she is punishing both herself and her double (Millie) for the oedipal crime of incest, just as Oedipus blinded himself. This portion of the film nicely illustrates the dream mechanism of dramatization, in that the dreamer, Pinky, can attribute incestuous sexual wishes to another character in the dream, Millie, rather than to herself.

After Willie rescues Pinky and becomes a new mother-surrogate, Millie undergoes a radical transformation as she seeks to do penance for her involvement in Pinky's trauma. We know the extent of Millie's transformation when she flatly rejects a sympathetic doctor who makes personal overtures outside Pinky's hospital room. Millie would have leapt at such an opportunity only the day before, but now her powerful desire to care for Pinky subsumes her previous longings. Her existence finally has a meaning greater than the one she created out of mail-order catalogs. She has found her true self in the role of Pinky's mother. Millie's selfless and guilt-ridden devotion to Pinky can be understood as an unconscious effort on her part to expiate her own guilt connected with the oedipal crime. Not only has she seduced father; she has almost killed off a female competitor in the process.

But when Pinky emerges from her coma, she first attempts to *become* Millie even as Millie begins to mother her in earnest. The first thing Pinky does upon awakening is disown her natural parents (Ruth Nelson and John Cromwell), whom Millie has summoned from Texas. At the top of her lungs she screams, "They're not my parents," and "I'm not Pinky," driving her parents from her hospital room. Here we see the family romance fantasy dramatically enacted. As Blum (1969) points out, when the child feels that his parents do not conform to the idealized and unconditionally loving roles he has attributed to them, he decides that his real parents, who have these features, have merely arranged for his adoption by those persons who claim to be his parents. This defense protects the child from the narcissistic injury of discovering that his parents do not love him in the way that he feels he should be loved. Moreover, Blum emphasizes how the genital/oedipal phase of development brings new significance to the family romance fantasy. By imagining himself to be a guest in the house of foster parents, the child eliminates the incest taboo in his relationship with his parents since biological relatedness is not an issue. The Oedipus myth would, of course, be the classical example of the family romance fantasy. Pinky's first words upon awakening from her coma, then, serve to announce the full flowering of this fantasy. Moreover, her words herald her passage from the pregenital quiescence of latency to the *reawakening* of the genital/oedipal phase of development associated with the onset of adolescence.

Back at the Purple Sage, Pinky takes over Millie's bed, her diary, her car, and her former lover, Edgar. In fact, Pinky is a great success at realizing the goals that eluded Millie: we see her at poolside attended by the same men who earlier scorned Millie. Meanwhile, Millie has changed from the impatient, disapproving big sister into the overindulgent, worried mother trying desperately to provide happiness and security for her child. Millie even loses her job to protect Pinky; she echoes Pinky's actions by rejecting *her* surrogate parents at the spa, Dr. Maas and Vivian. Since Millie has not seen her natural parents since she was eleven, Pinky is now the single focus of her familial life.

Pinky, on the other hand, wishes actually to replace Millie and in no way returns her devotion. Similarly, she seeks to replace both Willie and Millie by taking Edgar as her lover. Now Pinky acts like a daughter only in her wish to compete with Millie and Willie for the affection of Edgar, the father who by condensation is married to both Millie *and* Willie in Pinky's mind. Pinky's success in the competition for Edgar leaves Millie confused and humiliated, while Willie appears completely vanquished: after we see Pinky taking shooting lessons from an adoring Edgar, who utters the prophetic line "I'd rather face a thousand crazy savages than one woman who's learned how to shoot" (plate 40), the camera pans to the empty swimming pool where Willie lies unconscious amidst her paintings.

But Pinky cannot sustain her new role as the mother-vanquishing daughter, and after a bad dream she is again the insecure child asking to crawl into bed with Millie, whom she had earlier banished from the bedroom. At this moment an intoxicated Edgar enters and announces that Willie is in labor. Neither of the women has any interest in Edgar now (Millie shouts, "Don't touch her" as

PLATE 40. Edgar (Robert Fortier) teaching Pinky (Sissy Spacek) how to kill in *3 Women* (1977). Lion's Gate Films. The Museum of Modern Art/Film Stills Archive.

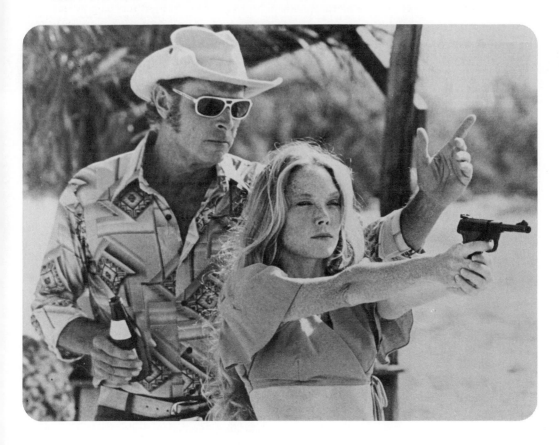

he reaches for the cowering Pinky), and they both dash off to help Willie. They arrive just as Willie is giving birth, and Millie orders Pinky to go for help. Pinky, however, remains: she watches while Millie attempts to deliver Willie's baby. After uttering what is perhaps the least encouraging series of lines ever delivered to a woman in labor in the history of film, Millie tells Willie that the baby is a boy and that it is dead. As Willie embraces the dead child, Millie sees that Pinky has not budged from her position outside the door. In a rage, Millie gives her the slap that should have gone to the newborn baby. After a brief period of trying to compete for men with the female rivals, Pinky has regressed to a phase of pregenital dyadic relationships in which she seeks to destroy baby brother in order to have sole possession of mother. Millie's displaced slap announces that Pinky has been reborn again, this time as the only child in the family.

The final scene of the film recalls the endings of Fellini's *Juliet of the Spirits* (1965) and Bergman's *Cries and Whispers* (1972), in which the scene changes provocatively from darkness to broad daylight. The three women are now comfortably ensconced in roles that complete their previously unfulfilled characters. When men arrive at Dodge City to deliver Coca-Cola, a gum-chewing, girlish Pinky tells them, "I'll get my mom." We see her go after a gray-robed figure who is not Willie but a stern-faced Millie. She is wearing the same hat and makeup that once belonged to Willie, and her hair is now dark and straight in Willie's old style. On the porch of the house behind the bar sits a new grandmotherly Willie without her old makeup and with full, graying, wavy hair. Free at last from reticence, she says she has just awakened from "the most wonderful dream." In the last moments of *3 Women,* Millie appears to dominate the other two, and Willie gently urges her not to be so mean to Pinky (who is now called "Millie"). The three women show a sense of domestic contentment that none of them every exhibited before. Edgar, by the way, has apparently died from a gunshot wound. Back in the bar, the Coca-Cola man remarks how odd it was that a man as expert with guns as Edgar should have died in what was presumably identified as a self-inflicted injury. The women, who are aloof to the personable young man, do not discuss the matter.

Although the script leaves the matter unresolved, it appears that all three women were involved in Edgar's death just as all three were involved in the death of Willie's child. They all had something to gain by both deaths. Indeed, Edgar's and the child's deaths serve a similar purpose, and in the dream work of condensation, they could be the same event. Altman has said as much to a *New York Times* interviewer: "The death of the male child was as much a murder as the death of Edgar, and maybe they were the same thing. And I don't think it makes any real difference" (Demby 1977, 17).

Both Edgar and the child represent the threat of the male and his genitality, which stand between the three women and their desire to form a sexless, mother/daughter relationship. Phallic symbols abound in this context. Edgar is first introduced as a malevolent-looking fellow who draws his gun and pulls a snake from under a rock the moment he sees Millie and Pinky. Like the overbearing male figure in Willie's murals, the penis is Edgar's most characteristic possession, and he has sexual relations with all three women.

Nevertheless, the three women all act out their wish to be rid of Edgar and his phallus. Willie, who is closest to Edgar, makes sand paintings of snakes, which she ornaments with bullet holes. At Dodge City, when Pinky asks Millie to identify one of these works of art, Millie explains it in the most matter-of-fact way although she suppresses the most important feature. "It's a sand painting with bullet holes," she says. Pinky too finds nothing unusual about the painting; in fact, she tells Willie that she likes it. Near the end of the film, after the Coca-Cola man leaves the bar, the camera comes to rest on the same sand painting hung on the wall as a kind of phallic trophy, indicating that Edgar and all other men in their lives have been effectively castrated. At one time or another, the film shows all three women on the shooting range putting bullet holes into the painted silhouette of a man, always in the phallic protrusion of the head. Edgar is further associated with phallic symbols when the sound of a rattlesnake accompanies the image of his face in Pinky's nightmare. Indeed Pinky speaks for all three women when she expresses the irrational fear that she may have been raped while she lay unconscious in her hospital bed.

In a more general sense, Edgar represents the male-oriented values of the society in which the women are expected to live. Edgar and his companions (many of whom are policemen) ride dirt bikes, drink beer from bottles, fire pistols, and take or ignore women at their whim. Millie's ex-roommate, Diedre, seems to be able to operate successfully in this world. Pinky, Millie, and Willie cannot. Pinky has a moment of success with men, which ends with her nightmare and her return to mother-Millie. Millie ineptly chases men through the first half of the film but never with the determination with which she later indulges Pinky after the suicide attempt. Willie is so frustrated in her marriage that she never speaks, expressing herself only by drawing bizarre caricatures of herself and Edgar and by shooting bullets into phallic snake paintings. While the three women are likely to be multidimensional characters, none of the male characters are represented as anything more than part-objects. In other words, there are no persons attached to the penises of the male characters, reflecting in part the anxiety and the inexperience in romantic matters of the pubescent girl dreaming the dream.

Only in the film's closing moments are the women free from male intrusions and able to lead the lives they had always been seeking in one way or another. Pinky has rejected her impossibly aged parents, who had brought her a plaque that urged her to become the traditional adult wife and mother. After also rejecting Millie's earlier conception of male-oriented adulthood, Pinky finds her true nature in perpetual childhood with not one but two mothers—one stern, the other beneficent. She will always have one mother to instruct her and another to indulge her. Altman's dream is unlike "Beauty and the Beast," however, because Beauty perseveres in the face of her genital anxiety to discover that men can be loving and three-dimensional human beings. Pinky retreats from the pressures intrinsic to fully genital, adult womanhood to a pregenital regressed state peopled with part-objects, symbolized by one good mother and one bad mother.

Millie has renounced her yellow-hued version of real life and accepted the role in which Pinky first cast her. In fact, Millie's brand of detached maternalism is something at which she had always excelled: at the spa, where the elderly occupants are treated like children, Vivian tells Pinky, "Millie's one of our best girls." Later, when she escorts Pinky's parents up the stairs to her apartment, she adopts a professional tone and tells them, "One hand on the rail." After Pinky's suicide attempt, Millie becomes more actively maternal, but she reverts after the death of the male child. As the stern mother-figure in the film's final scenes, Millie first appears in the same place where we first saw Willie, but it appears that Millie is washing away Willie's paintings. Millie has not lost her eye for how a place should look, and in the women's new life there is no need for sublimating emotions by means of art.

As for Willie, she has given up art for dreams, and pleasant dreams at that. She has rid herself of a male child, of Edgar, and of all his rowdy friends, and her personality has opened up. Early in the film she developed an empathy with Pinky when the younger girl admired her sand painting. When Pinky tried to take her own life, Willie was the first one in the water to save her, and she followed Pinky to her hospital room. Obviously Willie prefers Pinky to the male sibling whom Pinky helped destroy: she treats Pinky with tenderness in the final scenes.

As the film closes with Altman's camera panning away from the three women's house, we hear their voices as they conduct a day-to-day existence without men or threatening phallic symbols. In fact, in the film's final moments they have retreated into the womblike enclosure of the house behind the bar. Although they have apparently killed in order to achieve this peaceful existence, they do not seem to be haunted by guilt or disturbed by the fact that they will never know the love of the handsome prince. While the resolution of the dream may serve the proverbial function of guarding the dreamer's sleep, it may be the enemy of the dreamer's ultimate psychological growth. As Freud (1925) reflected in a later addition to his dream theory, when the solution to a problem of life is attempted in a dream, the dream solves the problem in the form of an irrational childhood wish rather than in a constructive rational manner. It would be interesting to speculate about what forces turned a fairy tale into the modernist vision of sex roles that *3 Women* represents. Altman has created a myth that speaks to cultural anxieties about the relations between the sexes as engagingly as it does to the secret wishes of the unconscious.

Epilogue

Filmmakers appear to be just as fascinated by psychiatry as psychiatrists are by movies. Psychiatrists and psychiatric matters have been regular subjects in films at least since 1904, and many writers have probed the mysteries of the cinema with psychoanalytically informed methodologies. Unlike other books about the interaction of movies and minds, this work has dealt with the relationship from both sides.

In part 1 we discussed some of the ways in which movies have stereotyped psychiatrists and appropriated them to serve the mechanical needs of plot and genre as well as the cinematic mythology of the day. In surveying over 250 American films, we have found only a handful that have not indulged in radically simplified or stylized portrayals of psychiatry, and more often than not, most of *these* films eventually turn from the examination of psychotherapeutic interactions toward familiar cinematic clichés: *Spellbound, One Flew over the Cuckoo's Nest,* and *Ordinary People* have little in common, but all three begin with themes relating to mental illness and ultimately end with highly conventionalized depictions of the psychiatrist saved by a lover, the clinical victimization of a Christ-like hero, or the climactic drama of a cathartic cure.

Psychiatrists are parodoxical figures for filmmakers. On the one hand, their work is extremely difficult to understand and has the potential to bring exciting action to a deadly halt. On the other hand, if psychiatrists are not observed too closely, they can conveniently provide the perfect forum for exposition and character development. They can also supply the legitimization of sexual themes, the rationalist contrast to supernatural "truths," the secular salvation of troubled souls, the romantic interest for misunderstood individuals, the convincing explanation for mysterious behavior, the commonsense solution for domestic crises, and the repressive opposition to free-spirited heroes. In addition, psychoanalysis's unsettling message—that we are not fully conscious of the motivations that direct our lives—has always been at odds with its image as a beneficent means to self-help, thus leaving itself open to polar opposites in its portrayal.

Few professions, ethnic groups, or social classes have been immune from a similar process of cinematic stereotyping, but psychiatrists may be unique for having occupied both the highest and lowest levels of prestige in their motion picture incarnations. We have charted these changes from the quacks of the early years through the secular saints of the Golden Age (1957–63), through the fools and criminals of the 1960s and 1970s, and finally to the more variegated group of movie psychiatrists that has begun to appear in the 1980s. In all of these periods, however, the needs of cinematic genres are almost always paramount: if they are not devalued beyond all reason, psychiatrists are usually idealized to an equally extreme degree. The need to see others as heroic and idealized—the celebrity phenomenon we described in chapter 9—is highly relevant in this context. Most movies demand idealized heroes because audiences demand them. These exaggerated figures give audiences hope, helping them weather their own individual existential storms, if only for two hours in a darkened theater.

We have found that only in the last few years have some filmmakers broken out of narrow generic conventions and put cinematic psychiatrists to imaginative uses. In particular, Woody Allen and Paul Mazursky have understood that mixtures of positive and negative traits are much more typical of human beings than heroism or villainy, and they have directed films in which psychiatry provides the means for examining this ambiguity. Their psychiatrists are seldom the Olympian healers of the Golden Age or the ridiculous figures of the late 1960s but rather the inhabitants of a world where difficult choices characterize human reality. Ironic comedy and gentle satire usually dominate the works of these directors, largely as a turning away both from the gravely serious social realism of the Golden Age as well as from the chic nihilism of the 1960s and 1970s.

In part 2 of this study, we discussed a number of films that can be better understood through the application of critical techniques derived from psychoanalysis. In the two chapters on narcissism in the cinema, we examined the manifestation of cultural patterns that dominate the themes of five recent films. Psychoanalytic methodologies can open up these works and lead to a larger view of contemporary American culture. After considering intrapsychic and cultural interactions in the adult world, we turned to the earliest experiences in the development of the child: a quite different methodology gives us insight into Ridley Scott's *Alien* and the genre of horror/science fiction films. Our reading of the film is designed to offer reasons for the primitive origins of horror film conventions as well as for the enduring appeal of these films. Finally, we hope that we have demonstrated how a knowledge of the dream work is essential to an understanding of the otherwise puzzling work of Robert Altman *3 Women.* Taken as a whole, part 2 of this book is meant as a brief introduction to the immense potential of psychoanalysis as a tool in film criticism. As psychoanalytic approaches to film study become more prevalent, it may soon be argued that cinema, more than fiction, poetry, or drama, is ideally suited to the kinds of analysis that Freud and his followers applied to the arts as well as to individuals and cultures. Moreover, the richness and complexity of the human psyche brought to light through psychoanalytic approaches illustrate the inadequacy of the one-dimensional stereotypical portraits of psychiatrists described in part 1. It is disconcerting to practitioners of depth psychology to see such superficial portraits of themselves painted in the medium of the cinema.

While it may be true that filmmakers and psychiatrists are mutually intrigued by one another, it is also true that there is a tendency toward mutual outrage. Filmmakers often react with incredulousness or even ridicule at what psychiatrists "read into" their movies, and psychiatrists are appalled at the film industry's portrayal of their therapeutic activities. Both sides feel misunderstood. The psychiatrist's reaction calls to mind the frequent response of the therapist who sees for the first time his videotaped interview of a patient. Typically, he or she gasps in disbelief, "Do I look like *that?*" or "I can't believe I said that," or "That's not what I meant." Clearly, there is a clash between how psychiatrists imagine themselves and what is actually recorded by the dispassionate eye of the camera. While the cinematic medium has an immense narcissistic appeal, as we noted in chapters 8 and 9, its power to inflict narcissistic injury is of equal strength. It may well be that those who select the vocation of psychotherapist are attracted to the privacy of the procedure, where they are insulated from the prying eyes and criticism of others who would seek to judge their work. The filmmaker's intrusion into the privacy of the consulting room may hence be viewed as an extraordinary violation. The well-known reluctance for psychotherapists to tape their work is undoubtedly related to more than the altruistic concern about the preservation of patient confidentiality. One suspects that most therapists are concerned that their technique is lacking in some respect and would not hold up to scrutiny by peers.

Beyond the anxiety about the quality of one's work, however, there may also be a sense among psychiatrists that the mere depiction of psychotherapy is almost obscene. Metz (1982) notes that there is a peculiar kind of voyeurism involved in the cinematic experience. What specifically defines this form of voyeurism is the absence of the object seen, not only contrary to true voyeurism as a clinical phenomenon but also in contrast to the theater, where the object is actually present on stage in front of the audience. In this sense, cinematic voyeurism is experienced as more unauthorized and more forbidden than the-atrical voyeurism, where the actors fully sanction the audience's desire to look at them. Metz argues that this differentiation provides for a more strongly established link to the primal scene in the cinematic audience than in the theatrical audience. Thus both the lure and the repugnance intrinsic to cinematic portrayals of psychiatric treatment may resonate with more primitive concerns about what is acceptable to see or to show.

The double-edged power of the cinema both to enhance and to devastate one's self-esteem is evident in the response of real-life therapists who have appeared in the movies. Dr. Penelope Russianoff, who appeared in Mazursky's *An Unmarried Woman,* is quite candid about the impact of her film experience (personal communication, 1984). She was not nearly as bothered by the movie's portrayal of her as a possible lesbian as she was by a few bad reviews. Six years after the movie she could still quote from them. Even though she was not an actress, the criticisms may have stung her because the film showed her at work as a psychotherapist. One can empathize with her reaction since it is difficult to divorce her performance as an actress from her performance as a therapist. As a woman of unusual height, she was accustomed to people staring at her on the street. After the film, she said that she was never sure if people were staring because she was tall or because she was in the movie. A few strangers spoke to her about the film, and some seemed incapable of separating her real character from the one they saw in the movie. These experiences, plus the bad reviews, eventually sent her back for a brief visit to her own therapist for refueling. Despite the emotional toll taken by her cinematic experience, she nevertheless longed to do more acting. She was disappointed when no subse-quent film offers were forthcoming, and she acknowledges that she would have liked to play the role of the Dr. Berger character in *Ordinary People,* a film that she believes her performance in *An Unmarried Woman* helped to make possible.

When Dr. Dean Brooks of the Oregon State Hospital in Salem was approached about playing a psychiatrist in *One Flew over the Cuckoo's Nest,* he had a number of misgivings. Although he knew that the film was only entertainment and not a documentary, he found it difficult to detach himself from the fact that it was being made in his hospital. He thought to himself, "Oh my God, my professional career is on the line. People will think that the hospital is really this way" (personal communication, 1985). Before he would agree to the filming at his hospital, he secured a commitment from producers Saul Zaentz and Michael Douglas that the film would in no way denigrate patients. During the first half of the filming, Brooks continued to go through internal struggles about his participation in the project. He reports that he was finally able to overcome these misgivings when he accepted that it was just a movie and decided to have fun. He commented that the movie actually hired eighty-nine patients, some of whom were paid more than he was. He described an extraordinary camaraderie between the cast and crew of the production and the hospital's patients, which he felt had a positive effect on many of the patients.

Ten years after the filming, Dr. Brooks feels that *One Flew over the Cuckoo's Nest* had no deleterious effect on his professional career. He also says that the hospital was in no way hurt. Initially, however, he experienced a number of criticisms from colleagues who felt that the film was "venal" or that it had "set psychiatry back twenty-five years." He defends his participation in the film, pointing out that the view of the movie as a negative portrayal of psychiatry is a narrow one. He believes that Ken Kesey was writing about institutions in general rather than about mental hospitals in particular, and that the film opened people's eyes to a number of concerns about institutions. Like Dr. Russianoff, he caught the acting bug as a result of *Cuckoo's Nest,* and he went on to act in another film, *Three Warriors,* which was never released theatrically but has appeared on cable television. He said that he never seriously considered leaving psychiatry to become an actor, but he unabashedly acknowledged that he loved being in front of the camera and enjoyed the celebrity that went along with the experience.

Donald Muhich, who has appeared in Mazursky's *Bob and Carol and Ted and Alice, Blume in Love, Willie and Phil,* and *Down and Out in Beverly Hills,* had acted even before he become a psychiatrist (personal communication, 1985). As a high school student in Minnesota, Muhich had been offered a scholarship to study acting at Northwestern University, a major proving ground for aspiring young actors. Although he eventually chose to accept an academic scholarship instead, Dr. Muhich has always kept his hand in as a producer and screenwriter as well as an actor. In addition to appearing in Mazursky's films, Muhich has participated in the writing of all ten of the director's movies, and he has produced a number of documentaries on his own. In 1970 he helped develop a short-lived television series, "Matt Lincoln," which brought "Ben Casey" star Vince Edwards back to television medicine, this time as a community psychiatrist. Muhich says that he terminated his brief career in commercial television when the producers of the struggling program brought in writers "to give the show heart."

The long and continuing association between Muhich and Mazursky began in the 1960s when the latter was writing jokes for Danny Kaye as well as the screenplay for Hy Averback's *I Love You, Alice B. Toklas* (1968). As Mazursky himself once acknowledged on the Johnny Carson show, he went to Muhich for treatment, knowing that the psychiatrist had a private practice in Beverly Hills primarily for creative people. Shortly afterward, when Mazursky learned that he would be allowed to direct *Bob and Carol and Ted and Alice,* he called Muhich and said, "I'm going to direct my first film. Come on out and we'll have a party!" Mazursky knew that Muhich had a good deal of acting experience and cast him for his knowledge of the performing arts as well as for his familiarity with the practice of psychiatry. In fact, Muhich has had a good deal of control over his appearances in Mazursky's films, and he continues to correspond with the director concerning all aspects of Mazursky's work. In both *Bob and Carol and Ted and Alice* and *Blume in Love,* Muhich worked closely with the director to achieve what he calls "the fine line between satire and realism." For example, the tight close-up in *Bob and Carol* that shows Muhich pinching his cheek while listening to Dyan Cannon was suggested by the psychiatrist as a means for capturing the slightly irreverent tone that he and the director intended. Muhich says that he never set out to represent the profession as it really is and certainly not to glorify it. If anything, Muhich believes that psychiatrists often claim more expertise than they are entitled to and that some chipping away at their image may not be an unworthy pursuit. He was amused by the number of mental health professionals who found his scene with Dyan Cannon to be an accurate presentation of psychotherapy, but he also admits that he stopped getting referrals from other psychiatrists after the film was released. Clearly, Muhich has derived immense pleasure from working with movie stars and filmmakers, and he recalls his acting experience in the movies as great fun. His continuing association with Mazursky suggests that he has succeeded in sustaining a dual commitment to what might be considered imcompatible professions.

The accounts from these three mental health professionals illustrate both the exhilaration of performance and the personal and professional vulnerability intrinsic to cinematic exposure. In the final analysis, the power of the cinema is probably multidetermined. The prospect of being preserved on celluloid is an immortality strategy that ensures one of surviving beyond the limitations of human mortality. The siren call of celebrity has a magnetic attraction that few of us can resist. Another determinant may be related to the Janus-faced dimension in all of us involving exhibitionism and scopophilia. While the actor in the movies may be sublimating exhibitionism, the psychotherapist in the privacy of his office sublimates his voyeuristic interests. While seemingly disparate in this respect, psychiatry and the cinema are both capable of offering a compelling glimpse into the human psyche. It is, of course, this point of convergence that will keep these two unlikely companions inextricably bound for years to come.

A Filmography for the Depiction of Psychiatry in the American Cinema

This list is by no means complete, omitting numerous low-budget movies of the horror and sex genres as well as any relevant films that we did not uncover in our research. As for European and other foreign films, we have listed only a few of the most important. Directors are identified immediately after a film's date, and the summary refers primarily to how each film characterizes psychiatrists or psychiatry.

The Accused (1949) William Dieterle. Loretta Young is psychology professor who commits murder for the right reasons.

After the Thin Man (1936) W. S. Van Dyke. George Zucco plays crackpot with Coke-bottle glasses who accuses nice young man (James Stewart) of being crazy. When Stewart turns out in fact to be quite mad, Zucco says, "Good heavens, I was right. The man is crazy."

Agnes of God (1985) Norman Jewison. Jane Fonda has personal problems, and she smokes too much, but her concern for patient (Meg Tilly) strongly recalls *Ordinary People's* Judd Hirsch. Since the film suggests with leaden ambiguity that a nun may have been impregnated by an angel (*sic*), Fonda may also be another rationalist who cannot appreciate The Unknown.

Airplane II: The Sequel (1982) Ken Finkleman. Testifying in court, John Vernon is asked to give his impression of the defendant. His reply: "I'm sorry, I don't do impressions. My expertise is in psychiatry."

The Amazing Dr. Clitterhouse (1938) Anatole Litvak. Absurd psychiatrist testifies in court against Edward G. Robinson but only creates confusion.

Anatomy of a Murder (1959) Otto Preminger. Fresh-faced Orson Bean is not exactly an oracular psychiatrist, but his presence plays against Viennese stereotypes.

Annie Hall (1977) Woody Allen. The eternal analysand's guide to life.

The Arrangement (1969) Elia Kazan. Analyst Harold Gould is one of several ineffectual characters involved in Kirk Douglas's midlife crisis.

Arsenic and Old Lace (1944) Frank Capra. In Capraland, only a psychiatrist would be so foolish as to think that these lovable eccentrics ought to be locked up.

The Bachelor and the Bobby Soxer (1947) Irving Reis. Court psychiatrist (Ray Collins) is a bit pontifical, but he gracefully solves the romantic problems of his two nieces (Myrna Loy and Shirley Temple).

Bad Timing: A Sensual Obsession (British; 1980) Nicholas Roeg. Theresa Russell drives Art Garfunkel, an American psychiatrist in Vienna, to distraction, to sodomy, and, finally, almost to necrophilia.

Bedlam (1946) Mark Robson. Boris Karloff, no less, is the sinister and cruel warden at the eighteenth-century institution to which courageous Anna Lee is committed.

Bedtime for Bonzo (1951) Frederick de Cordova. Amiable as ever, psychology professor Ronald Reagan proves his nurture-over-nature theories, instilling morality into a chimp.

Bedtime Story (1964) Ralph Levy. Con man David Niven poses as a Swiss psychiatrist in order to bilk Shirley Jones.

The Bell Jar (1979) Larry Peerce. Anne Jackson tries valiantly, but film grimly argues that no one as sensitive as Sylvia Plath (Marilyn Hassett) can survive in this world.

Bewitched (1945) Arch Oboler. Edmund Gwenn cures Phyllis Thaxter of schizophrenia.

Birdy (1985) Alan Parker. A double whammy on John Harkins: in his misguided treatment of bird-obsessed Vietnam vet (Matthew Modine), he exhibits worst stereotypes of psychiatry *and* the military.

Blind Alley (1939) Charles Vidor. Ralph Bellamy plays first godlike psychiatrist in an American film.

Blindfold (1966) Philip Dunne. "Dr. Bluebeard" Rock Hudson has trouble with women, but his powers of detection are beyond reproach.

The Bliss of Mrs. Blossom (1968) Joe McGrath. Bob Monkhouse is no help to Richard Attenborough, whose symptoms are actually caused by the man secretly kept in the attic by his wife (Shirley MacLaine).

Bluebeard's Eighth Wife (1938) Ernst Lubitsch. Stereotypical sanitarium director Professor Urganzeff (Lawrence Grant) appears briefly. Stock market fluctuations drive one of his patients to crow like a rooster.

Blume in Love (1973) Paul Mazursky. Real-life psychiatrist Donald F. Muhich sees George Segal through marital crisis.

Bob and Carol and Ted and Alice (1969) Paul Mazursky. Muhich again, this time in revealing exchange with Dyan Cannon.

The Boomerang (1925) Louis Gasnier. High jinks and romance among the staff at a sanitarium. First American movie to use the word *psychoanalyst*.

The Boston Strangler (1968) Richard Fleischer. Police inspector (Henry Fonda) knows how to handle killer with a split personality (Tony Curtis) much better than psychiatrist (Austin Willis).

Bringing up Baby (1938) Howard Hawks. Fritz Feld perfects the stereotype of the officious Viennese quack.

Bronco Billy (1980) Clint Eastwood. Woodrow Parfrey plays Dr. Canterbury, a buffoon-like asylum director who wears a pair of six-shooters over his white coat.

Butterfield 8 (1960) Daniel Mann. Prostitute heroine (Elizabeth Taylor) tells boyfriend, "I have to tell my psychiatrist everything. We're down to the smaller, starker details."

The Cabinet of Caligari (1962) Roger Kay. Dan O'Herlihy is benevolent healer, but disturbed patient Glynis Johns perceives him otherwise.

The Cabinet of Dr. Caligari (German; 1919) Robert Wiene. Expressionist masterpiece takes place in the mind of a mental patient who fantasizes that his psychiatrist is a malevolent mountebank sending a somnambulist (Conrad Veidt) on missions of murder.

The Caine Mutiny (1954) Edward Dmytryk. Pompous Whit Bissell is ultimately vindicated when he testifies that Captain Queeg (Humphrey Bogart) is not insane in spite of his ball bearings.

Call Me Bwana (1963) Gordon Douglas. Brief gag when Bob Hope flies past window of psychiatrist, who then lies down on couch and begins talking about his childhood.

Captain Newman, M.D. (1963) David Miller. Gregory Peck can heal his patients, but he cannot change the world.

Carefree (1938) Mark Sandrich. Fred Astaire sings, dances, and hypnotizes his way into Ginger Rogers's heart.

The Caretakers (1963) Hall Bartlett. Compassionate Robert Stack overcomes tough head nurse Joan Crawford and brings enlightened new order to a West Coast mental institution.

The Case of Becky (1921) Psychoanalytically oriented "nerve specialist" saves daughter from evil hypnotist.

The Cat People (1942) Jacques Tourneur. Simone Simon, who can actually turn into a panther, goes to suave, English psychiatrist (Tom Conway) who does not believe her. He substitutes seduction for therapy and pays with his life.

Caught (1949) Max Ophuls. Reclusive millionaire (Robert Ryan) marries fortune-hunting woman (Barbara Bel Geddes) largely to spite his officious analyst (Art Smith).

Chafed Elbows (1967) Robert Downey. Although his psychiatrist warns against it, protagonist marries his mother and lives happily ever after.

The Chapman Report (1962) George Cukor. Andrew Duggan, a thinly disguised Alfred Kinsey, is all business in this solemn sex exploitation film.

A Child Is Waiting (1963) John Cassavetes. Though untrained, Judy Garland is better at helping retarded children than professional Burt Lancaster.

Children of Loneliness (1939) Pompous psychiatrist narrates two pseudodocumentary accounts of homosexual "deviance."

A Clockwork Orange (1971) Stanley Kubrick. Whatever crimes Malcolm McDowell has committed, he surely does not deserve what the Skinnerian social engineers do to him.

Coast to Coast (1980) Joseph Sargent. Michael Lerner pays the price for conspiring with husband of free-spirited Dyan Cannon in effort to have her committed.

The Cobweb (1955) Vincente Minnelli. Melodrama among the troubled staff at a plush psychiatric hospital in the Midwest.

Cold Feet (1984) Bruce vanDusen. Slightly eccentric psychiatrist (Marcia Jean Kurtz) gives good advice in several sessions with romantically troubled heroine (Marissa Chibas).

Coming Apart (1969) Milton Moses Ginsberg. Rip Torn sets up hidden camera in his apartment to record himself doing just what title says.

Condemned Women (1938) Lew Landers. Prison psychologist (Louis Hayward) falls in love with inmate (Linda Wilson) and helps clear her of false charges.

Conflict (1945) Curtis Bernhardt. Sidney Greenstreet is omniscient psychologist using powers of detection to expose murderous scheme of Humphrey Bogart.

Coogan's Bluff (1968) Don Siegel. Tough-minded Clint Eastwood straightens out Susan Clark, a psychobabble-spouting parole officer.

The Couch (1962) Owen Crump. Grant Williams is a psychotic killer stalking both his psychiatrist (Onslow Stevens) and his pretty niece (Shirley Knight).

Cracking Up (1983) Jerry Lewis. Herb Edelman provides Jerry Lewis with an occasion to set up vignettes about life's absurdities. Parody of *Ordinary People* at conclusion. Rereleased in 1985 as *Smorgasbord*.

Crime Doctor (1943) Michael Gordon. After an amnesia attack, a mob boss (Warner Baxter) becomes a criminal psychologist with special talents for solving crimes. Itself based on a radio series, the film was followed by six sequels.

Crimes of Passion (1984) Ken Russell. Actors in close-up speak directly into camera at group therapy session with unseen, unheard therapist.

The Criminal Hypnotist (1909) D. W. Griffith. Hypnotist uses his psychological powers for evil purposes.

Dark Delusion (1947) Willis Goldbeck. Last of the Dr. Kildare movies, this time without Dr. Kildare. Dr. Tom Coalt (James Craig) uses narcosynthesis to help Dr. Gillespie (Lionel Barrymore) cure young girl's schizophrenia.

The Dark Mirror (1946) Robert Siodmak. With the help of Rorschach and free association tests, Lew Ayres solves the crime and wins himself a bride.

The Dark Past (1948) Rudolph Mate. Lee J. Cobb is oracular in faithful remake of *Blind Alley* (1939).

Dark Waters (1944) Andre de Toth. Franchot Tone is heroic doctor/detective/psychiatrist who helps Merle Oberon overcome villains trying to drive her crazy.

Daughters of Satan (1972) Hollingsworth Morse. Witches do not respond well to therapy.

David and Lisa (1962) Frank Perry. The title pair are lovable but seriously disturbed patients, and Howard da Silva's psychiatrist is wise and compassionate yet vulnerable.

Day of the Nightmare (1965) John Bushelman. Psychiatrist is killed by his transvestite son in retread of *Psycho*.

Dead Heat on a Merry-Go-Round (1966) Bernard Girard. Con man James Coburn seduces prison psychologist (Marian Moses) into arranging for his parole.

Dead of Night (British; 1946) Alberto Cavalcanti, Basil Dearden, Robert Hamer, and Charles Crichton. Best example of a film in which an absurdly rational psychiatrist consistently denies the reality of otherworldly phenomena.

Death Wish II (1982) Michael Winner. Unlike heroic vigilante Charles Bronson, prison psychologist does not know his right from his left.

Deep Throat (1972) Gerard Damiano. Harry Rheems spends a good deal of time having sex with his nurses, but he also has enough expertise to discover that Linda Lovelace's clitoris is in her throat.

The Deer Hunter (1978) Michael Cimino. Army psychiatrist fails to appreciate Christopher Walken's sufferings.

Desire (1936) Frank Borzage, produced by Ernst Lubitsch. Marlene Dietrich easily outwits "nerve specialist," played here by Alan Mowbray, who would later play a similarly inept psychiatrist in Lubitsch's *That Uncertain Feeling*.

The Detective (1968) Gordon Douglas. Pompous Lloyd Bochner conceals evidence sought by detective Frank Sinatra.

Dial 1119 (1950) Gerald Mayer. Sam Levene dies in a heroic attempt to reason with an escaped psychotic killer (Marshall Thompson).

Diary of a Mad Housewife (1970) Frank Perry. Upside-down psychiatrist urges Carrie Snodgress to be traditional wife and mother to intolerable husband and children. (Psychiatrist scenes are only in version of film shown on television.)

Dishonored Lady (1947) Robert Stevenson. Omniscient psychiatrist (Morris Carnovsky) clears Hedy Lamarr of murder charge.

Dr. Dippy's Sanitarium (1906) The psychiatrist makes his inauspicious debut on the American screen.

Doctor's Wives (1971) George Schaefer. Gene Hackman discovers that his wife is having a lesbian affair.

Down and Out in Beverly Hills (1986) Paul Mazursky. Donald F. Muhich continues his work with Mazursky by appearing as a delicately earnest psychiatrist attempting to treat the family dog.

Dracula (1931) Tod Browning. Unlike the wise Professor Van Helsing (Edward Van Sloan), sanitarium director Dr. Seward (Herbert Bunston) cannot see that Count Dracula is one of the Undead.

Dressed to Kill (1980) Brian De Palma. Michael Caine as the first homicidal transvestite psychiatrist in the American cinema.

The End (1978) Burt Reynolds. Carl Reiner drops dead immediately after inspiring Burt Reynolds with the joy of life.

End of the Road (1970) Aram Avakian. Although James Earl Jones's clinic is probably meant to be a metaphor, the patients in this institution are encouraged to have intercourse with chickens, and illegal abortions result in death.

The Entity (1983) Sidney J. Furie. If this film did not argue that invisible demon rapists really do exist, everything Ron Silver does for Barbara Hershey would make perfect sense.

Equus (1977) Sidney Lumet. Despairing Richard Burton cures psychotic boy (Peter Firth) but envies him for his bizarre horse religion.

The Evil (1978) Gus Trikonis. Richard Crenna rents haunted house for his clinic, but the previous inhabitants object.

The Exorcist (1973) William Friedkin. Psychiatry is no match for the Devil.

Exorcist II: The Heretic (1977) John Boorman. Especially when the psychiatrist is female (Louise Fletcher).

Face to Face (Swedish; 1976) Ingmar Bergman. Female psychiatrist in existential crisis.

Fear Strikes Out (1957) Robert Mulligan. Faceless Adam Williams cures baseball player Jimmy Piersall (Anthony Perkins). The film treats psychiatry so reverentially that even electroconvulsive therapy becomes benign.

The Fifth Floor (1980) Howard Avedis. Low-budget imitation of *Cuckoo's Nest* touches usual bases—a staff much sicker than patients uses ECT for punishment.

A Fine Madness (1966) Irvin Kershner. Motley crew of psychiatrists (Patrick O'Neal, Colleen Dewhurst, Clive Revill) lobotomize free-spirited poet (Sean Connery) but cannot tame him.

The Flame Within (1935) Edmund Goulding. Ann Harding as first female psychiatrist to lose her heart to a patient, in this case, Louis Hayward.

Fourteen Hours (1951) Henry Hathaway. Lovable cop (Paul Douglas) finally succeeds in coaxing suicidal Richard Basehart off ledge after two ineffectual psychiatrists fail.

Frances (1982) Graeme Clifford. Lane Smith can barely control himself during Jessica Lange's outbursts, and she pays dearly for her insolence.

Free Love (1930) Hobart Henley. Psychiatrist gives woman bad but expensive advice about her marriage.

Freud (1962) John Huston. Montgomery Clift is miscast, but the film comes very close to hagiography.

From the Terrace (1960) Mark Robson. Joanne Woodward's psychiatrist lover (Patrick O'Neal) is not very sympathetic, but then neither is anyone else in this melodrama.

The Front Page (1931) Lewis Milestone. Viennese quack hands gun to convicted murderer as part of examination. Remade in 1940 as *His Girl Friday* (directed by Howard Hawks) and in 1974 as *The Front Page* (directed by Billy Wilder) with little change in characterization of psychiatrist/alienist.

The Gay Intruders (1948) Ray McCarey. Married psychiatrists fail to cure quarreling stage couple—end up more confused than patients.

Girl of the Night (1960) Joseph Cates. Psychoanalyst Lloyd Nolan saves Anne Frances from a life of prostitution and then rescues her from her pimp.

Glen or Glenda? (1953) Edward D. Wood, Jr. Psychiatrist provides jargonistic introduction in attempt to legitimize this lame exploitation of transvestitism. A cult classic.

The Gnomemobile (1967) Robert Stevenson. Rationalist foil Jerome Cowan tells Walter Brennan that real-life gnomes are actually imaginary.

Grace Quigley (1985) Anthony Harvey. Chip Zien is a hip psychiatrist who tolerates, nay, rationalizes the work of professional hit man Nick Nolte.

The Group (1966) Sidney Lumet. Shirley Knight's first lover (Hal Holbrook) is hopelessly dependent on his manipulative analyst, but she eventually finds a good husband in James Broderick, an anti-Freudian hospital psychiatrist.

The Guilt of Janet Ames (1947) Henry Levin. Melvyn Douglas is a heavy-drinking newspaperman who nevertheless understands how to cure Rosalind Russell's hysterical paralysis. In one of several dream sequences, Sid Caesar broadly burlesques psychoanalysts.

Halloween (1978) John Carpenter. Unlike almost everyone else in this film, Donald Pleasence knows the Bogeyman when he sees him.

Hannah and Her Sisters (1986) Woody Allen. A silent analyst appears only briefly, but his patient (Michael Caine) appears to have benefited from the treatment.

Hard to Hold (1984) Larry Peerce. Child psychologist (Janet Eilber) is mostly competent and witty, but her relationship with rock star (Rick Springfield) is often more than she can handle.

Harold and Maude (1971) Hal Ashby. Absurd psychiatrist (G. Wood) cannot appreciate young Bud Cort's very real need to marry septuagenarian Ruth Gordon.

Harvey (1950) Henry Koster. James Stewart as the lovable drunk with the giant invisible rabbit who is saved at the last minute from the psychiatric interventions of Charles Drake and Cecil Kellaway.

Harvey Middleman, Fireman (1965) Ernest Pintoff. Mrs. Koogleman (Hermione Gingold) is too involved with her own sexual escapades to help hero.

Heartburn (1986) Mike Nichols. Maureen Stapleton plays no-nonsense leader of Meryl Streep's therapy group.

High Anxiety (1977) Mel Brooks. Hitchcock send-up casts Brooks as psychiatrist with vertigo.

High Wall (1947) Curtis Bernhardt. Audrey Totter functions as detective and lawyer as well as psychiatrist in order to save Robert Taylor from frame-up.

His Girl Friday (1940) Howard Hawks. See *The Front Page*.

Holiday for Lovers (1959) Henry Levin. Clifton Webb must supervise four troublesome daughters while on vacation in South America.

Hollow Triumph (1948) Steve Sekely. Paul Henreid kills a look-alike psychologist and then assumes his identity with initial success. Later released as *The Scar*.

Home Before Dark (1958) Mervyn LeRoy. Psychiatry is the solution to Jean Simmons's problems, but her unfaithful husband (Dan O'Herlihy) has other ideas.

Home Free All (1984) Stewart Bird. Daniel Benzalli is therapist who cancels treatment when antihero (Allan Nicholls) cannot pay his bills. It is just as well since Nicholls's problems are blamed on society.

Home of the Brave (1949) Mark Robson. Oracular Jeff Corey cures black serviceman (James Edwards) of hysterical paralysis.

The Hospital (1971) Arthur Hiller. David Hooks appears briefly at beginning so that George C. Scott can establish his character in a long confession.

House of Cards (1969) John Guillerman. Insufferably pompous psychiatrist (Keith Michell) is one of several right-wing conspirators. Heroine (Inger Stevens) refers to him as "the man who polices my psyche."

The Howling (1981) Joe Dante. Patrick Macnee seems like a good psychiatrist, but he is actually a werewolf.

I Never Promised You a Rose Garden (1977) Anthony Page. A character based on Frieda Fromm-Reichman (Bibi Andersson) struggles to save Kathleen Quinlan. One of the few sympathetic psychiatrists in seventies films.

I, the Jury (1953) Harry Essex. Mickey Spillane's Mike Hammer is seduced but not outwitted by murderous psychoanalyst Charlotte Manning (Peggie Castle). 1982 remake directed by Richard T. Heffron transformed Miss Manning into a sex therapist (Barbara Carrera).

I Was a Teenage Werewolf (1957) Gene Fowler, Jr. "Consulting psychologist" (Whit Bissell) unleashes the beast in Michael Landon.

I'm Dancing as Fast as I Can (1982) Jack Hofsiss. Dianne Wiest saves Jill Clayburgh after bad male psychiatrist (Joseph Maher) hooks her on Valium.

The Impossible Years (1968) Michael Gordon. University psychiatrist David Niven cannot control his teenage daughter.

Inside Daisy Clover (1966) Robert Mulligan. Faceless psychiatrist willingly submits to studio boss (Christopher Plummer) who exploits child-star Natalie Wood.

Interiors (1978) Woody Allen. E. G. Marshall and Diane Keaton deliver monologues to unseen psychiatrists.

The Interns (1962) David Swift. J. Edward McKinley is so eminent a psychiatrist that intern Michael Callan is willing to lie and cheat in order to study with him.

Invasion of the Body Snatchers (1956) Don Siegel. One psychiatrist (Whit Bissell) saves the world from alien invaders, while another (Larry Gates) is their agent. Remade by Philip Kaufman in 1978 with Leonard Nimoy as "pod" psychiatrist but without savior psychiatrist.

It's My Turn (1980) Claudia Weill. Briefly glimpsed psychiatrist at a party is a pompous boor.

Jagged Edge (1985) Richard Marquand. Bearded, rumpled psychiatrist appears briefly and offers a diagnosis of murder suspect that turns out to be wrong.

King's Row (1941) Sam Wood. Robert Cummings's great ambition is to study psychiatry in Vienna; Claude Rains is troubled psychiatrist who murders his schizophrenic daughter.

Klute (1971) Alan J. Pakula. Female psychiatrist Vivian Nathan gives Janes Fonda an opportunity to do some method acting, but she's not there when heroine needs her most.

Knock on Wood (1954) Norman Panama, Melvin Frank. Danny Kaye cures beautiful Mai Zetterling of her need to be a psychiatrist.

Kotch (1971) Jack Lemmon. Lovable old widower Walter Matthau submitted to absurd tests by young female psychologist.

Lady in a Jam (1942) Gregory La Cava. Heiress Irene Dunne convinces psychiatrist Patrick Knowles that he can cure her only by marrying her.

Lady in the Dark (1944) Mitchell Leisen. Barry Sullivan tells Ginger Rogers how to be a woman but mostly provides frame for production numbers.

The Last Embrace (1979) Jonathan Demme. Hitchcockian suspense/thriller includes brief scene with Jacqueline Brookes as white-coated therapist helping Roy Scheider recover from breakdown after his wife's death.

Let There Be Light (1946) John Huston. Documentary casts psychiatry as nearly infallible panacea for troubled veterans after World War II.

Let's Live a Little (1948) Richard Wallace. When "neuropsychiatrist" Hedy Lamarr falls for patient Robert Cummings, she acquires the same symptoms of love madness that once belonged to Cummings.

Lifeforce (1985) Tobe Hooper. Body of dour sanitarium director is temporarily invaded by naked woman vampire from outer space.

Lilith (1964) Robert Rossen. Warren Beatty plays a novice therapist who loses his heart and then his mind over a patient (Jean Seberg).

Lizzie (1957) Hugo Haas. Richard Boone cures Eleanor Parker of multiple personality. Released a few months before *Three Faces of Eve*.

The Locket (1946) John Brahm. Reflecting ambivalence typical of the 1940s, Laraine Day's psychiatrist husband (Brian Aherne) is first her victim, then her savior.

The Lonely Guy (1984) Arthur Hiller. Steve Martin speaks with his therapist exclusively through an intercom.

Lord Love a Duck (1966) George Axelrod. Sarah Marshall flies into hysterics because Roddy McDowall refuses to say that her Rorschach blots are dirty. She tells him he is being "hostile."

Love at First Bite (1979) Stan Dragoti. Richard Benjamin treats girlfriend Susan St. James only to find out if she is seeing other men.

Lover Come Back (1961) Delbert Mann. Richard Deacon dominates neurotic analysand (Tony Randall).

Lovesick (1983) Marshall Brickman. Dudley Moore is cute, but numerous other members of his profession are savaged.

Made for Each Other (1971) Robert B. Bean. Norman Shelly is caricatured therapist for couple who meet at an encounter group session.

The Magus (British; 1968) Guy Green. Anthony Quinn may or may not be a psychiatrist treating Michael Caine.

The Man Who Loved Women (1983) Blake Edwards. Julie Andrews somehow falls for neurotic womanizer Burt Reynolds.

The Man Who Saw Tomorrow (1922) Alfred E. Green. Psychologist hypnotizes patient so that he can see what his life would be like with each of two women he is considering marrying.

Manhunter (1986) Michael Mann. University of Chicago psychiatrist cautions cop (William L. Petersen) about dangers of taking his job too seriously. Another psychiatrist is a psychotic killer.

Marat/Sade (British; 1967) Peter Brook. Although the action takes place in a primitive nineteenth-century madhouse, treatment of patients is not unlike that shown in other films from this period.

The Mark (British; 1961) Guy Green. Rod Steiger cures Stuart Whitman of child-molesting and then saves him from those who would resurrect the past.

The Marriage of a Young Stockbroker (1971) Lawrence Turman. Patricia Barry wishes to emasculate healthy, normal American males.

The Medusa Touch (British; 1978) Jack Gold. Lee Remick eventually commits suicide after failing to destroy demons within the mind of Richard Burton.

Miracle on 34th Street (1947) George Seaton. In one of cinema's first attempts to distinguish psychologists from psychiatrists, Kris Kringle (Edmund Gwenn) scolds department store psychologist (Porter Hall) for practicing psychiatry.

Mirage (1965) Edward Dmytryk. Hostile psychiatrist (Robert H. Harris) is no help to amnesiac Gregory Peck.

Mr. Deeds Goes to Town (1936) Frank Capra. Gary Cooper realizes his humanitarian goals in spite of Viennese quack (Wyrley Birch) who testifies that he is crazy.

Moment to Moment (1966) Mervyn LeRoy. Jean Seberg drifts into a disastrous affair because psychiatrist husband (Arthur Hill) neglects her.

Movie Star, American Style or LSD, I Hate You (1966) Albert Zugsmith. Renegade headshrinker Del Moore gives lysergic acid to his patients.

Murder, My Sweet (1945) Edward Dmytryk. Hard-boiled Philip Marlowe (Dick Powell) has to cope with quack Otto Kruger.

My Favorite Wife (1940) Garson Kanin. Pedro de Cordoba appears briefly as a meddlesome psychiatrist, complete with goatee, rimless glasses, foreign accent, and the wrong diagnosis of why Cary Grant has been avoiding Gail Patrick.

The Naked Face (1984) Bryan Forbes. Roger Moore is a grieving widower, devoted to his patients, but unlike James Bond, he needs help when a Mafia don decides to silence him.

The Night Porter (Italian; 1974) Liliana Cavani. Psychiatrist is one of several ex-Nazis living secretly in postwar Vienna. They regularly meet for mock trials in which the defendant is "purged" of his guilt by denying accusations.

Nightmare Alley (1947) Edmund Goulding. Unscrupulous psychologist Helen Walker eventually turns "mentalist" Tyrone Power into a geek.

The Ninth Configuration. See *Twinkle, Twinkle, Killer Kane.*

Now Voyager (1942) Irving Rapper. Saintly Claude Rains shows Bette Davis how to live.

Oh God! Book II (1980) Gilbert Cates. Anthropomorphic god (George Burns) tries to enlighten a team of grossly caricatured psychiatrists.

Oh Men! Oh Women! (1957) Nunnally Johnson. Psychoanalyst David Niven is a great marriage counselor, but his dizzy fiancée (Barbara Rush) thinks him out of touch with his emotions.

Old Boyfriends (1979) Joan Tewkesbury. Stern-faced psychiatrist (John Houseman) is justified when he scolds psychologist (Talia Shire) for her disastrous attempts to treat Keith Carradine.

The Omen (1976) Richard Donner. Lee Remick goes to pompous John Strike for help, and although he arrives at a perfectly plausible diagnosis of her "fantasies," the patient's real problem is her son, Satan, who eventually kills her.

On a Clear Day You Can See Forever (1970) Vincente Minnelli. Yves Montand sets up production numbers when he discovers that Barbra Streisand can recall past lives.

One Flew over the Cuckoo's Nest (1975) Milos Forman. Christ-like sociopathic nonconformists beware! Lobotomy is the punishment for your attempts to bring salvation to emasculated males.

One Glorious Day (1922) James Cruze. Will Rogers is psychology professor who attempts to leave his body but is instead invaded by a mischievous spirit.

Ordinary People (1980) Robert Redford. Judd Hirsch hugs Timothy Hutton back to sanity.

Penelope (1966) Arthur Hiller. Dick Shawn is quack treating Natalie Wood.

The People Next Door (1970) David Greene. Nehemiah Persoff leads frustrating group therapy sessions for neurotic parents and their hippie children.

The Perfect Furlough (1958) Blake Edwards. Like most women who dare to practice psychiatry in fifties films, army psychologist (Janet Leigh) suffers several humiliations before Tony Curtis decides she is worthy of his affections.

Pillow Talk (1959) Michael Gordon. Tony Randall, betrayed by his best friend, says, "I should have listened to my psychiatrist. He told me never to trust anyone but him."

Plastered in Paris (1928) Benjamin Stoloff. "Famous specialist" fails to cure World War I veteran's kleptomania caused by war wound (*sic*).

Portnoy's Complaint (1972) Ernest Lehman. Psychiatrists are an essential part of modern life even though they never speak. One is even referred to as "Harpo."

Possessed (1947) Curtis Bernhardt. Oracular Stanley Ridges restores Joan Crawford's mental health after Van Heflin drives her crazy.

The President's Analyst (1967) Theodore J. Flicker. Eponymous hero (James Coburn) is not up to the assignment.

Pressure Point (1962) Hubert Cornfield. No other actor could have completed the early sixties trend toward idealization of the psychiatrist as well as Sidney Poitier.

Private Worlds (1935) Gregory La Cava. The complicated lives of an institution's staff. Claudette Colbert is one of the few female psychiatrists in the movies who is permitted to practice her trade after falling in love.

The Promise (1979) Gilbert Cates. Bibi Besch is pleasant enough, but she has only a small role in restoring Kathleen Quinlan to happiness.

Promise Her Anything (1966) Arthur Hiller. Bob Cummings is a prissy child psychologist who hates children and sucks his thumb.

Psycho (1960) Alfred Hitchcock. Simon Oakland is so extraordinarily acute and self-confident in his analysis of Anthony Perkins's psychosis that some critics believe Hitchcock intended the entire scene as a joke.

Psycho II (1983) Richard Franklin. Robert Loggia lets Anthony Perkins out of custody a little too early and pays for the mistake with his life.

Psycho III (1986) Anthony Perkins. Priest/psychiatrist is well-meaning but almost completely inconsequential.

Return to Oz (1985) Walter Murch. Nicol Williamson plays villainous Nome King as well as a psychiatrist about to subject the helpless Dorothy to ECT.

Reunion in Vienna (1933) Sidney Franklin. Viennese psychiatrist (Frank Morgan) represents enlightened alternative to decadent past when charming but overbearing Habsburg nobleman (John Barrymore) returns from exile to resume a romance with Diana Wynyard, now married to Morgan.

Revolution (1968) Jack O'Connell. Documentary about hippies pokes fun at psychiatrists' pious pronouncements.

St. Ives (1975) J. Lee Thompson. After an outburst that activates an analysand's worst fears, Maximillian Schell murders his only patient, a wealthy millionaire (John Houseman).

The Scar. See *Hollow Triumph*.

Schizoid (1980) David Paulsen. Klaus Kinski's patients are all being murdered. Guess who?

Secret Fury (1950) Mel Ferrer. When villains attempt to drive Claudette Colbert to insanity, a female therapist (Elisabeth Risdon) treats her in an institution not unlike the one in *The Snake Pit*.

Secrets of a Soul (German; 1926) G. W. Pabst. First serious treatment of psychoanalysis in film history, complete with German expressionism, sophisticated dream analysis, and talking cure supervised by Freud's disciples Abraham, Kaufmann, and Sachs.

The Sender (1982) Roger Christian. Kathryn Harrold is concerned and competent, but she cannot solve the supernatural problems of Zeljko Ivanek.

Serial (1980) Bill Persky. Richard Bonerz is laid-back California therapist who smiles helplessly through a child's hostile attacks.

The Seven-Per-Cent Solution (1976) Herbert Ross. Mildly satirized version of Sigmund Freud (Alan Arkin) helps greatly deromanticized version of Sherlock Holmes to kick the cocaine habit and then joins him in detective work.

The Seven Year Itch (1955) Billy Wilder. Creepy Oscar Homolka arrives early for an appointment, explaining nonchalantly that a patient just cut short his analytical hour by jumping out of the window.

The Seventh Veil (British; 1945) Compton Bennett. Herbert Lom speaks with unquestioned authority as he directs the life of concert pianist Ann Todd.

The Seventh Victim (1943) Mark Robson, produced by Val Lewton. As in *The Cat People* (also produced by Lewton), Tom Conway plays a smooth-talking psychiatrist with evil intentions.

Sex and the Single Girl (1964) Richard Quine. In spite of a doctorate in psychology, Helen Gurley Brown (Natalie Wood) quickly succumbs to the bogus charms of Tony Curtis.

Shadow on the Wall (1950) Patrick Jackson. Nancy Davis solves crime by helping traumatized child recall murder.

The Shaggy Dog (1959) Charles Barton. Disney farce includes another psychiatrist as rationalist foil. In this case he interprets Tommy Kirk's canine transformations as the "submerged second self" of his father (Fred MacMurray).

She Wouldn't Say Yes (1946) Alexander Hall. Rosalind Russell is another inadequate female therapist until she meets Lee Bowman.

Shining Victory (1941) Irving Rapper. Beautiful assistant (Geraldine Fitzgerald) to "nerve specialist" (James Stephenson) dies saving his important data from fire.

Shock (1946) Alfred L. Werker. Vincent Price kills wife and then uses psychiatric armamentarium to destroy witness.

Shock Corridor (1963) Samuel Fuller. In search of a murderer, journalist Peter Breck enters mental institution where maltreatment eventually drives him to psychosis. He does, however, win the Pulitzer Prize.

Shock Treatment (1964) Denis Sanders. Unscrupulous Lauren Bacall runs an institution for illicit financial gain but ends up a patient.

The Shrike (1955) Jose Ferrer. Most psychiatrists in a big-city institution are little more than jailers, but one oracular therapist saves the day for beleaguered hero.

Silent Madness (1985) Simon Nuchtern. The psychiatrist as damsel-in-distress.

Silent Rage (1982) Michael Miller. Ron Silver plays the therapist among a team of doctors who create a genetically engineered killer. Like Donald Pleasence in *Halloween,* he alone realizes the destructive potential of the monster, who is fortunately no match for Chuck Norris.

Since You Went Away (1944) John Cromwell. Supremely compassionate Viennese psychiatrist, bearing the formidable name Sigmund Gottlieb Golden, heals returning servicemen and consoles Jennifer Jones over the loss of her fiancé.

Sleep, My Love (1948) Douglas Sirk. George Coulouris is malevolent photographer posing as a psychiatrist in Don Ameche's plan to drive his wife (Claudette Colbert) to insanity. Ralph Morgan appears briefly but ineffectually as real psychiatrist.

The Sleeping Tiger (British; 1954) Joseph Losey. Alexander Knox reforms young criminal (Dirk Bogarde), but he fails miserably as Alexis Smith's husband.

Smile (1975) Michael Ritchie. Bruce Dern needs help, but his perfectly normal son is taken to the psychiatrist.

Smorgasbord (1983) Jerry Lewis. See *Cracking Up*.

The Snake Pit (1948) Anatole Litvak. Leo Genn cures Olivia de Havilland in spite of appalling conditions in New York institution.

So Young, So Bad (1950) Bernard Vorhaus. Humane Paul Henreid overcomes forces of reaction at a girls' reform school.

Some Kind of Hero (1982) Michael Pressman. Faceless psychiatrist is insensitive to mammoth problems of returning prisoner of war Richard Pryor.

Spellbound (1945) Alfred Hitchcock. Love for Gregory Peck transforms Ingrid Bergman from a mousy therapist into intrepid sleuth of the mind. Michael Chekhov is her irascible but lovable training analyst, and Leo G. Carroll is the psychiatrist/villain.

Splendor in the Grass (1961) Elia Kazan. Burgeoning adolescent sexuality drives Natalie Wood crazy—only psychiatry can help her.

Stardust Memories (1980) Woody Allen. Several gags about psychiatrists, including the classic line addressed to monster by Victor Truro: "I'm a psychoanalyst. This is my pipe."

Starting Over (1979) Alan J. Pakula. Burt Reynolds's psychiatrist brother (Charles Durning) sees him through a premarital crisis in a furniture store.

The Stepford Wives (1975) Bryan Forbes. Brief scene with female psychiatrist (Carol Rosson) who appears to be part of the conspiracy to replace suburban wives with automatons.

Still of the Night (1982) Robert Benton. Roy Scheider is either a typical Hitchcockian hero or a troubled psychiatrist out of control in a countertransference reaction.

The Stone Killer (1973) Michael Winner. Officious psychiatrist lectures tough cop (Charles Bronson) on how Vietnam War teaches American boys to be "psychopaths."

Strait Jacket (1964) William Castle. Joan Crawford's psychiatrist (Mitchell Cox) is victim of ax-murderer.

Suddenly, Last Summer (1959) Joseph L. Mankiewicz. Brain surgeon Montgomery Clift uses talking cure to save Elizabeth Taylor from villains wishing to lobotomize her.

Take the Money and Run (1969) Woody Allen. In parody of analyst, Don Frazier delivers elaborate psychosexual explanation for why hero (Allen) desires to play the cello. Earlier, Allen flunks Navy admission test when a Rorschach blot reminds him of two elephants having sex with a glee club.

Taking Off (1971) Milos Forman. Two scenes with psychiatrists are designed to drive home the message that middle-class adults are much stranger than their hippie children.

Teacher's Pet (1958) George Seaton. Gig Young, a psychology professor who seems to know everything without being pompous, helps Clark Gable get together with Doris Day.

10 (1980) Blake Edwards. Solemn therapist is no help to Dudley Moore in midlife crisis.

Tender Is the Night (1962) Henry King. Although Jason Robards, Jr., is a competent analyst, he never recovers from a countertransference reaction to the lovable Jennifer Jones.

The Terminal Man (1974) Mike Hodges. Team of doctors, including emotionally incompetent female psychiatrist (Joan Hackett), operates on mind of George Segal with disastrous results.

The Terminator (1984) James Cameron. Ridiculous "criminal psychologist" refuses to understand that man from the future is here to save humanity from Arnold Schwarzenegger.

The Testament of Dr. Mabuse (German; 1933) Fritz Lang. The last German film before the ascendancy of Hitler was about a power-mad psychiatrist.

That Touch of Mink (1962) Delbert Mann. Alan Hewitt treats Gig Young primarily for tips on the stock market.

That Uncertain Feeling (1941) Ernest Lubitsch. Blandly incompetent Alan Mowbray encourages Merle Oberon to question her marriage with Melvyn Douglas. Husband is preoccupied with business, but he eventually succeeds in regaining the affections he never deserved to lose.

They Might Be Giants (1971) Anthony Harvey. Joanne Woodward is a frumpy psychiatrist named Dr. Watson who finds fulfillment as the helpmate to George C. Scott, a schizophrenic who believes that he is Sherlock Holmes.

Third of a Man (1962) Robert Lewin. Whit Bissell saves institutionalized Simon Oakland from mob violence and then helps his brother to understand problems of the mentally ill.

The Three Faces of Eve (1957) Nunnally Johnson. Joanne Woodward has the part of a lifetime, but psychiatry and its domain remain mysterious. Though sympathetic, Lee J. Cobb is largely superfluous.

Three Nuts in Search of a Bolt (1964) Tommy Noonan. Three impoverished "nuts" in need of treatment send one person reporting symptoms of all three. Psychiatrist Ziva Rodann thinks she has found rare multiple personality case.

Three on a Couch (1966) Jerry Lewis. Janet Leigh is Ph.D., M.D., but her patients only need boyfriends.

The Thrill of It All (1963) Norman Jewison. Guidance counselor psychiatrist Paul Hartman provides James Garner with strategy for regaining the attentions of his wife (Doris Day).

Titicut Follies (1967) Fred Wiseman. Grim documentary on conditions in Massachusetts mental hospital.

Twinkle, Twinkle, Killer Kane (1980) William Peter Blatty. Stacy Keach runs weird mental hospital for shell-shocked marines. Also released as *The Ninth Configuration*.

An Unmarried Woman (1978) Paul Mazursky. Real-life psychologist Penelope Russianoff helps Jill Clayburgh face the troubling realities of modern relationships.

Vertigo (1958) Alfred Hitchcock. Psychiatrists patch up James Stewart after his breakdown, but his obsessions are beyond therapy.

A Very Special Favor (1965) Michael Gordon. Leslie Caron is a successful but unfulfilled therapist until she falls for Rock Hudson and motherhood.

Voyage to the Bottom of the Sea (1961) Irwin Allen. Joan Fontaine misinterprets scientific genius Walter Pidgeon and then attempts to sabotage submarine on its mission to save the world.

What a Way to Go! (1964) J. Lee Thompson. Bob Cummings, whose office includes a hydraulic couch, faints when he learns that Shirley MacLaine's wild stories are true.

What's New, Pussycat? (1965) Clive Donner. Peter Sellers with Viennese accent and Prince Valiant haircut is only interested in chasing women and running from his Wagnerian wife.

When the Clouds Roll By (1919) Victor Fleming. "Doctor of the mind" (Herbert Grimwood) turns out to be an escaped lunatic.

Where Were You When the Lights Went Out? (1968) Hy Averback. Terry-Thomas's analyst (Parley Baer) blandly responds "What do you think?" to his patient's questions but also manages to suggest that he is homosexual.

Whirlpool (1950) Otto Preminger. Neurotic wife (Gene Tierney) of renowned psychoanalyst (Richard Conte) is prey to evil hypnotist (Jose Ferrer) until Conte uses his scientific skills to save her.

Who Is Harry Kellerman and Why Is He Saying Those Terrible Things about Me? (1971) Ulu Grosbard. Psychiatrist Jack Warden is just another of rock singer Dustin Hoffman's delusions.

Who's Been Sleeping in My Bed? (1963) Daniel Mann. Martin Balsam cures Dean Martin of women problems.

Whose Life Is It, Anyway? (1981) John Badham. The doctors, nurses, physical therapists, and orderlies in this hospital are all dedicated, personable, and/or highly professional. Only the psychiatrists are caricatures.

Wild in the Country (1961) Philip Dunne. If you can accept Elvis Presley as a young Faulkner, you can accept Hope Lange as a successful therapist who saves her patient with a suicide attempt.

Willie and Phil (1980) Paul Mazursky's homage to *Jules and Jim* includes scene with oddball army psychiatrist at induction center.

Willy Wonka and the Chocolate Factory (1971) Mel Stuart. Brief scene with psychiatrist who is so anxious to find prize in chocolate bar that he interrogates a patient who dreams that he found it.

Woman Times Seven (1967) Vittorio De Sica. Shirley MacLaine's strange behavior leads psychiatrist Robert Morley to recommend long-term institutionalization, but Shirley is just trying to win her husband's attentions.

A Woman under the Influence (1974) John Cassavetes. Eccentric housewife (Gena Rowlands) is institutionalized and given ECT, but her supposedly normal husband (Peter Falk) exhibits a more destructive kind of craziness.

The Wrong Man (1956) Alfred Hitchcock. Werner Klemperer is competent and self-assured in brief scene with Henry Fonda.

Zelig (1983) Woody Allen. Mia Farrow parodies female psychiatrist in love. Newspaper headline reads: "Chameleon cured by woman doctor. She's pretty, too!"

Zotz! (1962) William Castle. Tom Poston has magic powers that James Millholin is unable to appreciate.

Chronology

1906
Dr. Dippy's Sanitarium

1909
The Criminal Hypnotist

1919
Cabinet of Dr. Caligari
When the Clouds Roll By

1921
The Case of Becky

1922
The Man Who Saw Tomorrow
One Glorious Day

1925
The Boomerang

1926
Secrets of a Soul

1928
Plastered in Paris

1930
Free Love

1931
Dracula
The Front Page

1933
Reunion in Vienna
The Testament of Dr. Mabuse

1935
The Flame Within
Private Worlds

1936
After the Thin Man
Desire
Mr. Deeds Goes to Town

1938
The Amazing Dr. Clitterhouse
Bluebeard's Eighth Wife
Bringing up Baby
Carefree
Condemned Women

1939
Blind Alley
Children of Loneliness

1940
His Girl Friday
My Favorite Wife

1941
King's Row
Shining Victory
That Uncertain Feeling

1942
The Cat People
Lady in a Jam
Now Voyager

1943
Crime Doctor
The Seventh Victim

1944
Arsenic and Old Lace
Dark Waters
Lady in the Dark
Since You Went Away

1945
Bewitched
Conflict
Murder, My Sweet
The Seventh Veil
Spellbound

1946
Bedlam
The Dark Mirror
Dead of Night
Let There Be Light
The Locket
She Wouldn't Say Yes
Shock

1947
The Bachelor and the Bobby Soxer
Dark Delusion
Dishonored Lady
The Guilt of Janet Ames
High Wall
Miracle on 34th Street
Nightmare Alley
Possessed

1948
The Dark Past
The Gay Intruders
Hollow Triumph (The Scar)
Let's Live a Little

Sleep, My Love
The Snake Pit

1949
The Accused
Caught
Home of the Brave

1950
Dial 1119
Harvey
Secret Fury
Shadow on the Wall
So Young, So Bad
Whirlpool

1951
Bedtime for Bonzo
Fourteen Hours

1953
Glen or Glenda?
I, the Jury

1954
The Caine Mutiny
Knock on Wood
The Sleeping Tiger

1955
The Cobweb
The Seven Year Itch
The Shrike

1956
Invasion of the Body Snatchers
The Wrong Man

1957
Fear Strikes Out
I Was a Teenage Werewolf
Lizzie
Oh Men! Oh Women!
The Three Faces of Eve

1958
Home before Dark
The Perfect Furlough
Teacher's Pet
Vertigo

1959
Anatomy of a Murder
Holiday for Lovers
Pillow Talk
The Shaggy Dog
Suddenly, Last Summer

1960
Butterfield 8
From the Terrace
Girl of the Night
Psycho

1961
Lover Come Back
The Mark
Splendor in the Grass
Voyage to the Bottom of the Sea
Wild in the Country

1962
The Cabinet of Caligari
The Chapman Report
The Couch
David and Lisa
Freud
The Interns
Pressure Point
Tender Is the Night
That Touch of Mink
Third of a Man
Zotz!

1963
Call Me Bwana
Captain Newman, M.D.

The Caretakers
A Child Is Waiting
Shock Corridor
The Thrill of It All
Who's Been Sleeping in My Bed?

1964
Bedtime Story
Lilith
Sex and the Single Girl
Shock Treatment
Strait Jacket
Three Nuts in Search of a Bolt
What a Way to Go!

1965
Day of the Nightmare
Harvey Middleman, Fireman
Mirage
A Very Special Favor
What's New, Pussycat?

1966
Blindfold
Dead Heat on a Merry-Go-Round
A Fine Madness
The Group
Inside Daisy Clover
Lord Love a Duck
Moment to Moment
Movie Star, American Style or LSD, I Hate You
Penelope
Promise Her Anything
Three on a Couch

1967
Chafed Elbows
The Gnomemobile
Marat/Sade
The President's Analyst

Titicut Follies
Woman Times Seven

1968
The Bliss of Mrs. Blossom
The Boston Strangler
Coogan's Bluff
The Detective
The Impossible Years
The Magus
Revolution
Where Were You When the Lights Went Out?

1969
The Arrangement
Bob and Carol and Ted and Alice
Coming Apart
House of Cards
Take the Money and Run

1970
Diary of a Mad Housewife
End of the Road
On a Clear Day You Can See Forever
The People Next Door

1971
A Clockwork Orange
Doctor's Wives
Harold and Maude
The Hospital
Klute
Kotch
Made for Each Other
The Marriage of a Young Stockbroker
Taking Off
They Might Be Giants
Who Is Harry Kellerman and Why Is He Saying Those Terrible Things about Me?
Willy Wonka and the Chocolate Factory

1972
Daughters of Satan
Deep Throat
Portnoy's Complaint

1973
Blume in Love
The Exorcist
The Stone Killer

1974
The Front Page
The Night Porter
The Terminal Man
A Woman under the Influence

1975
One Flew over the Cuckoo's Nest
St. Ives
Smile
The Stepford Wives

1976
Face to Face
The Omen
The Seven-Per-Cent Solution

1977
Annie Hall
Equus
Exorcist II: The Heretic
High Anxiety
I Never Promised You a Rose Garden

1978
The Deer Hunter
The End
The Evil
Halloween
Interiors
Invasion of the Body Snatchers
The Medusa Touch
An Unmarried Woman

1979
The Bell Jar
The Last Embrace
Love at First Bite
Old Boyfriends
The Promise
Starting Over

1980
Bad Timing: A Sensual Obsession
Bronco Billy
Coast to Coast
Dressed to Kill
The Fifth Floor
It's My Turn
Oh God! Book II
Ordinary People
Schizoid
Serial
Stardust Memories
10
Twinkle, Twinkle, Killer Kane
Willie and Phil

1981
The Howling
Whose Life Is It, Anyway?

1982
Airplane II: The Sequel
Death Wish II
Frances
I, the Jury
I'm Dancing as Fast as I Can
The Sender
Silent Rage

Some Kind of Hero
Still of the Night

1983
Cracking Up
The Entity
Lovesick
The Man Who Loved Women
Psycho II
Smorgasbord
Zelig

1984
Cold Feet
Crimes of Passion
Hard to Hold
Home Free All
The Lonely Guy
The Naked Face
The Terminator

1985
Agnes of God
Birdy
Grace Quigley
Jagged Edge
Lifeforce
Return to Oz
Silent Madness

1986
Down and Out in Beverly Hills
Hannah and Her Sisters
Heartburn
Manhunter
Psycho III

References

Agee, J. 1958. *Agee on film*. New York: McDowell Obolensky.

Alloway, L. 1971. *Violent America: The movies 1946–64*. New York: Museum of Modern Art.

Althusser, L. 1971. Ideology and ideological state apparatuses (notes towards an investigation). In *Lenin and philosophy and other essays*. Trans. Ben Brewster. London: New Left Books.

———. 1977. Marxism and humanism. In *For Marx*. Trans. Ben Brewster. London: New Left Books.

Altman, C. 1977. Psychoanalysis and the cinema: The imaginary discourse. *Quarterly Review of Film Studies* 2:257–72.

Ansen, D. 1983. Manhattan transfer. *Newsweek,* 21 February, 61.

———. 1986. Manhattan serenade. *Newsweek,* 3 February, 67–68.

Barthes, R. 1972. *Mythologies*. Trans. Annette Lavers. New York: Hill and Wang.

Becker, E. 1973. *The denial of death*. New York: Free Press.

Berman, J. 1985. *The talking cure: Literary representations of psychoanalysis*. New York: New York University Press.

Blum, H. 1969. A psychoanalytic view of *Who's Afraid of Virginia Woolf? Journal of the American Psychoanalytic Association* 17:888–903.

Bordwell, D. 1985. *Narration in the fiction film*. Madison: University of Wisconsin Press.

Bordwell, D., J. Staiger, and K. Thompson. 1985. *The classical Hollywood cinema: Film style and mode of production to 1960*. New York: Columbia University Press.

Braudy, L. 1968. Hitchcock, Truffaut, and the irresponsible audience. *Film Quarterly* 21:21–27.

———. 1977. *The world in a frame*. New York: Doubleday.

Brenner, C. 1982. *The mind in conflict*. New York: International Universities Press.

Bruccoli, M. 1963. *The composition of "Tender Is the Night."* Pittsburgh: University of Pittsburgh Press.

Burnham, J. 1978. The influence of psychoanalysis upon American culture. In *American Psychoanalysis: Origins and development,* edited by J. Quen and E. Carlson, 52–72. New York: Brunner/Mazel.

———. 1979. From avant-garde to specialism: Psychoanalysis in America. *Journal of the History of the Behavioral Sciences* 15:128–34.

———. 1982. American medicine's golden age: What happened to it? *Science* 215:1474–79.

Cagin, S., and P. Dray. 1984. *Hollywood films of the seventies: Sex, drugs, violence, rock 'n' roll and politics.* New York: Harper and Row.

Carroll, N. 1981. Nightmare and the horror film: The symbolic biology of fantastic beings. *Film Quarterly* 34:16–25.

Cavell, S. 1981a. *North by northwest. Critical Inquiry* 7:761–76.

———. 1981b. *Pursuits of happiness: The Hollywood comedy of remarriage.* Cambridge: Harvard University Press.

Ciment, M. 1977. Entretien avec Robert Altman. *Positif* 197 (September): 13–20.

Coltrera, J. T. 1981. Lives, events, and other players: Directions in psychobiography. In *Lives, events, and other players: Directions in psychobiography,* edited by J. T. Coltrera, 3–73. New York: Jason Aronson.

Crowther, B. 1946. Review of *Shock. New York Times,* 9 March, 10.

Davidson, V. 1977. Psychiatry's problem with no name: Therapist-patient sex. *American Journal of Psychoanalysis* 37:43–50.

de Lauretis, T. 1984. *Alice doesn't: Feminism, semiotics, cinema.* Bloomington: Indiana University Press.

Demby, B. J. 1977. Robert Altman talks about his life and his art. *New York Times,* 19 June, sec. 2.

Dervin, D. 1985. *Through a Freudian lens deeply.* Hillsdale, N.J.: Analytic Press.

Doane, M. A. 1982. Film and the masquerade: Theorizing the female spectator. *Screen* 23 (3–4): 74–87.

Durgnat, R. 1982. Review of *The imaginary signifier: Psychoanalysis and Cinema,* by Christian Metz. *Film Quarterly* 36 (2): 58–64.

Eber, M., and J. O'Brien. 1982. Psychotherapy in the movies. *Psychotherapy: Theory, Research and Practice* 19:116–20.

Ebert, R. 1978. Beyond narrative: The future of the feature film. In *The great ideas today 1978,* edited by M. J. Adler, 176–215. Chicago: Encyclopaedia Britannica.

Eberwein, R. T. 1984. *Film and the dream screen.* Princeton: Princeton University Press.

Eckert, C. 1974. The anatomy of a proletarian film: Warner's *Marked Woman. Film Quarterly* 27:10–24.

Ehrenburg, I. 1931. *Die Traumfabrik: Chronik des Films.* Berlin: Malik-Verlag.

Ellenberger, H. 1955. A comparison of European and American psychiatry. *Bulletin of the Menninger Clinic* 19:43–51.

Feldstein, R. 1985. The dissolution of the self in *Zelig. Literature/Film Quarterly* 13:155–60.

Feuer, J. 1982. *The Hollywood musical.* Bloomington: Indiana University Press.

Fink, P. J. 1983. The enigma of stigma and its relation to psychiatric education. *Psychiatric Annals* 13:669–90.

Fish, S. 1976. Interpreting the *Variorum. Critical Inquiry* 2:465–85.

Fitzgerald, F. S. 1934. *Tender is the night.* New York: Charles Scribner's Sons.

Frank, B., and B. Krohn. 1983. Entretien avec Martin Scorsese. *Cahiers du cinéma* 347 (May): 10–17.

Freedman, O., and R. Gordon. 1973. Psychiatry under siege: Attacks from without. *Psychiatric Annals* 3:10–34.

Freud, S. 1900. *The interpretation of dreams.* Vols. 4 and 5 of *The standard edition of the complete psychological works of Sigmund Freud* (hereafter *S.E.*). Trans. and ed. by J. Strachey. London: Hogarth Press.

———. 1910. Leonardo da Vinci and a memory of his childhood. *S.E.* 11:59–137.

———. 1914. On narcissism: An introduction. *S.E.* 14:73–102.

———. 1915. Observations on transference—Love. *S.E.* 12:157–71.

———. 1916. Those wrecked by success. *S.E.* 14:316–31.

———. 1920. Beyond the pleasure principle. *S.E.* 18:3–64.

———. 1923. The ego and the id. *S.E.* 19:3–66.

———. 1925. *Some additional notes on dream interpretation as a whole. S.E.* 19.

———. 1939. Moses and monotheism. *S.E.* 23:3–140.

Frye, N. 1957. *Anatomy of criticism.* Princeton: Princeton University Press.

Gabbard, G. 1979. Stage fright. *International Journal of Psycho-Analysis* 60:383–92.

———. 1983. Further contributions to the understanding of stage fright: Narcissistic issues. *Journal of the American Psychoanalytic Association* 31:423–41.

Gabbard, G., S. Twemlow, and F. Jones. 1981. Do "near-death experiences" occur only near death? *Journal of Nervous and Mental Disease* 169:374–77.

Gach, J. 1980. Culture and complex: On the early history of psychoanalysis in America. In *Essays in the history of psychiatry,* edited by E. Wallace and L. Pressley, 142–57. Columbia, S.C.: William S. Hall Psychiatric Institute of the South Carolina Department of Mental Health.

Gibson, W. 1954. *The cobweb.* New York: Knopf.

Greenberg, H. 1975. *The movies on your mind.* New York: Dutton.

———. 1983. The fractures of desire: Psychoanalytic notes on *Alien* and the contemporary "cruel" horror film. *Psychoanalytic Review* 70:241–67.

Grob, G. 1985. *The inner world of American psychiatry, 1890–1940.* New Brunswick, N.J.: Rutgers University Press.

Guthmann, H. 1969. The characterization of the psychiatrist in American fiction, 1859–1965. Ph.D. diss., University of Southern California.

Halliwell, L. 1983. *Halliwell's film guide.* 4th ed. New York: Charles Scribner's Sons.

Haskell, M. 1974. *From reverence to rape: The treatment of women in the movies.* New York: Holt, Rinehart, and Winston.

Heath, S. 1981. *Questions of cinema.* Bloomington: Indiana University Press.

Henry, M. 1983. Entretien avec Martin Scorsese. *Positif* 267 (May): 14–19.

Hillier, J., ed. 1985. *Cahiers du cinéma, the 1950's: Neo-realism, Hollywood, new wave.* Cambridge: Harvard University Press.

Holland, N. 1959. Psychiatry in pselluloid. *Atlantic Monthly,* February, 105–7.

Huss, R. 1986. *The mindscapes of art: Dimensions of the psyche in fiction, drama, and film.* Rutherford, N.J.: Fairleigh Dickinson University Press.

Huston, J. 1980. *An open book.* New York: Knopf.

Jacobs, D. 1982. . . . *But we need the eggs: The magic of Woody Allen.* New York: St. Martin's.

James, H. 1934. *The art of the novel.* New York: Charles Scribner's Sons.

James, W. 1958. *Varieties of religious experience: A study in human nature.* New York: Mentor.

Jameson, R., and K. Murphy. 1977. . . . They take on their own life. . . . *Movietone News,* 16 September, 2–12.

Jaques, E. 1965. Death and the mid-life crisis. *International Journal of Psycho-Analysis* 46:502–14.

Kael, P. 1973. Movieland—The bum's paradise. *New Yorker,* 22 October, 133–39.

———. 1980. The frog who turned into a prince, the prince who turned into a frog. *New Yorker,* 27 October, 183–90.

Kaminsky, S. 1978. *John Huston: Maker of magic.* Boston Houghton Mifflin.

Kaplan, A. E., ed. 1980. *Women in film noir.* London: British Film Institute.

Kawin, B. 1978. *Mindscreen: Bergman, Godard, and first-person film.* Princeton: Princeton University Press.

Kernberg, O. 1965. Notes on countertransference. *Journal of the American Psychoanalytic Association* 13:38–56.

———. 1974. Further contributions to the treatment of narcissistic personalities. *International Journal of Psycho-Analysis* 55:215–40.

———. 1975. *Borderline conditions and pathological narcissism.* New York: Jason Aronson.

———. 1980. *Internal world and external reality.* New York: Jason Aronson.

Kinder, M. 1980. The adaptation of cinematic dreams. *Dreamworks* 1:54–68.

Kirk, G. S. 1970. *Myth: Its meaning and functions in ancient and other cultures.* Cambridge: Cambridge University Press.

Knight, A. 1963. Who's morbid? *Saturday Review,* 10 August, 34.

Kohut, H. 1971. *The analysis of the self.* New York: International Universities Press.

———. 1977. *The restoration of the self.* New York: International Universities Press.

———. 1984. *How does analysis cure?* Chicago: University of Chicago Press.

Kramm, J. 1952. *The shrike.* New York: Random.

Kuhn, A. 1982. *Women's pictures: Feminism and the cinema.* London: Routledge and Kegan Paul.

Lacan, J. 1977. *Ecrits: A selection.* Trans. Alan Sheridan. New York: Norton.

Laplanche, J., and J.-B. Pontalis. 1973. *The language of psychoanalysis.* Trans. Donald Nicholson-Smith. New York: Norton.

Lasch, C. 1979. *The culture of narcissism.* New York: Norton.

Lehmann, H. 1980. Unusual psychiatric disorders, atypical psychoses, and brief reactive psychoses. In *Comprehensive textbook of psychiatry,* 3d ed., edited by H. Kaplan, A. Freedman, and B. Sadock. Baltimore: Williams and Wilkins.

Linter, J. 1979. Reflections on the media and the mental patient. *Hospital and Community Psychiatry* 30:415–16.

Lundberg, F., and M. Farnham. 1947. *Modern woman: The lost sex.* New York: Harper.

MacCabe, C. 1985. *Tracking the signifier, theoretical essays: Film, linguistics, literature.* Minneapolis: University of Minnesota Press.

Mast, G. 1976. *A short history of the movies.* 2d ed. Indianapolis: Bobbs-Merrill.

Mast, G., and M. Cohen, eds. 1985. *Film theory and criticism.* 3d ed. New York: Oxford University Press.

Melosh, B. 1983. Doctors, patients, and "big nurse": Work and gender in the postwar hospital. In *Nursing History: New perspectives, new possibilities,* edited by E. Lagemann, 157–79. New York: Teachers College Press.

Metz, C. 1982. *The imaginary signifier: Psychoanalysis and the cinema.* Trans. Celia Britton et al. Bloomington: Indiana University Press.

Miller, M., and R. Sprich. 1981. The appeal of *Star Wars:* An archetypal-psychoanalytic view. *American Imago* 38:203–19.

Monaco, J. 1979. *American film now.* New York: Oxford University Press.

———. 1981. *How to read a film: The Art, technology, language, history and theory of film and media.* Rev. ed. New York: Oxford University Press.

Moss, R. 1980. Woody Allen. *Saturday Review,* November, 40–44.

Münsterberg, H. [1916] 1970. *The film: A psychological study.* New York: Dover.

Nichols, B., ed. 1976. *Movies and methods: An anthology.* Berkeley: University of California Press.

Nielsen, A. 1980. Choosing psychiatry: The importance of psychiatric education in medical school. *American Journal of Psychiatry* 137:428–31.

Niver, K. 1971. *Biograph bulletins 1896–1908.* Los Angeles: Artisan Press.

Oudart, J.-P. 1978. Cinema and suture. *Screen* 18 (4): 35–47.

Pardes, H., and H. Pincus. 1983. Challenges to academic psychiatry. *American Journal of Psychiatry* 140:1117–26.

Piersall, J., and A. Hirshberg. 1955. *Fear strikes out.* Boston: Little, Brown.

Plank, R. 1956. Portraits of fictitious psychiatrists. *American Imago* 13:259–67.

Ray, R. B. 1985. *A certain tendency of the Hollywood cinema, 1930–1980.* Princeton: Princeton University Press.

Rickey, C. 1982. Frances Farmer's dark victory. *Village Voice,* 30 November, 73ff.

Rieff, P. 1966. *The triumph of the therapeutic.* New York: Harper and Row.

Russo, V. 1981. *The celluloid closet: Homosexuality in the movies.* New York: Harper and Row.

Samuels, L. 1985. Female psychotherapists as portrayed in film, fiction and nonfiction. *Journal of the American Academy of Psychoanalysis* 13:367–78.

Sarris, A. 1980. Woody doesn't rhyme with Federico. *Village Voice,* 1–7 October, 49.

Sartre, Jean-Paul. 1986. *The Freud scenario.* Ed. J.-B. Pontalis; trans. Quintin Hoare. Chicago: University of Chicago Press.

Sayre, N. 1982. *Running time: Films of the cold war.* New York: Dial Press.

Schatz, T. 1982. *Annie Hall* and the issue of modernism. *Literature/Film Quarterly* 10:180–88.

Schneider, I. 1977. Images of the mind: Psychiatry in the commercial film. *American Journal of Psychiatry* 134:613–20.

———. 1985. The psychiatrist in the movies: The first fifty years. In *Psychoanalytic study of literature,* edited by J. Reppen and M. Charney, 53–67. Hillsdale, N.J.: Analytic Press.

Segal, H. 1964. *Introduction to the work of Melanie Klein.* New York: Basic Books.

Self, R. 1984. Review of *American Skeptic: Robert Altman's Genre-Commentary Films,* by Norman Kagan. *Wide Angle* 6 (1): 66–68.

———. 1985. Robert Altman and the theory of authorship. *Cinema Journal* 25 (1): 3-11.

Sharpe, E. 1937. *Dream analysis.* New York: Brunner/Mazel.

Silverman, K. 1983. *The subject of semiotics.* New York: Oxford University Press.

Sizemore, C. 1977. *I'm Eve.* Garden City, N.Y.: Doubleday.

Sklar, R. 1975. *Movie-made America.* New York: Random House.

Steinberg, C. 1980. *Film facts.* New York: Facts on File, Inc.

Stine, W. 1974. *Mother Goddam.* New York: Hawthorn Books.

Thomas, A., and S. Chess. 1984. Genesis and evolution of behavioral disorders from infancy to early adult life. *American Journal of Psychiatry* 141 (1): 1–9.

Truffaut, F. 1984. *Hitchcock.* Rev. ed. New York: Simon and Schuster.

Vernet, M. 1975. Freud: Effects spéciaux/mise en scène: U.S.A. *Communications* 23:223–34.

Walsh, A. 1984. *Women's film and female experience 1940–1950.* New York: Praeger.

Ward, M. 1946. *The snake pit.* New York: Random House.

Williams, L. 1981. *Figures of desire: A theory and analysis of surrealist film.* Urbana: University of Illinois Press.

Winick, C. 1963. The psychiatrist in fiction. *Journal of Nervous and Mental Disorders* 136:43–57.

Wolfenstein, M., and N. Leites. 1970. *The movies: A psychological study.* New York: Atheneum.

Wood, M. 1975. *America at the movies.* New York: Basic Books.

Wood, R. 1977. *Hitchcock's films.* Cranbury, N.J.: A. S. Barnes.

———. 1986. *Hollywood from Vietnam to Reagan.* New York: Columbia University Press.

Wouk, H. 1951. *The Caine mutiny: A novel of World War II.* Garden City, N.Y.: Doubleday.

Yager, J., K. Lamotte, A. Nielsen, and J. Eaton. 1982. Medical students' evaluation of psychiatry: A cross-country comparison. *American Journal of Psychiatry* 139:1003–9.

Yager, J., and S. Scheiber. 1981. Why psychiatry is recruiting fewer residents: The opinions of medical school deans and psychiatric department chairmen. *Journal of Psychiatric Education* 5:258–68.

Index

Abbott, Diahnne, 207
Achilles, 15
Adam's Rib, 13
Adler, Alfred, 51
Aeschylus, 163, 165
After the Thin Man, 57, 58
Agee, James, 73
Agnes of God, 19, 144
Aiello, Danny, 220, 221
Albert, Eddie, 111
Alcoholism, 35, 113, 114
Alda, Alan, 114, 238
Alex in Wonderland, 190
Alien, 108, 188, 226, 229–39, 253
Alienists, 48, 49
Aliens, 238, 239
Allen, Irwin, 100
Allen, Nancy, 118
Allen, Woody, xix, 16, 25, 27, 28, 131–36, 144, 148, 187, 190, 191, 194–203, 206, 215–25, 231, 253
Alloway, Lawrence, 88
All That Jazz, 187, 189–97, 200, 201, 203
Allyson, June, 76, 77
Althusser, Louis, 5, 178, 185
Altman, Robert, 31, 135, 154, 158, 188, 240–51, 254
Amadeus, 140
Amazing Dr. Clitterhouse, The, 57, 58
American psychiatry, history of, 44, 47, 60, 72, 78, 82, 84–86, 111–14, 122, 123, 128, 144, 171, 172

Anagnorisis, 163
Anatomy of a Murder, 87, 88
Andersson, Bibi, 25, 143
Andrews, Dana, 5
Andrews, Julie, 27
Annie Hall, 25, 131–33, 148, 200, 202
Anorexia nervosa, 114
Ansen, David, 149
Anspach, Susan, 135
Anti-Semitism, 68, 69
Apartment, The, 152, 154
Arbus, Alan, 114
Aristotle, 45
Arkin, Alan, xi, 142
Arthur, 114, 153
Arthur, Robert Alan, 190
Ashby, Hal, 140
Ashley, Elizabeth, 120, 121
Astaire, Fred, 14, 31, 55–57, 223, 225
Auteurism, 178, 241
Avakian, Aram, 17, 142
Averback, Hy, 256
Awful Truth, The, 56
Ayres, Lew, xvii, 68, 69, 75, 87

Bacall, Lauren, 78–80, 124
Bachrach, Burt, 135
Back Street, 12
Bad and the Beautiful, The, 77
Baker, Elliot, *A Fine Madness,* 127
Balsam, Martin, 110
Bananas, 200

Bancroft, Anne, 112
Band Wagon, The, 77
Barrault, Marie-Christine, 197
Barretts of Wimpole Street, The, 51
Barry, Patricia, 120, 121, 142
Barrymore, John, 50, 51
Barth, John, *End of the Road,* 128
Barthes, Roland, 5, 6, 13, 178
Bartlett, Hall, 111–13
Baxter, Warner, 8
Bazin, André, 178
Bean, Orson, 87
Beatty, Warren, 85, 124, 216
"Beauty and the Beast" (fairy tale), 240, 250
Becker, Ernest, 204, 205, 214
Bedlam, 72
Bedtime for Bonzo, 75
Bellamy, Ralph, 17, 40, 53–56, 60, 86, 130
Bell Jar, The, 128, 156
Bellow, Saul, 216–18; *Seize the Day,* 128
Benjamin, Richard, 20, 119–21, 142, 148
Bennett, Joan, 52
Benton, Robert, 144, 148, 158–62
Benzedrine, 157
Bergen, Polly, 112
Bergman, Ingmar, xvii, 195, 248
Bergman, Ingrid, 4, 19, 22, 24, 29, 61–64,
    67, 124, 144, 146, 147, 150, 159
Bergren, Eric, 154
Berkeley, Busby, 14, 183
Berman, Jeffrey, 103, 127, 187
Bernhard, Sandra, 209, 213, 214
Bernhardt, Curtis, xix, 6, 67
Best Years of Our Lives, The, 5
Bettelheim, Bruno, 216, 217
Biehn, Michael, 238
Big Fix, The, 134
Bill of Divorcement, A, 49
Birch, Wyrley, 58
Bissell, Whit, 74, 75, 80–84, 87, 94
Blade Runner, 231–33
Blair, Linda, 228
Blind Alley, xv, 17, 32, 40, 53–55, 60, 63,
    67, 80, 86, 109, 114, 130, 132

Blindfold, 20, 21, 32, 124
Bloch, Robert, 99
Bloom, Claire, 34
Blow Out, 118
Bluebeard's Eighth Wife, 57, 58
Blum, Harold, 246
Blum, John Morton, 216, 218
Blume in Love, 134–38, 256, 257
Bob and Carol and Ted and Alice, 134–36, 256,
    257
Body Double, 118
Bogart, Humphrey, 4, 80, 81, 126
Bond, James, 164
Bonnie and Clyde, 127, 158
Boomerang, 47
Boorman, John, 33, 142
Bordwell, David, xix, 181
Born Yesterday, 152
Boston Strangler, The, 32, 130, 131
Bottome, Phyllis, 51
Boyer, Charles, 23, 51, 52, 78–80
Braudy, Leo, 31, 105
Breathless, 127
Breen Office, 49, 51; *see also* Production Code
Brenner, Charles, 165
Brickman, Marshall, 19, 101, 115, 144, 148,
    150–52
Bridges, Jeff, 88
Bridges, Lloyd, 39
Brill, A. A., 85
Bringing up Baby, 18, 58, 130, 152
Broderick, James, 126
Bronson, Charles, 121, 122, 126, 145
Brooks, Dean, 139, 255, 256
Brooks, Mel, 161
Brother from Another Planet, The, 220
Brown, Helen Gurley, 25, 26
Browning, Tod, 32
Bruce, Lenny, 200
Buffalo Bill and the Indians, 241
Bunston, Herbert, 32
Burnham, John, 47, 54, 85, 114, 122, 123,
    136
Burrow, Trigant, 85

Burton, Richard, 25, 33, 141
Busby, Gerald, 243
Butch Cassidy and the Sundance Kid, 127

Cabinet of Caligari, The, 99
Cabinet of Dr. Caligari, xvii, 46, 63, 81, 99
Cahiers du cinéma (journal), 95, 178, 181, 185
Caine, Michael, 19, 115, 116, 118, 119, 133,
    169, 170
Caine Mutiny, The, 80, 81, 84, 88, 98, 126
Callan, Michael, 94
Callenbach, Ernest, 109
Call Me Bwana, 101
Cambridge, Godfrey, 129
Camera Obscura (journal), 178
Cameron, James, 238
Cannibalism, 104
Cannon, Dyan, 134, 135, 257
Capgras' Syndrome, 229, 236
Capra, Frank, 5, 58, 59, 65, 76
Captain Newman, M.D., 19, 110, 111, 113
Carefree, 25, 31, 55–57
Caretakers, The, 111–13
Caron, Leslie, 23, 24, 124
Carpenter, John, 33, 220, 226, 228, 236
Carrera, Barbara, 75
Carrie, 119
Carroll, Leo G., 63
Carroll, Noël, 226
Carson, Johnny, 207, 208, 211, 225, 256
Casablanca, 4, 81
Case of Becky, The, 47
Castle, Peggie, 19, 75
Castle, William, 101, 124
Cates, Gilbert, 19
Cates, Joseph, 94
Catharsis, 163
Cathartic cure, 15, 36–42, 60, 63, 64, 79,
    104, 109, 111, 169, 252
Cat People, The, 21, 32
Cavani, Liliana, xvii
Cavell, Stanley, 56, 158, 185
Cavett, Dick, 207, 208
Centaurs, 15

Chabrol, Claude, 178
Chafed Elbows, 128
Chandler, Raymond, 65
Chaplin, Charlie, 198
Chapman Report, The, 34, 94
Charles, Ray, 207
Chase, Mary, 75
Chekhov, Anton, 200
Chekhov, Michael, 61–63, 103, 146, 147, 150
Chess, Stella, 42
Chien andalou, Un, 63
Child Is Waiting, A, 80
Children of Loneliness, 59, 60
Chiron, 15
Christian, Roger, 25
Christ symbolism, 18, 107–9, 140, 156, 221,
    222, 252
Cimino, Michael, 11, 142
CinemaScope, 77, 91, 130
Clark, Kendall, 77
Classical Hollywood cinema, xix, 4, 5, 12, 35,
    51, 81, 95, 122, 126, 153, 178, 181–85
Clayburgh, Jill, 25, 137, 138, 143
Clifford, Graeme, 17, 148, 154, 157, 158
Clift, Montgomery, 104, 106–9, 126, 182,
    183
Closeup (journal), xii
Cobb, Lee J., 38, 40, 90, 91
Coburn, James, 129, 130, 142
Cobweb, The, 77–80, 87, 88, 92, 113
Colbert, Claudette, 14, 51–53, 99
Coming Apart, 19
Communications (journal), 178
Communists in America, 86; *see also* McCarthy
    Era
Condemned Women, 25
Connery, Sean, 127, 231
Conrad, Joseph, 232; *Heart of Darkness,* 233;
    Nostromo, 232
Conte, Richard, 21
Conway, Tom, 21, 32
Cooke, Alistair, 90, 91
Cool Hand Luke, 126, 127, 156
Cooper, Gary, 5, 58, 59

Copernicus, 108
Coppola, Francis, 135
Corey, Jeff, 39
Cornell University, 54
Cornfield, Hubert, 97
Cort, Bud, 140, 141
Corti, Axel, 108
Countertransference, xvii, 20–32, 55, 56, 62–
    64, 97, 98, 101–3, 142, 145–62, 163,
    164, 168
Cracking Up, 41
Crawford, Joan, 6, 14, 112, 124
Cries and Whispers, 248
Crimes of Passion, 17
Cromwell, John, 17, 246
Crossfire, 68, 69
Crowther, Bosley, 72, 73
Cukor, George, 34, 49
Culbert, David, 73
Culp, Robert, 134, 135
Cummings, Robert, 23, 124
Current Opinion (journal), 85
Curtis, Tony, 24–26, 111, 130

Daily, Dan, 92, 93
Dali, Salvador, 63
Dane, Clarence, 49
Daniels, Jeff, 220–23
Darin, Bobby, 97, 98, 111, 150
Dark Mirror, The, xvii, 25, 32, 68, 69, 75,
    82, 87, 91, 114
Dark Past, The, 40, 67
Darwin, Charles, 108
da Silva, Howard, 95–97, 119, 143
David and Lisa, xv, 17, 35, 79, 95–97, 101,
    103, 110, 111, 113, 119, 120, 143
da Vinci, Leonardo, 186
Davis, Bette, 41, 60, 61, 95, 97
Day, Doris, 101, 110
Dayan, Daniel, 179, 182, 184
Days of Wine and Roses, 113
Deacon, Richard, 82, 101
Dead Heat on a Merry-Go-Round, 27, 125, 130
Dead Ringer, 68
Death Wish, 126, 211
Death Wish II, 121, 122, 126

de Broca, Philippe, 95
de Cordova, Frederick, 75
Deer Hunter, The, 11, 142
de Havilland, Olivia, 19, 36, 68–72, 101
Dekker, Albert, 104, 182
de Lauretis, Teresa, 182
Delphi, Temple at, 115
Demedicalization of psychiatry in the movies,
    xvii, 19, 22, 28, 30, 36, 37, 46, 52–54,
    64, 68, 85, 165
DeMille, Cecil B., 47
Demme, Jonathan, 25
De Niro, Robert, 56, 206, 207, 209, 210,
    211, 212
De Palma, Brian, 43, 68, 115–19, 161, 237
Derepression, 7, 37–39, 74, 169
Derrida, Jacques, 178
Dervin, Daniel, 188
De Salvo, Albert, 130
de salvo, Anne, 202
de Saussure, Ferdinand, 178
Detective, The, 32
Deutsch, Helene, 13
Devore, Christopher, 154
Dewhurst, Colleen, 127
Diary of a Mad Housewife, 13, 16, 119, 120,
    128, 156
Diazepam, 151
Dickinson, Angie, 19, 111, 116, 117
Dirty Harry, 126, 156
Displacement, xii, 4, 39, 40, 104, 105, 140,
    161, 166, 177, 240, 248
Disputed Passage, 52
Dmytryk, Edward, xix, 80
Doane, Mary Ann, 182
Dr. Dippy's Sanitarium, xii, xvi, 44, 45
Dr. Strangelove, or How I Learned to Stop Worrying
    and Love the Bomb, 123
Documentary film, 73, 107, 123
Dolby film sound, 230, 232
Donner, Clive, 20
Donner, Richard, 142
Douglas, Gordon, 74
Douglas, Michael, 255
Dourif, Brad, 140
Dow, Peggy, 31

Down and Out in Beverly Hills, 134, 256
Downey, Robert, 128
Dracula, 32
Dragoti, Stan, 20, 142
Drake, Charles, 31, 87
Dream of a Rarebit Fiend, 46
Dreams and dream analysis, xii, xv, 8, 9, 40, 47, 51, 54, 63, 92, 107, 109, 145, 158, 160, 161, 169, 170, 177, 185, 188, 240–51, 253
Dream screen, 185
Dressed to Kill, 19, 43, 115–19, 146, 169, 170, 237
Dreyer, Carl, 158
Dreyfuss, Richard, 92
Drury, James, 94
Duck Soup, 133
Duellists, The, 232
Duggan, Andrew, 34, 94
Duke, Patty, 112, 113
Dullea, Keir, 79, 95, 97
Dunne, Philip, 20, 99
Durgnat, Raymond, 184
Durning, Charles, 19
Duvall, Robert, 111
Duvall, Shelley, 242, 243

Eastmancolor, 92
Eastwood, Clint, 205, 206
Easy Rider, 126, 127
Eber, Milton, 37
Ebert, Roger, 241
Eberwein, Robert, 185
Eckert, Charles, 4, 177
Edelman, Herb, 41
Edwards, Blake, 27, 75, 100, 113, 142
Edwards, James, 39
Edwards, Vince, 256
8 1/2, 190, 191, 194, 195, 197
Eisenstein, Sergei, 178
Electroconvulsive therapy (ECT), 35–37, 41, 42, 70, 88, 112, 121, 122, 139, 140, 146, 156, 164, 167, 168
Eliot, T. S., *The Cocktail Party,* 127
Ellenberger, Henri, 122
Elvira Madigan, 41

End of the Road, 142
Entity, The, 32
Equus, 141
Erikson, Erik, 123
Escape from Alcatraz, 156
Escaped Lunatic, The, 44, 45
est, 134
E.T., 220
Exorcist, The, 226–28, 236
Exorcist II: The Heretic, 33, 142

Faceless psychiatrist, 7, 9, 10, 11, 12, 15, 16, 34, 35, 42, 80, 81, 88, 89, 93, 94, 130, 143
Face to Face, xvii
Fail-Safe, 123
Fairbanks, Douglas, 46, 47
Falk, Peter, 97, 98, 150
Family Plot, 158
Farmer, Frances, 154–57
Farnham, Marynia, 13, 63
Farrow, John, 49
Farrow, Mia, 27, 28, 133, 216, 220, 223
Fear Strikes Out, 16, 35, 37, 42, 88–90, 92, 93, 121
Feld, Fritz, 18–20, 58, 130
Feldstein, Richard, 188
Fellini, Federico, 190, 191, 195, 248
Female psychiatrists, 3, 15, 21–30, 51, 52, 61–67, 75, 99, 100, 120, 121, 124, 125, 138, 142–44, 146, 147, 152, 160, 216, 217, 219
Feminist analysis, xviii, 12–14, 21–29, 41, 52, 119, 120, 139, 140, 180, 182–84
Ferrer, Jose, 21, 36, 76, 77, 80, 81
Ferrer, Mel, 124
Feuer, Jane, 185
Field, Sally, 113
Fields, W. C., xi
Fifth Floor, The, 35
Film genres, xii, xv–xvii, xix, 14, 29, 30–36, 42, 43, 45, 47, 54, 66, 68, 77, 82, 94, 110, 118, 123, 148, 152, 156–58, 161, 162, 185, 226, 253
Film music, 63, 68, 108, 109, 115, 137, 195, 212, 222, 229, 230, 232, 233, 243

Film noir, 64–68, 84, 158
Film Quarterly (journal), 109
Fine Madness, A, 27, 126–28, 155
Fink, Paul, 164–66, 173
Firth, Peter, 141
Fish, Stanley, 14
Fitzgerald, F. Scott, 101–3
Fitzgerald, Geraldine, 153
Fitzgerald, Zelda, 103
Five Easy Pieces, 126
Flame Within, The, 26
Flashbacks, 6, 27, 39, 42, 82, 87, 97, 124, 136, 159, 190
Fleischer, Richard, 130
Fleming, Rhonda, 62, 93
Fleming, Victor, 19, 46
Fletcher, Louise, 33, 139, 140
Flicker, Theodore J., 128
Fonda, Henry, 56, 105, 130, 131
Fonda, Jane, 7, 19, 34, 144
Fontaine, Joan, 14, 100, 102
Forbes, Bryan, 142, 144
Forbidden Planet, The, 228
Ford, Joh, xix, 95
Foreman, Carl, 39
Forman, Milos, 17, 138, 155
Fortier, Robert, 242, 247
Fosse, Bob, 187, 189–97, 200, 202, 203, 212
Fourteen Hours, 75
Frances, xv, 17, 35, 36, 148, 154–57, 162, 164, 167
Francis, Anne, 94
Francis, Robert, 80
Frankenstein, 104
Franklin, Sidney, 50
Franz, Dennis, 116, 118
Free Love, 54–56, 85
Freeman, Howard, 72
Freud, Anna, 109
Freud, Sigmund, xii, xviii, 4, 8, 22, 30, 37, 50, 54, 68, 70, 85, 92, 106–9, 115, 126, 133, 141, 142, 146, 148, 150–54, 160, 177–80, 185–87, 230, 240, 251, 254
Freud, 34, 73, 92, 104, 106–10, 113, 115
Freudianism, 13, 47, 60, 63, 123, 127, 132, 218

Frings, Ketti, 76
Fromm-Reichmann, Frieda, 25
Front Page, The (1931), 11, 31, 48, 49, 54, 166
Front Page, The (1974), 45
Frye, Northrop, 152
Fuller, Samuel, 121
Funny Girl, 155
Furie, Sidney J., 32

Gabbard, Glen O., 189, 201
Gach, John, 47
Garland, Judy, 121
Garner, James, 110
Gates, Larry, 81, 87
Gavin, John, 116, 183
Gay Intruders, The, 31, 72
Gazzara, Ben, 87, 88
Geer, Will, 129
Geffner, Deborah, 189
Genn, Leo, 35, 70, 71, 77, 78, 88, 91
Gentleman's Agreement, 68
Gershwin, Ira, 7
Gibson, William, 77, 113
Gigi, 77
Gilgamesh, 204
Gillespie, Dizzy, 129
Gilman, Charlotte Perkins, "The Yellow Wallpaper," 127
Gingold, Hermione, 124
Girl of the Night, 34, 94
Gish, Lillian, 78, 79
Glen or Glenda? 60, 74
Godard, Jean-Luc, xii, 127, 178
Gold, Jack, 25, 142
Golden Age of psychiatry in the movies, 3, 12, 16, 17, 28, 29, 37, 43, 72, 77, 84–114, 115, 118, 119, 121–24, 131, 137, 138, 142, 144, 147, 150, 156, 171, 182, 253
Golden Boy, 126
Goldsmith, Jerry, 108, 232
Gone with the Wind, 46
Gordon, Keith, 116
Gordon, Michael, 22
Gordon, Ruth, 140

Gordon, Steve, 113, 153
Gorman, Cliff, 200
Goulding, Edmund, 17
Gowland, Gibson, xi
Graduate, The, 123, 129, 152–54, 162
Grahame, Gloria, 78, 79
Grant, Cary, 154
Grant, Lawrence, 58
Greed, xi
Greek mythology, 15, 196
Green, Guy, 94
Greenberg, Harvey R., xviii, 12, 105, 106, 231
Griffith, D. W., 178
Grimwood, Herbert, 46
Group, The, 125, 126
Guillerman, John, 123
Guinness, Alec, 148

Habsburgs, 50, 51
Hack, Shelley, 208
Hall, Jon, 8, 9
Halloween, 33, 226
Hammett, Dashiell, 65
Hannah and Her Sisters, 133, 134
Harold and Maude, 140, 141, 155
Harris, Robert H., 124
Harrold, Kathryn, 25, 143, 144
Hart, Moss, 7, 11
Harvey, Anthony, 24
Harvey, 32, 75, 76, 87
Harvey Middleman, Fireman, 124
Haskell, Molly, 12–14
Hassett, Marilyn, 128
Hawks, Howard, 18, 48, 56, 58, 126
Hays Office, 49; *see also* Production Code
Hearst, Patty, 164, 212
Heath, Stephen, 185
Hecht, Ben, 48
Heflin, Van, 4
Hefner, Hugh, 212, 213
Heller, Joseph, *Catch-22,* 128
Henley, Hobart, 54
Henn, Carrie, 238, 239
Henreid, Paul, 4, 60, 61, 67, 68, 95, 97, 126

Hepburn, Katharine, 14, 20, 24, 58, 104, 130, 154
Hershey, Barbara, 32, 133
Hi! Mom, 118
High Anxiety, 31, 161
High Noon, 232
High Wall, 26, 32, 67
Hill, Arthur, 125
Hill, Lister, 112
Hiller, Arthur, 7, 17
Hinckley, John, 164, 208
Hippies, 123, 129, 130
Hirsch, Judd, 18, 40, 41, 144, 168, 170
His Girl Friday, 13, 48, 49, 56
Hitchcock, Alfred, xix, 17, 19, 48, 61–64, 90, 94, 99, 104–6, 115–19, 146, 158, 159, 161, 183, 184, 237
Hitler, Adolf, 214
Hoffman, Dustin, 56, 152–54, 162, 225
Hofsiss, Jack, 25, 143
Holbrook, Hal, 125, 126
Holden, William, 40
Holiday, 152, 154
Holland, Norman, xv
Hollow Triumph, 67
Holm, Ian, 236
Holmes, Oliver Wendell, Sr., 44
Holmes, Sherlock, 24, 142
Holmes, Taylor, 64
Home before Dark, 93, 94, 113
Home of the Brave, 35, 39, 70, 73, 80, 86, 97, 98
Homer, 204
Homosexuality, 23, 35, 59, 60, 104, 138, 255
Hooks, David, 7
Hooper, Tobe, 227
Hope, Bob, xi, 101
Horton, Edward Everett, 48
Hospital, The, 7, 35
House Committee on Un-American Activities, 95
Houseman, John, 77, 145
House of Cards, 123
Howard, Ron, 220
Howard, Sidney, 54
Howe, Irving, 216, 225

Howling, The, 32
Huckleberry Finn, 126
Hudson, Rock, 20, 21, 23, 101, 124, 225
Humoresque, 126
Hurd, Gale Ann, 238
Hurt, John, 234, 235
Huss, Roy, 120
Huston, John, 34, 73, 106–10, 114, 115, 148, 150, 153
Hutton, Timothy, 40, 41, 168
Hypnosis, 37, 38, 46, 47, 55, 56, 73, 75, 109, 169

I, the Jury (1953), 19, 25, 32, 75, 146
I, the Jury (1982), 25, 32, 75
Ibsen, Henrik, xviii; *Rosmersholm,* 8; *The Wild Duck,* 6
I Love You, Alice B. Toklas, 256
Images, 154
I'm Dancing as Fast as I Can, 25, 143
I Never Promised You a Rose Garden, 17, 25, 112, 142, 143
Inflated genre film, 86, 91, 100
Inside Daisy Clover, 121, 125
Interiors, 17, 200
Intermezzo, 12
Interns, The, 35, 94
Invaders from Mars (1953), 227
Invaders from Mars (1986), 227
Invasion of the Body Snatchers (1956), 32, 80–82, 87, 227, 228, 236
Invasion of the Body Snatchers (1978), 32, 227
Invisible psychiatrist, 16, 17
Ireland, John, 28
It Happened One Night, 152
It's My Turn, 138, 166
Ivanek, Zeljko, 25
I Was a Teenage Werewolf, xv, 74, 75, 80

Jackson, Anne, 128
Jacobs, Diane, 194, 197, 199
Jagged Edge, 88
James, Henry, 7
James, William, 204
Jaques, Elliot, 199, 200
Jason, 15

Jerome, Edwin, 90
Jewison, Norman, 16, 110, 144
Johnny Belinda, 37
Johns, Glynis, 34, 99
Johnson, Nunnally, 37, 90, 91
Johnson, Van, 80
Jones, Fowler C., 201
Jones, James Earl, 17, 142
Jones, Jennifer, 17, 101–3, 147
Jones, Jim, 214
Jorgensen, Christine, 60
Juliet of the Spirits, 248

Kael, Pauline, 190, 240
Kaminsky, Stuart, 108
Kaplan, Ann E., 66
Karloff, Boris, 72
Kaufman, Charles, 108
Kaufman, Philip, 32, 227
Kaufman, Sue, 119
Kawin, Bruce, 185
Kay, Roger, 99
Kaye, Danny, 21, 22, 256
Kazan, Elia, 16, 85, 94
Kazan, Nicholas, 154
Keaton, Diane, 132
Keith, Ian, 64
Kelland, Clarence Budington, 58
Kellaway, Cecil, 76
Keller, Helen, 112
Kennedy, John F., 127
Kernberg, Otto, 146, 191, 192, 194, 198, 199, 207, 212
Kerr, John, 78, 79
Kershner, Irvin, 126
Kesey, Ken, 127, 256
Kinder, Marsha, 185
King, Henry, 19, 101
King of Comedy, 187, 206–13, 214, 215, 218, 219, 224, 225
King of Hearts, 95
Kinsey, Alfred, 34
Kirk, G. S., 15
Kismet, 77
Kitty Foyle, 12, 14

Klein, Melanie, 188, 199, 200, 226, 228, 229, 233, 234–39
Klemperer, Werner, 105
Klugman, Jack, 113
Klute, 7
Knight, Arthur, 112
Knight, Shirley, 125, 126
Knock on Wood, 21, 22, 24, 27, 30, 75
Kohut, Heinz, 42, 191, 195, 207, 213, 224
Koster, Henry, 32, 75
Kotch, 142
Kotto, Yaphet, 232
Kracauer, Siegfried, 178
Kramer, Stanley, 35, 39, 80, 81, 86, 97, 98
Kramer vs. Kramer, 158
Kramm, Joseph, 76, 77
Kristeva, Julia, 178
Kristofferson, Kris, 135
Kübler-Ross, Elisabeth, 200
Kubrick, Stanley, 123, 229
Kuhn, Annette, 182

Lacan, Jacques, xviii, 178–81, 183, 184–86, 188
La Cava, Gregory, 25, 51
Ladd, Alan, 4
Lady in the Dark, 7–14, 17, 30, 42, 43, 55, 56, 61, 63, 71, 86, 120
Lady Sings the Blues, 155
Lady Vanishes, The, 158
Laing, R. D., 95
Lake, Veronica, 195
Lamarr, Hedy, 22, 23
La Motta, Jake, 210
Landon, Michael, 74, 75
Lang, Fritz, xvii, xix, 65, 158
Lange, Hope, 28–30, 99, 100
Lange, Jessica, 154–57, 192, 193
Langella, Frank, 119
Lasch, Christopher, 187, 189, 197, 205, 206, 212, 218
Last Embrace, The, 25
Late Show, The, 158
Laugh-In, 129
Laurel and Hardy, 244
Leather, Derrick, 232

Left cycle/right cycle, 126–28, 130, 144, 153, 156
Lehman, Ernest, 142
Leigh, Janet, 24, 27, 100, 116–18, 125, 183
Leisen, Mitchell, 7
Leites, Nathan, xviii
Lemmon, Jack, 113, 142, 154
Lennon, John, 198, 214
Lenny, 190
LeRoy, Mervyn, 93
Leslie, Bethel, 111
Let's Live a Little, 22, 23, 26, 63
Let There Be Light, 70, 73, 107, 108
Levant, Oscar, 79
Lévi-Strauss, Claude, 15, 178, 180, 185
Lewin, Robert, 94
Lewis, Jerry, 27, 41, 207, 208, 211, 214
Lie-detector tests, 68
Life magazine, 84
Lilith, 26
Lincoln, Abraham, 4
Little Big Man, 126
Litvak, Anatole, xix, 19, 57
Lobotomy, 35, 36, 104, 127, 139, 140, 156, 157, 182
Logan's Run, 231
Lonely Guy, The, 17
Lord Love a Duck, 125
Lorre, Peter, 100
"Lost Generation," 103
Lost Weekend, 113
Love at First Bite, 20, 26, 142, 148, 149
Lover Come Back, xv, 101
Lovesick, 19, 26, 32, 101, 115, 144, 148–57, 161, 162, 164, 168
Loves of a Psychiatrist, 34
LSD, 125
Lubitsch, Ernst, 57
Lugosi, Bela, 48, 74
Lukas, Paul, 101, 102, 147
Lumet, Sidney, 123, 125, 141
Lundberg, Ferdinand, 13, 63
Lust for Life, 77

MacArthur, Charles, 48
MacCabe, Colin, 185

McCallum, David, 109
McCarey, Leo, 56
McCarthy, Kevin, 81, 82, 87
McCarthy Era, 81, 227, 228
McCrea, Joel, 52, 194
McDowall, Roddy, 125
McGovern, Elizabeth, 32, 40, 41, 148–51, 168
McGuire, Dorothy, 37
McKinley, J. Edward, 94
MacLaine, Shirley, 124
MacMurray, Fred, 80, 81
Macnee, Patrick, 32
Madame X, 12
Mafia, 144
Magnificent Obsession, 52
Maher, Joseph, 143
Making Love, 59
Malden, Karl, 42
Manhattan, 148, 200
Mankiewicz, Joseph L., 104
Mann, Daniel, 110
Mann, Delbert, 101
Manoff, Dinah, 40
Manson, Charles, 212
Man Who Knew Too Much, The, 158
Man Who Loved Women, The, 27
Man Who Saw Tomorrow, The, 6, 47
Marat/Sade, 36, 128
Marathon Man, xi
Margolin, Janet, 79, 101
Marguiles, David, 118
Mark, The, 35, 94
Marnie, xix
Marriage of a Young Stockbroker, The, 120, 121, 128, 142, 152
Marshall, Sarah, 125
Martin, Dean, 110
Martin, Steve, 17
Marx Brothers, 133
Marxism, xviii, 180, 185, 218
M*A*S*H, 22
"M*A*S*H" (television series), 114
Mason, Marsha, 135
"Masterpiece Theatre" (television series), 91
Mastroianni, Marcello, 191

Mate, Rudolph, 40
Matthau, Walter, 142
"Matt Lincoln" (television series), 114, 256
Mazursky, Paul, 131, 134–38, 144, 190, 220, 253, 255–57
Medusa Touch, The, 25, 32, 142
Melodrama, 4, 5, 31, 34, 47, 51, 52, 63, 66, 68
Melosh, Barbara, 22
Men in White, 35
Menninger Clinic, 77
Mental Health and Mental Retardation Act, 112
Methaqualone, 151
Method acting, 7
Metz, Christian, xv, 178, 179, 181, 185, 254, 255
Midnight Express, 156
Miles, Vera, 105, 117
Milestone, Lewis, 48
Milland, Ray, 8, 9
Miller, David, 110
Miller, J. P., 113
Miller, M., 231
Minnelli, Liza, 153, 207
Minnelli, Vincente, 9, 10, 77, 78
Miracle on 34th Street, 32, 72
Miracle Worker, The, 112, 113
Mirage, 32, 124
Mirror-stage, 180
Miserables, Les, 51
Mr. and Mrs. Smith, 158
Mr. Deeds Goes to Town, 5, 58, 59, 69, 75
Moment to Moment, 125
Monaco, James, 137, 178
Monroe, Marilyn, 109, 110,170, 225
Montand, Yves, 9, 10
Moore, Dudley, 19, 32, 113, 115, 142, 144, 148, 149–54, 168
Moore, Mary Tyler, 18, 40, 41
Moore, Norman, 89
Moore, Roger, 144
Morgan, Frank, 50, 51
Morning Glory, 12
Morris, Chester, 40, 54, 55
Morse, Susan, 215

Moscow on the Hudson, 220
Moses, Marian, 130
Mother films, 31, 41
Movie Star, American Style or LSD, I Hate You, 125
Mozart, Wolfgang Amadeus, 229, 230
Muhich, Donald F., 134–38, 256, 257
Mulligan, Robert, 16, 88, 121
Multiple personality syndrome, 38, 39, 113, 114, 116, 118, 130, 131
Mulvey, Laura, 14, 182–84
Munchkins, 8, 12
Münsterberg, Hugo, xi, xii, xviii
Murder, My Sweet, 72, 86
Murdoch, Iris, *A Severed Head,* 128
Murphy, Michael, 137
Musical comedy, 14, 31, 77, 185
My Favorite Wife, 72

Nabokov, Vladimir, *Pnin,* 128
Nagel, Conrad, 54
Naked Face, The, 144
Napier, Alan, 29
Narcissism, 187, 189–225, 253, 254
Narcosynthesis, 6, 8, 70, 73
Nathan, Vivian, 7
National Institute of Mental Health, 112, 171
Nelson, Ruth, 246
New Deal, 50
Newsweek (journal), 149
New York, New York, 209
Nichols, Mike, 152
Nicholson, Jack, 18, 126, 139, 140
Nietzsche, Friedrich, 133
Night of the Living Dead, 226, 228
Night Porter, The, xvii
Nightmare Alley, 17, 25, 64–67, 71, 75
Niven, David, 92, 93
Niver, Kemp, 44
Nixon, Richard, 141
Nolan, Lloyd, 94
North by Northwest, 106, 158
Notorious, 158
Novak, Kim, 105, 184
Now Voyager, xv, 12, 17, 41, 60, 61, 69, 70, 79, 80, 82, 86, 91, 95, 97, 170

Nursing, history of, 22
Nyby, Christian, 228

Oakland, Simon, 17, 87, 94, 105, 106, 117–19, 130
O'Brien, J., 37
Obsession, 118
O'Connell, Arthur, 87
O'Connell, Jack, 123
Odets, Clifford, 28
Oedipus, 161, 165
Oedipus complex, 108, 109, 160, 181, 245, 246
O'Herlihy, Dan, 93, 94, 99
Oh God! Book II, 19, 32
Oh Men! Oh Women! 56, 91–93, 101
Old Maid, The, 12
Olivier, Laurence, xi
Omen, The, 142
"Omnibus" (television series), 90
On a Clear Day You Can See Forever, 9, 10
O'Neal, Patrick, 127
O'Neal, Ryan, 154
One Flew over the Cuckoo's Nest, 17, 18, 22, 35, 36, 121, 127, 128, 138–40, 155, 156, 167, 168, 252, 255, 256
One Glorious Day, 47
Oracular psychiatrist, 16, 17, 32, 40, 53–55, 60, 61, 77, 80, 86, 87, 117–19, 130, 166, 172
Ordinary People, 17, 18, 40, 41, 43, 112, 114, 115, 138, 143, 144, 164, 168, 169, 252, 255
O'Toole, Peter, 125
Oudart, Jean-Pierre, 181, 184
Outland, 231
Outlaw hero/official hero, 4, 126, 127, 139, 140, 144, 151, 153

Pabst, G. W., xvii
Page, Anthony, 25
Pakula, Alan, 7, 121, 231
Panama, Norman, and Melvin Frank, 21
Papillon, 156
Parallax View, The, 231
Paramount Pictures, 88

Paul VI, 141

Peck, Gregory, 19, 24, 62–64, 110, 111, 124, 146, 147

Peerce, Larry, 128

Penelope, 125

Penn, Arthur, 112, 158

Perfect Furlough, The, 24, 27, 34, 75, 100

Perkins, Anthony, 42, 87–89, 116, 117, 183, 184

Perkins, Millie, 29

Perry, Eleanor, 119, 120

Perry, Frank, 119, 120

Peters, Werner, 127

Phantom of the Paradise, 119

Pickles, Vivian, 140

Pidgeon, Walter, 100, 228

Piersall, Jim, 16, 42, 88–90

Pillow Talk, 101, 110, 123

Pinky, 68

Pirandello, Luigi, 220

Places in the Heart, 158

Plan Nine from Outer Space, 74

Plastered in Paris, xv, 47

Plath, Sylvia, 128

Playboy magazine, 212, 213

"Playhouse 90" (television series), 112, 113

Pleasence, Donald, 33

Plummer, Christopher, 121

Poitier, Sidney, 97, 98, 150

Pollack, Sydney, 231

Pornography, 34

Porter, Edwin S., 46

Portnoy's Complaint, 142

Possessed, 6, 8, 61, 70

Poston, Tom, 101

Powell, William, 58

Power, Tyrone, 64–67

Preminger, Otto, 21, 79, 87

President's Analyst,The, 128–30, 142

Presley, Elvis, 28, 29, 30, 99, 214, 225

Pressman, Michael, 11

Pressure Point, 35, 80, 97, 98, 103, 110, 111, 113, 142, 150

Price, Vincent, 72

Private Worlds, 25, 49, 51, 53, 54, 62, 77, 91, 99

Production Code, 29, 34, 49, 50, 52, 91

Prostitution, 34, 94, 117, 118

Proust, Marcel, 135

Pryor, Richard, 11

Psychiatric education, 171–72

"Psychiatrist, The" (television series), 114

Psychiatrist as *ficelle,* 7, 10, 11, 14, 124

Psychiatrist as rationalist foil, 25, 32, 33, 100, 101, 132, 142, 144, 252

Psychiatrists in love, 19–32, 51, 52, 55, 56, 62–64, 67, 68, 75, 92, 99–104, 147–53, 252

Psycho, 17, 87, 94, 99, 105, 106, 115–19, 130, 131, 182–84, 237

Psychoanalytic movement, history of, 37, 47, 48, 54, 171, 172

Psychobiography, 186

Psychopharmacology, 36

Pudovkin, Vsevolod I., 178

Purple Rose of Cairo, The, 187, 206, 219–25

Quinlan, Kathleen, 25, 143

Racism, 35, 39, 94, 97, 98

Ragina's Secrets, 34

Raging Bull, 210

Rains, Claude, 41, 60, 61, 70, 91, 170

Rampling, Charlotte, 197

Randall, Tony, 92, 101

Ray, Robert B., 5, 15, 35, 57, 63, 81, 86, 91, 106, 126, 177, 185, 211, 212

Reagan, Ronald, 75, 205, 208

Rear Window, 158

Redford, Robert, 18

Red River, 126

Reds, 216

Reefer Madness, 59

Reinhardt, Wolfgang, 108

Reinking, Ann, 192

Reiser, Paul, 239

Remick, Lee, 25, 142

Reunion in Vienna, 49–51, 54, 56

Revill, Clive, 127

Revolution, 123

Reynolds, Burt, 19, 27

Rickey, Carrie, 157

Riskin, Robert, 58
Rivers, Larry, 152
Rivette, Jacques, 178
Robards, Jason, Jr., 19, 101–3, 147
Roberts, Eric, 212
Robson, Mark, xix, 39, 73
Rogers, Ginger, 8–10, 13, 14, 31, 55–57, 92, 93, 225
Rogers, Will, 47
Rohmer, Eric, 178
Romero, George, 228
Romm, May E., 62
Rorschach tests, 68, 108, 125, 217
Rose, The, 155
Ross, Herbert, 142
Ross, Katharine, 154
Roth, Philip, *Portnoy's Complaint,* 142
Rothman, William, 179
Rowe, Bill, 232
Royal Family of Broadway, The, 12
Rozsa, Miklos, 63
Rule, Janice, 241, 242
Rush, Barbara, 92
Russell, Ken, 17
Russell, Kurt, 228
Russell, Rosalind, 24, 49
Russianoff, Penelope, 138, 255, 256
Russo, Vito, 60, 104
Ryan, Robert, 69

Sachs, Hans, xii
Safra, Jaqui, 202
St. Ives, 19, 145, 146
Samuels, Laurel, 25
Sanders, Denis, 121
Sarafian, Richard, 113
Sarris, Andrew, 190
Sartre, Jean-Paul, 106–9; *Freud Scenario, The,* 108
Sayles, John, 220
Sayre, Nora, 39
Schatz, Thomas, 133
Scheider, Roy, 144, 159–61, 189, 190, 194
Schell, Maximillian, 19, 145
Schenck, Aubrey, 73

Schneider, Irving, xv, xvi, 11, 13, 44, 135
Science fiction and horror films, 32, 33, 74, 75, 81, 100, 188, 226–39, 253
Scorsese, Martin, 135, 187, 206, 208–12
Scott, George C., 7, 24
Scott, Ridley, 108, 188, 226, 230–38, 253
Screen (journal), 178, 185
Sears, Heather, 37
Seberg, Jean, 124, 125, 127
Secrets of a Soul, xii, xvii
Segal, George, 135
Segal, Hanna, 234, 235, 237
Sekely, Steve, 67
Self, Robert, 31, 241
Sellers, Peter, 20, 80, 124, 125, 147
Selznick, David O., 63, 147
Semiotics, xii, xviii, xix, 177, 179–87
Semi-Tough, 134
Senate Committee on Labor and Public Welfare, 112
Sender, The, 25, 32, 143, 144
Seven-Per-Cent Solution, The, 142
Seventh Veil, The, 61
Seven Year Itch, The, 75
Sex and the Single Girl, 25–27, 30, 34, 124
Sexuality in the movies, xvi, 33–35, 49–52, 59, 60, 65–67, 91, 94, 112, 118, 134–36, 140, 252
Shadow of a Doubt, 158
Shadow on the Wall, 27
Shaffer, Peter, 141
Shaid, Nick, 53
Shakespeare, William, xviii, 63, 79
Shane, 4
Sharpe, Ella F., 240, 242
Shaw, Anabel, 72
Shaw, George Bernard, 222
Shawn, Dick, 23, 125
Shawn, Wallace, 148
Sherwood, Robert E., 50
She Wouldn't Say Yes, 26
Shields, Jim, 232
Shimkus, Joanna, 120, 121
Shock, 72–74
Shock Corridor, 35, 121
Shock Treatment, 25, 35, 121, 124

Shrike, The, 36, 76, 77, 81, 87
Siegel, Don, 32, 81, 82
Silent Night, Deadly Night, 229
Silver, Ron, 32
Silverman, Kaja, 180, 183, 184
Simmons, Jean, 93, 94
Simon, Simone, 21, 32
Simon, 148
Since You Went Away, 12, 17, 61, 82, 84
Sin of Madelon Claudet, The, 12
Siodmak, Robert, 68
Sisters, 68, 118
Sizemore, Chris Costner, 38, 39, 90
Skerritt, Tom, 229
Sklar, Robert, 5, 6, 49, 51, 58, 59
Sleeper, 231
Sleeping Tiger, The, 79
Smith, Kent, 21
Smith, Lane, 17, 155
Snake Pit, The, 19, 35, 36, 68–72, 77–80,
    88, 91, 101, 104, 111
Snodgress, Carrie, 13, 119, 120
Social problem film, 35, 68, 69, 84, 86, 92,
    94, 97, 98, 106, 112–14, 123
Socrates 133,
Some Kind of Hero, 11
Sommer, Josef, 159
Sondheim, Stephen, 166
Sontag, Susan, 216, 217
Sophocles, xviii, 163, 165
Spacek, Sissy, 242–44, 247
Spellbound, 12, 19, 22, 24, 26, 29, 48, 61–
    63, 66, 67, 69, 71, 82, 90, 91, 103, 105,
    144, 146, 147, 150, 158, 159, 161, 162,
    252
Spielberg, Stephen, 220
Spillane, Mickey, 75
Spiral Staircase, The, 37
Splash, 220
Splendor in the Grass, 16, 34, 85, 94, 113, 156
Split-screen editing, 130, 132
Sprich, R., 231
Spock, Benjamin, 84
Stack, Robert, 111, 113
Stanley, Kim, 154–56
Stanton, Harry Dean, 232

Stardust Memories, 132, 187, 190, 191, 194–
    203, 219, 223
Star 80, 212, 213
Starman, 220
Starting Over, 19, 142
Star Wars, 144, 230, 231
Steiger, Rod, 94, 144
Stella Dallas, 12, 31, 41
Stepford Wives, The, 142
Stevens, George, 4
Stevens, Inger, 123
Stevens, Mark, 70
Stewart, James, 58, 75, 76, 87, 88, 105
Still of the Night, 32, 144, 148, 158–62
Stone, George E., 48
Story of Esther Costello, The, 37
Story of Louis Pasteur, The, 52
Stradner, Rose, 55
Strait Jacket, 124
Strasberg, Susan, 79, 101
Stratten, Dorothy, 212
Streep, Meryl, 159–61
Streisand, Barbra, 9, 10, 154
Structural anthropology, 15, 178
Sturges, Preston, 194, 195
Suburbia Confidential, 34
Suddenly, Last Summer, 104, 182
Sullivan, Annie, 112, 113
Sullivan, Barry, 8–11, 13
Sullivan's Travels, 194, 195
Supreme Court rulings, 34
Surrealism, xv
Survivor guilt, 40
Suture, 180–85
Sybil, 113

Take the Money and Run, 199, 216
Tale of Two Cities, A, 51
Tandy, Jessica, 159
Tate, Sharon, 212
Taxi Driver, 208, 211, 212
Taylor, Elizabeth, 104, 182, 183
Taylor, Robert, 67
Tea and Sympathy, 77
Technicolor, 92
Telekinesis, 25

Television, xvii, 31, 68, 86, 90, 91, 103, 112–
    14, 119, 129, 204, 206, 225, 256
10, 142
Tender Is the Night, 19, 25, 101–4, 110, 147,
    150
Terminator, The, 32, 238
Testament of Dr. Mabuse, The, xvii
Texas Chain Saw Massacre, The, 226
That Touch of Mink, 101, 110
That Uncertain Feeling, 72
Them! 74
Theremin, 63
They Might Be Giants, 24, 25, 27, 142
Thing, The (1951), 228
Thing, The (1982), 228, 236
Third of a Man, 80, 94
Thirty-nine Steps, The, 158
Thomas, Alexander, 42
Thompson, J. Lee, 124, 145
Three Days of the Condor, 231
Three Faces of Eve, The, 17, 35, 37, 38, 39,
    42, 90–92, 113, 156, 170
Three Nuts in Search of a Bolt, 34
Three on a Couch, 27, 125
Three Warriors, 256
3 Women, 188, 240–51, 254
Thrill of It All, The, 16, 110
Tierney, Gene, 21
Tilly, Meg, 19, 144
Tiomkin, Dmitiri, 68
Titicut Follies, 36, 128
Tobin, Genevieve, 54
To Each His Own, 12
Together Again, 12
Torn, Rip, 19
Totter, Audrey, 67
Tourneur, Jacques, 32
Transference, 21, 22, 27, 29, 37, 66, 97, 146,
    165, 166, 168–70, 172, 186, 214, 224
Transsexuals, 116, 118
Transvestism, 74, 116
Travers, Henry, 51
Truffaut, François, 27, 64, 117, 178
Truro, Victor, 132
Turman, Lawrence, 120
Twemlow, Stuart W., 201

Twins, 244
Twisted Sex, The, 34
2001: A Space Odyssey, 229–31

Under the Volcano, 114
Universal-International Studios, 110
Unmarried Woman, An, 112, 137, 138, 142,
    255

Valium, 143
Van Dyke, Dick, 225
Van Dyke, W. S., 57
Vanlint, Derek, 232
Van Sloan, Edward, 32
Veidt, Conrad, 4
Verdon, Gwen, 190
Vereen, Ben, 201
Vernet, Marc, xix, 37
Vertigo, 105, 184
Very Special Favor, A, 23–25, 27, 30, 34, 124
Vidor, Charles, 17, 40
Vietnam War, 127
Vinson, Helen, 52
von Eltz, Theodore, 53
von Sternberg, Josef, xix, 183
von Stroheim, Eric, xi
Voyage to the Bottom of the Sea, 100
Voyeurism, 34, 74, 94, 105, 120, 121, 181,
    183, 184, 254, 255, 257

Wagner, Richard, 137
Walken, Christopher, 11, 142
Walker, Helen, 17, 64–67
Walking Tall, 126
Walsh, Andrea, 13, 14, 61
Wanger, Walter, 51
Warwick, James, 53
Washington, George, 4
Wayne, John, 56, 126, 170
Weaver, Sigourney, 229, 238
Webb, Charles, 152
Weill, Claudia, 138, 166
Weill, Kurt, 7
Weld, Tuesday, 29
Welles, Orson, xix
Wengraf, John, 92

West, Adam, 121
West Side Story, 166
What a Way to Go! 124
What's New, Pussycat? 20, 26, 80, 124, 125, 148, 149
What's up, Doc? 154
When the Clouds Roll By, 19, 44, 46, 47
Whirlpool, 21, 79
Whitman, Stuart, 94
Who's Been Sleeping in My Bed? 34, 110
Whose Life Is It, Anyway? 92
Widmark, Richard, 77–80, 88, 92
Wiene, Robert, xvii
Wiest, Dianne, 25, 143
Wilde, Oscar, 173
Wilder, Billy, 45, 113
Wild in the Country, 27–30, 99, 100
Williams, Adam, 16, 42, 88, 89
Williams, Linda, xv
Williams, Tennessee, 6, 104; *The Glass Menagerie,* 6; *Suddenly, Last Summer,* 104
Williamson, Nicol, 143
Willie and Phil, 134, 256
Willis, Austin, 130, 131
Willis, Gordon, 215
Wind, Bodhi, 242
Winner, Michael, 121, 211
Winters, Shelley, 34
Wizard of Oz, The, 12, 46, 99
Wolfenstein, Martha, xviii

Woman under the Influence, A, 156
Women's films, 12–14, 61, 82, 94, 95, 97, 155
Wood, Edward D., Jr., 74
Wood, G., 141
Wood, Michael, 3, 4, 5, 11, 15, 56, 95
Wood, Natalie, 25, 26, 34, 85, 94, 121, 124, 125, 134
Wood, Robin, 33, 41, 49, 50, 105, 184, 185
Woodward, Joanne, 24, 25, 38, 90, 91, 113, 142
Woolf, Virginia, *Mrs. Dalloway,* 127
Wouk, Herman, 80, 81
Wrong Man, The, 105, 158
Wyman, Jane, 37
Wynyard, Diana, 50, 51

York, Susannah, 34, 106, 108, 109
Young Dr. Freud, 108
Young Mr. Lincoln, 95

Zaentz, Saul, 255
Zelig, 27, 28, 187, 188, 206, 215–20, 223, 225
Zetterling, Mai, 21, 22, 24
Zimbalist, Efram, Jr., 94
Zimmerman, Paul D., 206, 211, 212
Zotz! 32, 101
Zucco, George, 58